An Evidence-Based Practice in Nursing and Healthcare

An Evidence-Based Practice in Nursing and Healthcare

Editor: Eric MacGregor

STATES
ACADEMIC PRESS
www.statesacademicpress.com

www.statesacademicpress.com

STATES
ACADEMIC PRESS

Cataloging-in-Publication Data

An evidence-based practice in nursing and healthcare / edited by Eric MacGregor.
p. cm.
Includes bibliographical references and index.
ISBN 978-1-63989-790-2
1. Evidence-based nursing--Practice. 2. Nurse practitioners--Practice. 3. Nursing--Practice.
4. Nursing services. 5. Medical care. I. MacGregor, Eric.
RT42 .E85 2023
610.73--dc23

States Academic Press,
109 South 5th Street,
Brooklyn, NY 11249, USA

ISBN 978-1-63989-790-2 (Hardback)

Contents

Preface

Evidence-based practice (EBP) refers to a method through which practitioners in the healthcare industry review and analyze the current researches to facilitate the delivery of care. Nursing is a profession within the healthcare sector that utilizes EBP for providing care to individuals and their families by helping them recover from illnesses, and maintain optimal health and quality of life. The EBP in nursing comprises three components, which involve utilizing the best accessible external advice, drawing on the clinical expertise, and taking into account the expectations and values of the patients. Furthermore, EBP allows the assessment of research for understanding the effectiveness and risks of the diagnostic tests and treatments. This book is a guide to evidence-based practice in nursing and healthcare. For all readers who are interested in nursing, the studies included herein will serve as an excellent guide to develop a comprehensive understanding.

All of the data presented henceforth, was collaborated in the wake of recent advancements in the field. The aim of this book is to present the diversified developments from across the globe in a comprehensible manner. The opinions expressed in each chapter belong solely to the contributing authors. Their interpretations of the topics are the integral part of this book, which I have carefully compiled for a better understanding of the readers.

At the end, I would like to thank all those who dedicated their time and efforts for the successful completion of this book. I also wish to convey my gratitude towards my friends and family who supported me at every step.

Editor

1

Health Professionals' Perspectives on the Efficacy of Using Comprehensive Care to Improve Outcomes in Patients with Traumatic Injury

Hsing-Ju LU[1] • Hsiu-Mei HUANG[2] • Tsai-Yun HSIAO[3] • Chang-Chiao HUNG[4] • Wei-Ting LIN[5] • Bih-O LEE[6*]

ABSTRACT

Background: Barriers related to comprehensive posttrauma care and health outcome monitoring exist. The insights and perspectives of health professionals on this issue may help integrate care experiences to provide continuous care to patients with traumatic injury.

Purpose: The purpose of this study was to explore the perspectives of health professionals with regard to comprehensive care to improve the outcomes of patients with traumatic injury.

Methods: Data were collected at two teaching hospitals in Taiwan. In total, 28 health professionals across various disciplines were interviewed in five focus groups.

Results: Six themes were delineated, including "wound care is a primary concern for patients," "ineffective health education during the hospital stay," "patients and families worry about postinjury conditions," "current continuity of care is not effective," "lack of standards for discharge planning," and "incorporation of interdisciplinary care to improve patient outcomes."

Conclusions: The experiences of health professionals are useful to the establishment of a foundation for trauma case management and interdisciplinary care for hospitals.

Key Words:
focus groups, traumatic injury outcomes, health professionals.

Introduction

Survivors of traumatic injury may experience permanent disabilities that are associated with high medication and rehabilitation costs in addition to potentially tremendous homecare and nonofficial care expenses (Haagsma et al., 2016; Ministry of Health and Welfare, Taiwan, ROC, 2016). Surveys conducted in Taiwan indicate that the average age of survivors of major trauma is 45.1 years (Lee et al., 2010). The national productivity losses, demand for medical resources, and economic and emotional stresses imposed on affected families as a result of traumatic injury have become a major medical and economic burden for Taiwan (Lee et al., 2010).

Traumatic injury is generally defined as sudden-onset, physical injuries that are sufficiently severe to require systemic and immediate medical treatment (University of Florida Health, 2019). Traumatic injuries are diverse and heterogeneous in nature, reflecting the body regions involved as well as the severity of trauma (Meerding et al., 2004). Some studies have used the type of traumatic injury, such as musculoskeletal injury, as inclusion criterion for participants (Torgbenu et al., 2019). The Injury Severity Score is an international scoring system that is commonly used to evaluate and categorize traumatic injuries (Baker & O'Neill, 1976). Lee et al. (2008) conducted a study in which patients with Injury Severity Score values of 9–15 and greater than 15 were categorized as having moderate and severe traumatic injuries, respectively.

Studies exploring the outcomes of moderate-to-severe traumatic injury have found that physical function may be decreased at 3 months after injury (Lee et al., 2008), physical and functional disabilities may be present at 6 months after blunt thoracic injury (Baker et al., 2018) or musculoskeletal injuries (Torgbenu et al., 2019), and patients with multiple traumas may have difficulty with physical mobility at 12 months after injury (Dimopoulou et al., 2004). Moreover, psychosocial and cognitive disabilities have been associated with return to work (RTW) in patients with multiple traumatic injuries (Lee et al., 2018; Opsteegh et al., 2009). For example, only 40% of patients were able to work at 3 months after traumatic injury

[1]*MSN, RN, Supervisor, Department of Nursing, Chiayi Chang Gung Memorial Hospital, Taiwan, ROC* • [2]*MSN, RN, Supervisor, Tzu-Yuan Hospital, Taiwan, ROC* • [3]*MSN, RN, Lecturer, Chung-Jen Junior College of Nursing, Health Sciences and Management, Taiwan, ROC* • [4]*PhD, RN, Associate Professor, Department of Nursing, Chang Gung University of Science and Technology, and Associate Research Fellow, Department of Nursing, Chiayi Chang Gung Memorial Hospital, Taiwan, ROC* • [5]*PhD, RN, Associate Professor, College of Nursing, Kaohsiung Medical University, Taiwan, ROC* • [6]*PhD, RN, Professor, College of Nursing, Neuroscience Research Center, Kaohsiung Medical University, Taiwan, ROC.*

(Clay et al., 2012; Lin et al., 2013; Zieger et al., 2011). Approximately 60%–80% took more than 12 months to RTW or to find a new job. Another 20%–30% did not RTW because of disabilities (Clay et al., 2012; Lin et al., 2013).

Various studies have attempted to improve the health outcomes of patients with traumatic injury. For example, Lee et al. (2015) found that traumatic-injury-related physical symptoms and perceptions of control regarding trauma were positively affected by a nursing intervention at 3 months after injury, although the intervention did not change any other health outcomes. Vranceanu et al. (2015) conducted a study that examined "a mind body skills-based intervention" that used cognitive and behavioral treatments to help patients recover from traumatic injury over a period of 1–2 months. The findings indicate that disability and pain outcomes were changed and that the intervention affected participants' psychological and cognitive outcomes. Zatzick et al. (2013) conducted a study that involved patients who developed posttraumatic stress disorder after experiencing traumatic injury. The study used interdisciplinary case management combined with behavioral activation therapy, and the intervention significantly reduced posttraumatic stress disorder symptoms in comparison with a control group. Although previous research has accumulated substantial evidence regarding the improvement of trauma care, barriers related to comprehensive care and health outcome monitoring still exist, including the lack of trauma case management in most of Taiwan's hospitals (Lee et al., 2018) and the lack of specific discharge managers in hospitals who regularly follow up on postdischarge conditions and outcomes (Kimmel et al., 2016).

There is a lack of consensus regarding the intervention and outcome measures used for patients with traumatic injury because previous studies were conducted by a variety of different healthcare providers, including nurses (Lee et al., 2015), medical clinicians (Vranceanu et al., 2015), and psychologists (Zatzick et al., 2013). Furthermore, the timelines of past studies for intervention and follow-up of patients with traumatic injury have ranged from the acute stage (Vranceanu et al., 2015) to 12 months after injury (Zatzick et al., 2013). Therefore, integrating care across the trauma continuum may lead to improved short- and long-term health outcomes for individuals with traumatic injury. At the same time, limited research regarding the experiences of patients with traumatic injury at the acute and very early stage has been conducted. For example, only one previous qualitative study used individual interviews to assess the early recovery experiences of patients with traumatic injury (Chou et al., 2014). The findings of that study indicated that the traumatic injury itself traumatized patients. Themes from the research indicate that patients experienced acute pain and the inability to fulfill daily needs after traumatic injury and that recovery took a long time (Chou et al., 2014). Thus, appropriate interventions that meet the needs of patients with traumatic injuries are important for short- and long-term outcomes.

Clinician discussions have been used to integrate the disparate perceptions of healthcare providers to provide comprehensive care (Jelinek et al., 2014; Rowe et al., 2012). However, these studies have not typically been conducted in trauma care settings. Through clinician discussions, a number of possible improvements to continuous care have been suggested, including improvements to clinic-based interventions, assessments of patient and family needs, and implementation of related health education (Jelinek et al., 2014; Rowe et al., 2012). In this study, a comprehensive care model is defined as an integrated model that provides interdisciplinary professional practices, roles, and collaborative relationships in clinical practice (Ramont & Niedringhaus, 2012). This study used focus groups to obtain health professionals' perspectives regarding comprehensive care to improve the outcomes of patients with traumatic injury.

Methods

This study explored the perspectives of health professionals regarding comprehensive care to improve the outcomes of patients with traumatic injury.

Data Collection

Data were collected from November 2016 to October 2017. The researchers invited groups of health professionals from two teaching hospitals in Taiwan. These two hospitals both have 900–1,000 beds, treat 1,500–2,000 patients with traumatic injury each year, and maintain "Trauma Blue Teams." However, neither uses an independent trauma specialist to liaise with interdisciplinary care providers and monitor postinjury patients. Patients with injury receive general surgical care in both hospitals.

Purposive sampling was used to approach potential study participants. The inclusion criteria required that participants be health professionals who had worked in surgical ward units and/or surgical intensive care units for at least 1 year. Two nursing supervisors recruited participants at each hospital based on these inclusion criteria. As suggested by Carey (1994), each focus group was composed of five to six participants. Semi-structured and audiotaped interviews were adopted as the data collection method (McLafferty, 2004), and the suggestions of Doody et al. (2013) were followed in conducting the focus group discussions. The interview questions were developed based on the research purpose. The interview questions were as follows: (a) "Please talk about your experiences caring for patients with traumatic injury"; (b) "Please share some information regarding the traumatic-injury-related facilities, resources, and characteristics in your hospital"; (c) "What kinds of difficulties patients with traumatic injury or their families typically face?"; (d) "Please provide your perspective regarding comprehensive care for patients with traumatic injury"; and (e) "Please contribute some thoughts based on your medical expertise about how to refine care for patients with traumatic injury."

In the focus group interviews, the principal investigator shared the results from two previous projects that studied nursing interventions. Each focus group began by introducing the moderator and gathering informed consent signatures, which included consent to audiotape the group discussion to facilitate analysis. A research team member moderated the focus group interviews, as she was an experienced qualitative researcher. First, the researcher introduced the interview questions, and then the participants were invited to share their perspectives and experiences based on the interview questions.

Data Analysis

The interview content was analyzed using content analyses (Merriam & Associates, 2002). The following steps were used: (a) The transcribed recordings were read repeatedly to understand the perceptions of the participants, (b) particular sentences and any sentences that were mentioned repeatedly were marked, (c) perceptions with common features were generalized to form a theme, (d) the relationships of each theme were explored cautiously, (e) all of the themes were generalized to form the context, (f) the themes of the perceptions were formed, and (g) findings were returned to 60% of the participants to make sure the themes reflected their perceptions. Focus group interviews were discontinued when new themes ceased to emerge and after each group had been interviewed at least once.

Four standards from Lincoln et al. (1985) and Kidd and Parshall's (2000) guidance were used to achieve rigor. Credibility was established by continuous verification of the findings with the participants and researchers. The research team held discussions to ensure the credibility of the interview data. Percent agreement was applied to determine the interrater reliability between two persons based on suggestions from Feng (2014). The interrater agreement focused on the number of themes that were considered for their necessary data chunks by each independent rater (Zhao et al., 2013). Interrater agreement ranged from 78% to 84% for each theme, indicating that the level of agreement was acceptable overall. Two researchers analyzed the data independently, and then two research meetings were held to check the preliminary analysis and reach consensus with regard to the findings. Meanwhile, the participants helped clarify and confirm the emerging findings. To ensure dependability, the interviews were conducted and transcribed verbatim by the same researcher. The abundant data reflecting the participants' perceptions represented study transferability.

Ethical Considerations

Institutional review board approval was obtained from the study hospital (Approval No. 201600766B0). The purpose of the study and the process of the interviews were explained to each participant, and written consent was obtained.

Results

Twenty-eight health professionals were interviewed in five focus groups. Each focus group consisted of five to six participants, with 16 and 12 participants, respectively, participating from the two study hospitals. Eight participants (28.6%) were male, and 20 (71.4%) were female, including nine senior surgical nurses, five surgeons, five surgical nurse practitioners, three surgical nursing supervisors, three physical therapists, two social workers, and one trauma manager. The average job tenure and age of the participants were 15.6 (*SD* = 3.5) and 48.6 (*SD* = 10.2) years, respectively. The six themes are presented in the following sections.

Wound Care Is a Primary Concern for Patients

Several participants said that most of their patients were concerned about the condition of their wound and wound healing. Although participants would have already provided the patients with instructions related to wound care in hospitals, patients still generally had problems with wound care. Some patients could not care for their wounds well and would call the hospital or return to a nurse station to ask for help.

One participant reported:

I feel that patients are most concerned about their wounds. Trauma patients feel anxious about the condition they are in when they get discharged from the hospital. They worry about the care they will receive after returning home. Patients are particularly worried about how the bandage on the wound should be changed at home when the stitches have yet to be removed, and about how they should seek medical attention in case of problems with the wound.

Another said:

Within the first week or two after the date of discharge, we often receive calls from patients who try to describe their wound but usually cannot do so clearly. For example, "My wound is very swollen, painful, and red and has some secretions." Such a description makes it difficult for us to determine whether there is inflammation or whether the wound is healing. So we have to ask the patient to come see a physician. If an appointment is not possible, we will request that he or she seek emergency treatment.

Ineffective Health Education During the Hospital Stay

The participants perceived that they generally offered sufficient health instructions to patients and their families based on postinjury conditions. The medical staff members sometimes needed to repeat their instructions several times when patients and their families could not quickly understand the content. However, patients still often failed to follow instructions after hospital discharge.

One participant stated:

I am often surprised when patients fail to listen no matter how much you tell them. You tell the patient what to pay attention to after the surgery and, the next day, the problem occurs again. Or you tell a patient not to apply too much force when walking after the surgery. The patient then goes home and has his or her family take care of him or her. The family is confused and problems occur with the wound, or the patient does not move correctly....

Another participant said:

I often think that our health instructions are clear, but, in fact, patients sometimes do not understand and many difficulties occur. Patients are informed about what to pay attention to after a fracture surgery in which metal screws are used. Also, we repeat the instructions to their family.... Trauma patients and their family members may be upset and fail to focus on care-related issues, in which case we also do not know what to do.

Patients and Families Worry About Postinjury Conditions

The participants said that patients and their families were concerned about a variety of problems after experiencing a traumatic injury. Patients worried about physical symptoms such as pain, dizziness, and other injury complications. Other concerns focused on nursing facility arrangements and the timing of resuming work. The participants felt that patients generally had multiple problems that needed to be solved.

One participant said:

Patients worry about how to return to their previous lifestyles after the injury. We often see that family members are reluctant to tell patients that there will be no one to take care for them after they go home. Some patients want to go to special institutions (nursing homes) after being discharged from the hospital and the selection of such an institution is another major issue. Families demand that the institution must be close to home and the quality of care must be good.

Another participant said:

Most trauma patients are relatively young—20 ~ 60 years old. Patients worry about their future recovery and working ability. They are concerned about whether they can continue to work. Some patients worry about financial problems that can be caused by the injury, including medical treatment expenses and daily life expenditures. They worry about how they will cope if they cannot work in the future....

Current Continuity of Care Is Not Effective

More than half of the participants expressed the view that they were usually very busy and needed to put aside their work to evaluate patient needs. This may place an extra burden on medical personnel. The participants understood that patients with traumatic injury have complicated conditions and that some care needs are not effectively addressed. Greater consensus among medical staff is necessary to build up continuity of care.

One participant said that:

The late implementation of rehabilitation for trauma can cause many problems and increase the number of hospital visits, wasting medical treatment resources. The time at which post-trauma rehabilitation is started is very important and can affect the patient's prognosis. However, clinicians do not have a clear understanding or consensus regarding the timing of trauma rehabilitation during the emergency treatment stage. For instance, some surgeons may prescribe rehabilitation and include this in the treatment plan, while some surgeons may believe that rehabilitation should take place after hospital discharge.

Another participant stated:

The rehabilitation period after trauma is long. The needs of trauma patients differ from those of other patients. Students, workers, and those who live alone face more problems. Patients who live alone are often unable to come to rehabilitation regularly, which results in poorer prognoses. Also, many hospitals do not provide rehabilitation services in the evenings. Insufficient rehabilitation leads to the inability to reach initial rehabilitation goals and achieve functional recovery, which causes concern among patients. The inability to fully recover makes them worry.

Lack of Standards for Discharge Planning

Most participants stated that they usually provide health education 2–3 days before hospital discharge. Providers in the participating hospitals generally inform patients on matters requiring attention after discharge based on professional judgment. Patients usually did not have any questions during the discharge preparation period. Nonetheless, patients or family members frequently call the hospital after discharge to ask about what they should do in a particular situation. The participants suggested that hospital discharge preparation services should be standardized.

One participant said:

The difficulty lies in the fact that we do not know the best time for carrying out hospital discharge health education. Also, other than the patient, who else should be included? In many cases, family members take turns to provide care and we do not know exactly whom we need to speak to. In some cases, foreign workers provide care, and their understanding of the health education content is limited.

Another participant stated:

Patients do not actively voice their needs before going home. Often, just before their discharge, patients inform medical personnel that they do not have anyone to take care of them at home and that they do not know how their home environment should be prepared. Nowadays, each hospital has a specialist responsible for discharge preparation. However, the specialist cannot fully manage all the issues that patients have and can assist only some patients with homecare. Thus, current discharge preparation services require improvement....

Incorporation of Interdisciplinary Care to Improve Patient Outcomes

More than two thirds of the participants reported that the care currently provided from the preoperative to postoperative stages is not comprehensive and expressed hope for improvement. Points of consensus among most of the participants included the need to set up a discharge referral unit, to integrate an interdisciplinary medical team, and to construct a systematic healthcare manual for injured patients and their families.

One participant stated:

Current health education leaflets and manuals are insufficient to prepare patients for hospital discharge and require improvements. The care provided by discharge referral centers must also be included. This is because these referral centers will evaluate patients but then not provide us (nurses) with clear updates on their situations. Subsequently, the patients will contact the related care units and the centers will conduct follow-ups. Thus, the nurses will not have a clear understanding of what is going on and what they must do.

Another participant said:

The post-trauma care that is provided may be not comprehensive. The content of a systematic healthcare manual for trauma patients should include wound care, diet, rehabilitation, psychological recovery, social resources, and insurance. Audiovisual materials could be provided to foreign caregivers and patients and family members who cannot read. These materials could then be viewed in the hospital or on a phone. It is important for interdisciplinary medical personnel to jointly discuss more comprehensive content for health education.

Discussion

The findings of this study corresponded with the stated research purpose. The participants provided detailed information about patient and family concerns. Those concerns may not have been fully understood by health professionals in the past, and yet they are important for patients. The results of this study may reflect the fact that few studies have explored the early recovery experiences of patients with traumatic injuries, even as some have followed patients for up to 12 months after traumatic injury (Clay et al., 2012; Lee et al., 2008, 2010).

Of the various themes revealed in this study, most were associated with the complications, concerns, and difficulties perceived by patients with traumatic injuries during the early recovery stage. The participants reported facing several problems in helping patients to cope with postinjury situations. The first theme was that wound care was a primary concern for most patients with traumatic injury, suggesting that health professionals may want to focus more on different aspects of wound care, including the differences between wounds caused by accidents and those stemming from operations. Wound care for patients with traumatic injury may be either simple or complicated. Under Taiwan's National Health Insurance system, patients may be restricted to relatively short hospital stays. Standard wound care instructions tailored for wounds associated with different types of traumatic injuries may thus be important for patients and their families.

Previous research has shown that factors such as acute and chronic pain, poor physical function, cardiovascular complications, and mental problems cause postinjury disabilities (Perkins et al., 2012). However, this study found that patients and their families generally seemed not to pay attention to health education from providers. This may be because each traumatic injury was a shocking event for the patient and his or her family. Thus, the patient or family members may focus on the adjustment to the new realities of life and work before hospital discharge. In addition, most health professionals working in hospitals are very busy. Providing health education has become a routine aspect of medical work. Moreover, traumatic injuries are heterogeneous, and postinjury conditions may be complicated. Given the above factors, it may be difficult to offer effective education and instructions to prevent complications of traumatic injury. If a surgical unit does not establish systematic instructions for an injury on topics such as wound care, providers may offer relevant instructions based on their own experiences. Thus, the themes "ineffective health education during hospital stay" and "patients and families worry about postinjury conditions" also emerged in this study. These themes may result from patients and their families not having integrated postinjury care knowledge and information before hospital discharge.

The theme "current continuity of care is not effective" corresponds with the finding in Chou et al. (2014) that patients may have problems dealing with the consequences of traumatic injury. According to the theme, postinjury rehabilitation seems troublesome because therapy requires an extended amount of time to improve patient outcomes, and rehabilitation outcomes depend on the patient's condition. Meanwhile, if rehabilitation is slower than the patient expects, the patient may feel more anxious and experience other symptoms of mental and emotional distress. The best strategy may thus be to arrange a rehabilitation plan for each patient before hospital discharge. A patient with traumatic injury may either return to the hospital or go to a rehabilitation clinic for the therapy. However, one major problem is that Taiwan's National Health Insurance system does not cover rehabilitation and psychological consultation fees for all patients with traumatic injuries. Whether a patient with traumatic injury needs to consult a rehabilitation therapist or psychologist depends largely on the judgment of the patient's attending physician, but the needs of some patients may be ignored during the hospital stay, with the consequences of a traumatic injury emerging after discharge.

There was consensus among the participants regarding the first to fourth findings, which were rooted in the theme "lack of standards for discharge planning." Furthermore, the participants perceived that the best solution for patients with traumatic injury may be encapsulated in the last theme: "incorporation of interdisciplinary care and patient education materials to improve patient outcomes." Previous research has demonstrated a lack of consensus among health professionals regarding intervention protocols (Lee et al., 2015; Vranceanu et al., 2015; Zatzick et al., 2013). The findings of this study support the view that adopting standards for discharge preparation, interdisciplinary care, and integrated patient education materials will improve the quality of care provided to patients with traumatic injury.

Hospital care and rehabilitation programs must be based on evidence to provide the greatest benefits. Case management has been applied comprehensively to help patients with traumatic injury regain functionality in countries such as Australia (Arnold & Elder, 2013) and China (Kong et al., 2012). In addition, recently generated evidence on trauma care has touched on issues such as wound care (Virani et al., 2016), pain management (Jennings et al., 2014), postinjury rehabilitation (Faux et al., 2015), psychological and cognitive interventions (Vranceanu et al., 2015), and multidisciplinary recovery programs (Zatzick et al., 2013).

This study obtained detailed information related to provider perceptions of patient concerns and then reached consensus among the participating health professionals on establishing a standard for discharge planning using interdisciplinary care. This provides a window of opportunity to integrate all appropriate ideas into trauma care that may result in better health outcomes for patients with traumatic injury. The findings of this study may best be applied in medium-sized hospitals that do not assign a health professional such as a liaison case manager to provide postdischarge follow-up.

Conclusions

The aim of this study was to explore the experiences of health professionals in using comprehensive care to improve outcomes for patients with traumatic injury. The findings suggest that the concerns of these patients and their families may not be fully understood. The health professionals may encourage patients and their families to participate actively in the process of care planning. Moreover, the detailed information that emerged from the health professionals' experiences may be useful in establishing an essential foundation for trauma case management and interdisciplinary care in hospitals in Taiwan and other countries.

Implications for Practice

Interdisciplinary trauma case management should be organized and planned by hospital administrators. First, collaboration appears to have a positive impact on postinjury care. Trauma case management should establish a process for coordinating comprehensive healthcare services after a traumatic injury. Second, interdisciplinary teamwork, including efforts aimed at wound care, pain management, rehabilitation planning, and psychological interventions, should be integrated from the acute stage to an extended period of follow-up for individuals with injury. Third, interdisciplinary care may take time to succeed. Thus, surgical units should seek to establish or integrate educational and instructional materials for patients and their families. A dedicated contact window at each hospital may also be set up for patients to ask questions about postinjury care after hospital discharge. Last, as direct providers of healthcare, nurses should encourage patients to participate actively in their discharge planning.

Limitations

This study highlighted the perceptions of health professionals regarding the care provided to patients with traumatic injury. Future studies should also assess the concerns and perceived care needs of these patients and their families. Furthermore, the focus group interviews in this study were conducted at two regional hospitals in southern Taiwan only. Thus, the findings may be specific to this region and may not be applicable throughout Taiwan.

Acknowledgments

This work was supported by the National Science Council (grant number: NSC 101-2314-B-255-005-MY3), Chang Gung Memorial Hospital (grant number: CMRPF6F0041), and Kaohsiung Medical University Neuroscience Research Center (grant number: KMU-TC108B01) in Taiwan. Furthermore, we thank all of the participants for sharing their precious patient-care experiences.

Author Contributions

Study conception and design: BOL
Data collection: HJL
Data analysis and interpretation: BOL, HMH, TYH
Drafting of the article: HJL, HMH, WTL
Critical revision of the article: BOL, CCH

References

Arnold, S., & Elder, M. (2013). Case management: The allocation of hours and influencing factors in the management of survivors of traumatic brain injury. *Care Management Journals, 14*(1), 2–10. https://doi.org/10.1891/1521-0987.14.1.2

Baker, E., Xyrichis, A., Norton, C., Hopkins, P., & Lee, G. (2018). The long-term outcomes and health-related quality of life of patients following blunt thoracic injury: A narrative literature review. *Scandinavian Journal of Trauma, Resuscitation and Emergency Medicine, 26*(1), Article No. 67. https://doi.org/10.1186/s13049-018-0535-9

Baker, S. P., & O'Neill, B. (1976). The injury severity score: An update. *Journal of Trauma and Acute Care Surgery, 16*(11), 882–885. https://doi.org/10.1097/00005373-197611000-00006

Carey, M. A. (1994). The group effect in focus groups: Planning, implementing, and interpreting focus group research. In J. Morse (Ed.) *Critical issues in qualitative research methods* (pp. 225–241). Sage.

Chou, P. L., Chien, C. S., Lee, B. O., Bai, Y. L., & Hung, C. C. (2014). Early recovery experience of patients with injury in Taiwan. *Journal of Nursing Scholarship, 46*(4), 245–252. https://doi.org/10.1111/jnu.12084

Clay, F. J., Fitzharris, M., Kerr, E., McClure, R. J., & Watson, W. L. (2012). The association of social functioning, social relationships and the receipt of compensation with time to return to work following unintentional injuries to Victorian workers. *Journal of Occupational Rehabilitation, 22*(3), 363–375. https://doi.org/10.1007/s10926-012-9354-4

Dimopoulou, I., Anthi, A., Mastora, Z., Theodorakopoulou, M., Konstandinidis, A., Evangelou, E., Mandragos, K., & Roussos, C. (2004). Health-related quality of life and disability in survivors of multiple trauma one year after intensive care unit discharge. *American Journal of Physical Medicine & Rehabilitation, 83*(3), 171–176. https://doi.org/10.1097/01.PHM.0000107497.77487.C1

Doody, O., Slevin, E., & Taggart, L. (2013). Preparing for and conducting focus groups in nursing research: Part 2. *British Journal of Nursing, 22*(3), 170–173. https://doi.org/10.12968/bjon.2013.22.3.170

Faux, S. G., Kohler, F., Mozer, R., Klein, L. A., Courtenay, S., D'Amours, S. K., Chapman, J., & Estell, J. (2015). The ROARI project – Road Accident Acute Rehabilitation Initiative: A randomized clinical trial of two targeted early interventions for road-related trauma. *Clinical Rehabilitation, 29*(7), 639–652. https://doi.org/10.1177/0269215514552083

Feng, G. C. (2014). Intercoder reliability indices: Disuse, misuse, and abuse. *Quality & Quantity, 48*(3), 1803–1815. https://doi.org/10.1007/s11135-013-9956-8

Haagsma, J. A., Graetz, N., Bolliger, I., Naghavi, M., Higashi, H., Mullany, E. C., Abera, S. F., Abraham, J. P., Adofo, K., Alsharif, U., Ameh, E. A., Ammar, W., Antonio, C. A., Barrero, L. H., Bekele, T., Bose, D., Brazinova, A., Catalá-López, F., Dandona, L., ... Vos, T. (2016). *The global burden of injury: Incidence, mortality, disability-adjusted life years and time trends from the Global Burden of Disease study 2013. Injury Prevention, 22*(1), 3–18. https://doi.org/10.1136/injuryprev-2015-041616

Jelinek, G. A., Boughey, M., Marck, C. H., Phillip, J., Weil, J., Lane, H., & Weiland, T. J. (2014). "Better pathways of care": Suggested improvements to the emergency department management of people with advanced cancer. *Journal of Palliative Care, 30*(2), 83–89. https://doi.org/10.1177/082585971403000203

Jennings, P. A., Cameron, P., Bernard, S., Walker, T., Jolley, D., Fitzgerald, M., & Masci, K. (2014). Long-term pain prevalence and health-related quality of life outcomes for patients enrolled in a ketamine versus morphine for prehospital traumatic pain randomised controlled trial. *Emergency Medicine Journal, 31*(10), 840–843. https://doi.org/10.1136/emermed-2013-202862

Kidd, P. S., & Parshall, M. B. (2000). Getting the focus and the group: Enhancing analytical rigor in focus group research. *Qualitative Health Research, 10*(3), 293–308. https://doi.org/10.1177/104973200129118453

Kimmel, L. A., Holland, A. E., Hart, M. J., Edwards, E. R., Page, R. S., Hau, R., Bucknill, A., & Gabbe, B. J. (2016). Discharge from the acute hospital: Trauma patients' perceptions of care. *Australian Health Review, 40*(6), 625–632. https://doi.org/10.1071/AH15148

Kong, W., Tang, D., Luo, X., Yu, I. T., Liang, Y., & He, Y. (2012). Prediction of return to work outcomes under an injured worker case management program. *Journal of Occupational Rehabilitation, 22*(2), 230–240. https://doi.org/10.1007/s10926-011-9343-z

Lee, B. O., Chaboyer, W., & Wallis, M. (2008). Predictors of health-related quality of life three months after traumatic injury. *Journal of Nursing Scholarship, 40*(1), 83–90. https://doi.org/10.1111/j.1547-5069.2008.00210.x

Lee, B. O., Chien, C. S., Hung, C. C., & Chou, P. L. (2015). Effects of an in-hospital nursing intervention on changing illness perceptions in patients with injury. *Journal of Advanced Nursing, 71*(11), 2540–2550. https://doi.org/10.1111/jan.12716

Lee, B. O., Fan, J. Y., Chan, P. T., & Hung, C. C. (2018). Illness perceptions and return to work in patients with moderate to severe injuries. *Rehabilitation Nursing, 43*(5), 297–304. https://doi.org/10.1097/rnj.0000000000000101

Lee, J. L., Chen, R. J., Chen, W. Y., Liang, Y. W., & Chen, T. C. (2010). Factors associated with disability after major trauma. *Taiwan Journal of Public Health, 29*(6), 518–517. https://doi.org/10.6288/TJPH2010-29-06-06 (Original work published in Chinese)

Lin, K. H., Guo, N. W., Shiao, S. C., Liao, S. C., Hu, P. Y., Hsu, J. H., Hwang, Y. H., & Guo, Y. L. (2013). The impact of psychological symptoms on return to work in workers after occupational injury. *Journal of Occupational Rehabilitation, 23*(1), 55–62. https://doi.org/10.1007/s10926-012-9381-1

Lincoln, Y., Guba, E., & Pilotta, J. J. (1985). *Naturalistic inquiry* (Vol. *9*, pp. 438–439). International Journal of Intercultural Relations.

McLafferty, I. (2004). Focus group interviews as a data collecting strategy. *Journal of Advanced Nursing, 48*(2), 87–194. https://doi.org/10.1111/j.1365-2648.2004.03186.x

Meerding, W. J., Looman, C. W., Essink-Bot, M. L., Toet, H., Mulder, S., & van Beeck, E. F. (2004). Distribution and determinants of health and work status in a comprehensive population of injury patients. *The Journal of Trauma Injury, Infection, and Critical Care, 56*(1), 150–161. https://doi.org/10.1097/01.TA.0000062969.65847.8B

Merriam, S. B., & Associates. (2002). *Qualitative research in practice: Examples for discussion and analysis* (1st ed.) Jossey-Bass.

Ministry of Health and Welfare, Taiwan, ROC. (2016). *2014 Health and national health insurance annual statistics information service.* http://www.mohw.gov.tw/CHT/Ministry/Index.aspx\

Opsteegh, L., Reinders-Messelink, H. A., Schollier, D., Groothoff, J. W., Postema, K., Dijkstra, P. U., & van der Sluis, C. K. (2009). Determinants of return to work in patients with hand disorders and hand injuries. *Journal of Occupational Rehabilitation, 19*(3), 245–255. https://doi.org/10.1007/s10926-009-9181-4

Perkins, Z. B., De'Ath, H. D., Sharp, G., & Tai, N. R. (2012). Factors affecting outcome after traumatic limb amputation. *The British Journal of Surgery, 99*(1, Suppl.), 75–86. https://doi.org/10.1002/bjs.7766

Ramont, R. P., & Niedringhaus, D. (2012). *Comprehensive nursing care. Revised second edition* (2nd ed.). Pearson Education.

Rowe, S., Goldsmith, G., Price, R., Brooks, A., & Harvey, A. (2012). Health care providers' perspectives of an intervention designed to improve colorectal cancer screening rates in family medicine residency clinics: A qualitative study. *Journal of Cancer Education, 27*(4), 695–702. https://doi.org/10.1007/s13187-012-0393-5

Torgbenu, E. L., Ashigbi, E. Y. K., Opoku, M. P., Banini, S., & Prempeh, E. B. A. (2019). Rehabilitation and management outcomes of musculoskeletal injuries in a major referral hospital in Ghana. *BMC Musculoskeletal Disorders, 20*(1), 40. https://doi.org/10.1186/s12891-019-2423-5

University of Florida Health. (2019). *Traumatic injury.* https://ufhealth.org/traumatic-injury

Virani, S. R., Dahapute, A. A., Bava, S. S., & Muni, S. R. (2016). Impact of negative pressure wound therapy on open diaphyseal tibial fractures: A prospective randomized trial. *Journal of Clinical Orthopaedics and Trauma, 7*(4), 256–259. https://doi.org/10.1016/j.jcot.2016.05.007

Vranceanu, A. M., Hageman, M., Strooker, J., ter Meulen, D., Vrahas, M., & Ring, D. (2015). A preliminary RCT of a mind body skills based intervention addressing mood and coping strategies in patients with acute orthopaedic trauma. *Injury, 46*(4), 552–557. https://doi.org/10.1016/j.injury.2014.11.001

Zatzick, D., Jurkovich, G., Rivara, F. P., Russo, J., Wagner, A., Wang, J., Chris, D., Lord, S. P., Petrie, M., O'Connor, S., & Katon, W. (2013). A randomized stepped care intervention trial targeting posttraumatic stress disorder for surgically hospitalized injury survivors. *Annals of Surgery, 257*(3), 390–399. https://doi.org/10.1097/SLA.0b013e31826bc313

Zhao, X., Liu, J. S., & Deng, K. (2013). Assumptions behind intercoder reliability indices. *Annals of the International Communication Association, 36*(1), 419–480. https://doi.org/10.1080/23808985.2013.11679142

Zieger, M., Luppa, M., Meisel, H. J., Günther, L., Winkler, D., Toussaint, R., Stengler, K., Angermeyer, M. C., König, H. H., & Riedel-Heller, S. G. (2011). The impact of psychiatric comorbidity on the return to work in patients undergoing herniated disc surgery. *Journal of Occupational Rehabilitation, 21*(1), 54–65. https://doi.org/10.1007/s10926-010-9257-1

2

Person-Centered Care Environment Associated with Care Staff Outcomes in Long-Term Care Facilities

JiSun CHOI[1] • Da Eun KIM[2] • Ju Young YOON[3*]

ABSTRACT

Background: Although a general implementation of person-centered care in Korean long-term care delivery systems would be challenging, person-centered care has the potential to improve resident and staff outcomes through changes in current care services. However, little empirical evidence currently supports a positive relationship between person-centered care environments and staff outcomes.

Purpose: This study was designed to examine the relationship between person-centered care environments and staff outcomes, including job satisfaction and turnover intention, among care staff in Korean long-term care facilities.

Methods: This descriptive, correlational study used data from 235 care staff (94 nursing staff and 141 personal care workers) in 13 long-term care facilities in Korea. Data were collected using structured survey questionnaires, including items related to the person-centered care environment, job satisfaction, and turnover intention. Multilevel linear and logistic regression analyses were performed using Mplus Version 7.0.

Results: After controlling for individual (age, education, monthly income, position, shift work, and job tenure) and organizational (type of facility, location, ownership, bed size, and staffing levels) characteristics, a significant relationship was found between the person-centered care environment and job satisfaction and turnover intention among staff in Korean long-term care facilities.

Conclusions/Implications for Practice: The study findings indicate that working in a person-centered care environment is key to higher job satisfaction, which is a significant predictor of turnover intention among staff in long-term care facilities. To recruit and retain qualified staff to provide high-quality person-centered care in long-term care facilities, a supportive work environment is crucial. Fostering a person-centered care environment will ultimately improve quality of care for residents.

KEY WORDS:
intent to leave, job satisfaction, nursing home, nurse staffing, person-centered care.

Introduction

The rapid increase in the aging population worldwide has led to a growing demand for long-term care facilities such as nursing homes and skilled nursing facilities for older adults who experience cognitive or functional impairment (McGilton et al., 2016). However, the chronic shortage of long-term care staff, including registered nurses (RNs), certified nursing assistants (CNAs), and personal care workers (PCWs), who are essential caregivers in these facilities, is a pressing concern (Bethell et al., 2018; Radford et al., 2015; Zhang et al., 2019). Research findings have shown a significant and negative association between a high rate of turnover for long-term care staff and the quality of resident care in terms of outcome variables such as frequency of nursing care deficiencies and incidence of pressure ulcers (Lerner et al., 2014; Trinkoff et al., 2013). Thus, stability in the nursing care workforce is vital to the improvement of care quality in long-term care settings.

Considering the complex care needs of residents living in long-term care facilities, it is commonly recognized that work in these facilities presents physical and emotional challenges (McGilton et al., 2016). Factors related to turnover and turnover intention among staff in long-term care settings include job satisfaction, supportive supervision, work shift, demographic characteristics (e.g., age and education), and organizational characteristics (e.g., staffing levels, bed size, and location; Karantzas et al., 2012; Zhang et al., 2019). Job dissatisfaction is one of the most cited predictors of turnover intention among long-term care staff (Choi & Johantgen, 2012; Karantzas et al., 2012; Kuo et al., 2014). Interestingly, however, several researchers have found that CNAs and care aides working in long-term care facilities, although generally satisfied with their work, are less satisfied with their working

[1]*PhD, RN, Associate Professor, College of Nursing Science, Kyung Hee University, Seoul, Republic of Korea* • [2]*PhD, RN, Assistant Professor, College of Nursing, Research Institute of Nursing Science, Kyungpook National University, Daegu, Republic of Korea* • [3]*PhD, RN, Associate Professor, College of Nursing, Research Institute of Nursing Science, Seoul National University, Seoul, Republic of Korea.*

conditions, which include heavy workloads, lack of appreciation and recognition, and lack of the resources necessary to provide quality care (Chamberlain et al., 2016; Choi & Johantgen, 2012; Squires et al., 2015). Moreover, job satisfaction is a significant mediator in the relationship between work stress and turnover intention among long-term care nurses (Kuo et al., 2014).

In addition to job satisfaction, researchers have investigated work environments for long-term care staff, showing a significant relationship between a supportive work environment, job satisfaction, and lower turnover intention (Chamberlain et al., 2016; Choi & Johantgen, 2012; Gilster et al., 2018; Squires et al., 2015). A person-centered care environment consists of care delivery systems that facilitate individualized care based on a holistic approach through a therapeutic relationship (Edvardsson et al., 2009) and is crucial for job satisfaction among long-term care staff (McCormack et al., 2010). In addition, there have been great efforts to create a more person-centered care environment as a key element of quality care for residents in long-term care facilities (Edvardsson et al., 2017; McCormack et al., 2010; McCormack & McCance, 2006).

The previously discussed trends apply to Korea, which has experienced the most rapid growth in aging population in the world, with 14.3% of the population older than 65 years old in 2018 (Statistics Korea, 2018). The consequent rapid growth in new, long-term care facilities for vulnerable older adults in Korea has raised serious concerns such as nursing staff shortage, poor working conditions, and poor quality of resident care (H. Y. Lee et al., 2015, M. Lee et al., 2013). In response to the demand for higher quality care in long-term care facilities, there has been growing interest in person-centered care approaches that involve shifting the focus from caregiver tasks to individual residents (McCormack & McCance, 2006). Although developing person-centered care delivery systems in all Korean long-term facilities would be a difficult challenge, successful implementation of person-centered care into practice may improve the current state of long-term care services as well as resident and staff outcomes in Korea. In one study, a significant association was found between person-centered care and nursing care quality in Korean long-term care hospitals (Sagong & Lee, 2016). However, little empirical evidence is currently available to confirm the positive effect of person-centered care environments on staff outcomes in Korean long-term care hospitals. Therefore, this study was conducted to investigate the relationship between person-centered care environments and staff outcomes, including job satisfaction and turnover intention, among staff working in long-term care facilities in Korea.

Methods

Study Design

The data in this descriptive, correlational survey study were collected between November 2016 and February 2017 from a convenience sample of care staff, including nursing staff (RNs and CNAs) and PCWs, who had worked for more than 1 month in their current facility.

Study Sample and Data Collection

In long-term care facilities in Korea, both RNs and CNAs are considered nursing staff and provide nursing care to residents. PCWs assist residents with most direct care and daily activities such as feeding, bathing, toileting, and other personal needs. The parent study identified the overall relationships among person-centered care and care outcomes from the perspectives of "residents" and "staff" and conducted psychometric testing of person-centered care instruments in a Korean cultural setting. This study, part of the parent study, focused on person-centered environment and staff outcomes. For this study, the minimum sample size of 150 was calculated based on the rule of thumb for regression analysis of at least 10 cases per estimated parameter (Waltz et al., 2017), with 15 predictors included in our regression models. The final analytical sample consisted of 235 staff, including 94 nursing staff and 141 PCWs in 13 long-term care facilities in Korea (IRB No. E1811/001-001).

Measures

Staff outcomes

The two staff outcome variables considered in this study were job satisfaction and turnover intention. Job satisfaction was measured using the job satisfaction subscale of the Korean version of the Copenhagen Psychological Questionnaire II (COPSOQ II-K; June & Choi, 2013). The COPSOQ II was originally developed by the National Institute of Occupational Health Research in Denmark as a comprehensive measure of the psychosocial working environment (Pejtersen et al., 2010). In the COPSOQ-K, the job satisfaction subscale consists of four items that are scored on a 4-point Likert scale, with higher scores indicating higher job satisfaction. Good reliability and validity were established for the subscale, with a Cronbach's alpha of .78, and concurrent validity, using correlation analysis with Korean job stress, was assessed as −.67 in a psychometric testing study of the COPSOQ-K (June & Choi, 2013). The Cronbach's alpha was .88 in this study. Turnover intention was measured using a single, dichotomously scored item (1 = *yes*, 0 = *no*), asking whether the respondent planned to leave within 1 year.

Person-centered care environment

Person-centered care environment was measured using the Korean version of the Person-centered Climate Questionnaire-Staff version (PCQ-S), translated by Sagong et al. (2018). The PCQ-S was originally developed in Sweden by Edvardsson and colleagues to measure the care environment as perceived by staff in healthcare settings in which person-centered care is provided (Edvardsson et al., 2009). The PCQ-S comprises 14 items in three subdomains: "climate of safety," "climate of everydayness," and "climate of community." The items are rated on a 6-point Likert scale, with higher scores indicating a more person-centered care environment. The reliability and validity of the Korean version of the PCQ-S were established, with strong evidence of internal consistency reliability (Cronbach's alpha = .91) and construct validity in a sample of staff working in Korean long-term care facilities (Sagong et al., 2018). The Cronbach's alpha was .92 in this study.

Demographic and organizational characteristics

Demographic characteristics included age (in years), marital status (with or without spouse), educational level (high school or lower, college diploma, or bachelor's degree or higher), type of job (nursing staff or PCW), shift work (yes or no), and job tenure (number of months working at the current facility). Organizational characteristics included type of facility (long-term care hospital or nursing home), location (urban or rural), ownership (not-for-profit [incorporated] or for-profit), years in operation, number of beds, and staffing levels (resident-to-nursing staff ratio and resident-to-PCW ratio).

Statistical Analysis

Descriptive statistics were used to summarize the characteristics of the staff and long-term care facilities. To examine the relationships between the person-centered care environment and the two staff outcomes (job satisfaction and turnover intention), multilevel analyses were used with Mplus Version 7.0 (Muthén & Muthén, Los Angeles, CA, USA), adjusted for the nested data structure, with individual care staff nested in their respective facilities. Specifically, two-level linear regression analysis was performed for job satisfaction, and two-level logistic regression analysis was performed for turnover intention. In these multilevel modeling analyses, the first level was individual care staff and the second level was long-term care facilities. Maximum likelihood estimation with robust standard errors was used to consider the nonnormal distribution of the two staff outcome variables.

Results

General Characteristics of the Long-Term Care Facility Sample

The characteristics of the 13 long-term care facilities included in this study are presented in Table 1. Of these facilities, nine were nursing homes and four were long-term care hospitals. Eleven were located in urban areas, and seven were for-profit facilities. The average number of years in operation was 10.9, the average resident-to-nursing staff ratio was 16.2, and the average resident-to-PCW ratio was 3.8.

General Characteristics of the Care Staff Sample

In Table 2, the 235 staff participants included 94 nursing staff (RNs and CNAs) and 141 PCWs. The average age was approximately 52.9 years, and most (98.3%) were female. Almost two thirds of the respondents (56%) had a high school diploma or lower, and the average tenure at their current facility was 45.6 months (3.8 years). The mean scores for person-centered care environment and job satisfaction were 4.7 and 2.9, respectively. Almost 17.3% of the respondents reported that they intended to leave (turnover intention) within 1 year.

Results of Multilevel Regression Analyses

The results of multilevel regression analysis for job satisfaction and turnover intention are presented in Table 3. In the two-level linear regression model for job satisfaction, person-centered care environment was statistically associated with job satisfaction. For each one-unit increase in person-centered care environment, job satisfaction among care staff increased 0.49 points, on average. For other individual care staff and organizational characteristics, facility type (long-term care hospitals compared with nursing homes) and the resident–nursing staff ratio were found to be statistically and negatively associated with job satisfaction.

In the two-level logistic regression model for turnover intention, which included both person-centered care environment and job satisfaction, person-centered care environment was statistically associated with turnover. For each one-unit increase in person-centered care environment, the care staff participants were 11% less likely to respond affirmatively to the turnover intention question. In addition, job satisfaction was statistically and negatively associated with turnover intention. Among individual staff, those holding a bachelor's degree or higher were more likely to respond affirmatively to the turnover intention question than those holding a high school diploma or lower. With regard to organizational characteristics,

Table 1

General Characteristics of the Long-Term Care Facilities Sample (N = 13)

Variable	Total (*N* = 13)		NH (*n* = 9)		LTCH (*n* = 4)	
	n	%	*n*	%	*n*	%
Location						
Urban	11	84.6	7	77.8	4	100.0
Rural	2	15.4	2	22.2	0	0.0
Ownership						
Not-for-profit (incorporate)	6	46.2	5	55.6	1	25.0
For-profit	7	53.8	4	44.4	3	75.0
Variable	***M***	***SD***	***M***	***SD***	***M***	***SD***
Operating period (years)	10.9	6.0	12.2	6.7	7.8	2.2
Number of beds	111.7	81.4	72.8	38.3	199.3	88.3
Resident-to-nursing staff ratio	16.2	9.6	21.5	5.9	4.3	0.1
Resident-to-personal care worker ratio	3.8	2.3	2.7	0.4	6.2	3.1

Note. NH = nursing home; LTCH = long-term care hospital.

Table 2

General Characteristics of the Study Participants (N = 235)

Variable	Total		Job Satisfaction				Turnover Intention			
	n	%	*M*	*SD*	*t/F*	*p*	*n*	%	χ^2	*p*
Age[a] (years; *M* and *SD*)	52.9	9.4			2.711	.046			6.854	.077
21–40	27	11.7	2.8	0.5			9	33.3		
41–50	47	20.3	2.9	0.4			9	19.1		
51–60	114	49.4	2.9	0.4			14	12.3		
61–70	43	18.6	3.1	0.5			5	11.6		
Gender[a]					−1.688	.186			9.501	.002
Female	228	98.3	2.9	0.5			35	15.4		
Male	4	1.7	2.6	0.4			3	75.0		
Marital status[a]					0.813	.420			0.210	.646
With spouse	202	86.3	2.9	0.5			34	16.8		
Without spouse	32	13.7	3.0	0.4			4	12.5		
Educational level[a]					1.361	.258			6.075	.048
High school diploma or lower	131	56.0	3.0	0.5			14	10.7		
College diploma	54	23.1	2.8	0.4			11	20.4		
Bachelor's degree or higher	49	20.9	2.9	0.4			13	26.5		
Type of job					2.891	.004			2.950	.086
Nursing staff	94	40.0	2.8	0.4			21	22.3		
Personal care worker	141	60.0	3.0	0.5			17	12.1		
Shift work[a]					−0.099	.921			0.081	.776
Yes	84	36.1	2.9	0.5			23	27.4		
No	149	63.9	2.9	0.4			15	10.1		
Monthly income[a] ($; *M* and *SD*)	1,635.0	341.4			0.843	.471			1.835	.607
< 1,500	93	40.3	3.0	0.5			13	14.0		
1,500–1,999	89	38.5	2.9	0.5			15	16.9		
2,000–2,499	43	18.6	2.8	0.4			9	20.9		
≥ 2,500	6	2.6	2.9	0.3			0	0.0		
Job tenure (months; *M* and *SD*)	45.6	38.4								
Person-centered care environment (*M* and *SD*)	4.7	0.6								
Job satisfaction (*M* and *SD*)	2.9	0.5								
Turnover intention (*n* and %)	38	16.2								

[a]Missing data.

turnover intention was statistically higher in long-term care hospitals, in facilities located in a rural area, and in facilities with higher resident-to-nursing staff ratios.

Discussion

This study was conducted to investigate the relationship between person-centered care environment and, respectively, job satisfaction and turnover intention among RNs, CNAs, and PCWs working in long-term care facilities in Korea. The findings of this study indicate a significant association between person-centered care environments and job satisfaction and turnover intention among nursing staff after adjusting for individual and organizational characteristics such as age, educational level, ownership type, and staffing levels. Consistent with the results of a previous study on the development of person-centered care environments in nursing homes (McCormack et al., 2010), this study revealed that increasing the person-centric nature of care environments contributes significantly to higher job satisfaction among long-term care staff. Moreover, this study was the first to provide empirical evidence regarding the importance of person-centered care environments to the improvement of staff outcomes in Korean long-term care facilities such as increased job satisfaction and decreased turnover intention.

As regards the underlying mechanism, a prior study used mediation analysis to explore how person-centered care environments influence positive staff outcomes, including job satisfaction and burnout (te Boekhorst et al., 2008), finding that in small-scale living homes, care staff felt they had more work control, perceived fewer job demands, and received more social support from their coworkers. Reducing job

Table 3

Results of Hierarchical Linear/Logistic Regression Analysis

Variable	Job Satisfaction (n = 230)			Turnover Intention (n = 220)	
	β	*SE*	*p*	*OR*	CI
Job satisfaction	—	—	—	0.847	[0.739, 0.971]
Person-centered care environment	0.49	0.05	<.001	0.890	[0.796, 0.995]
Individual factors					
Age (years)	0.13	0.07	.070	0.877	[0.754, 1.020]
Educational level (ref: high school or lower)					
College diploma	0.04	0.09	.664	1.082	[0.932, 1.255]
Bachelor's degree or higher	−0.01	0.07	.848	1.157	[1.029, 1.301]
Monthly income ($)	−0.04	0.07	.525	0.931	[0.822, 1.053]
Nursing staff (ref: personal care worker)	−0.11	0.06	.072	1.066	[0.921, 1.234]
Shift work (ref: fixed work)	−0.09	0.05	.069	1.089	[0.940, 1.261]
Job tenure (months)	0.04	0.06	.496	0.953	[0.850, 1.068]
Organizational factors					
Long-term care hospital (ref: nursing home)	−0.62	0.25	.012	2.192	[1.315, 3.655]
Urban location (ref: rural)	0.20	0.14	.157	0.638	[0.459, 0.884]
For-profit (ref: not-for-profit)	−0.02	0.09	.802	1.005	[0.946, 1.066]
Number of beds	0.32	0.22	.144	1.110	[0.827, 1.489]
Resident-to-nursing staff ratio	−0.67	0.21	.001	2.199	[1.339, 3.615]
Resident-to-personal care worker ratio	−0.21	0.21	.310	0.837	[0.620, 1.130]

Note. β = standardized coefficient; *SE* = standard error; *OR* = odds ratio; CI = confidence interval; ref = reference.

demands in a care setting increases the likelihood that care staff support colleagues and experience less emotional exhaustion. Moreover, staff empowerment is an important component of person-centered care (Koren, 2010). Nursing staff who work in person-centered care environments are more likely to control their work and actively participate in care practices, which increases job satisfaction (Rokstad et al., 2015).

To enhance job satisfaction among nursing staff, who play a vital role in providing better resident care (McGilton et al., 2016), long-term care facility administrators should consider implementing person-centered care. In this study, the reported average score for person-centered care environments was slightly lower than the score from a previous study that applied the same PCQ-S (Edvardsson et al., 2009) to nurse assistants working in residential care settings in southern Sweden (Wallin et al., 2012). Although much attention has been given to the person-centered care model, and some nursing home administrators have attempted to develop a person-centered culture in Korea (M. Lee et al., 2013), much work remains ahead to create a care environment that provides individualized and person-centered care to accommodate the unique needs, preferences, and dignity of each resident in the very limited number of long-term care facilities in Korea.

Turnover intention was examined in a separate regression model that included both person-centered care environment and job satisfaction as potential predictors. As expected, a statistically significant relationship was found between person-centered care environment and turnover intention. In the regression model, there was a significant association between job satisfaction and turnover intention among nursing staff, which corroborates the findings of previous studies, indicating a strong link between job satisfaction and turnover intention among long-term care staff (Choi & Johantgen, 2012; Karantzas et al., 2012; Kuo et al., 2014). As was shown by Kuo et al. (2014), job satisfaction had a significant, mediating effect on the relationship between work stress and turnover intention (Kuo et al., 2014). The question of whether job satisfaction mediates the relationship between person-centered care environment and turnover intention is beyond the scope of this study. Given that our findings showed a positive association between person-centered care environment and job satisfaction and, in a separate regression model, a significant association between this environment and turnover intention, further research is needed to explore the comprehensive relationships among person-centered care environment, job satisfaction, and turnover intention among long-term care staff.

With regard to care staff characteristics, age and educational level were found to be significantly and positively related, respectively, to job satisfaction and turnover intention. These results are consistent with the findings of a previous study on job satisfaction and turnover intention among CNAs working in nursing homes in the United States (Choi & Johantgen, 2012). Particularly in Korea, although these two demographic characteristics are the most basic qualifications when hiring staff in long-term care settings, facility administrators must sensibly consider these characteristics in addition to personal needs and motivators during employment interviews.

With regard to organizational characteristics, as expected, on the basis of results of previous studies (Donoghue, 2010;

Karantzas et al., 2012; Zhang et al., 2019), a significant association was found between staffing level and job satisfaction as well as turnover intention. Specifically, the resident-to-nursing staff ratio was significantly associated with job satisfaction as well as turnover intention in this study. In addition, location was significantly related to turnover intention but not to job satisfaction. In this study, nursing staff working in urban long-term care facilities were less likely than their counterparts in rural settings to report turnover intention. This result may be related to the relatively poorer quality of care and working conditions often experienced in long-term care facilities in rural areas in Korea (B. R. Lee, 2016).

Limitations

This study may have been affected by several limitations. Data were gathered from a convenience sample of nursing staff working in 13 long-term care facilities. In addition, the sample size was relatively small for multilevel regression analysis, which may reduce its statistical power, as it is usually recommended to have as many observations as possible at the top level of the multilevel model (Snijders, 2005). Thus, the results should be interpreted with caution and may not be generalizable to staff working in long-term care facilities throughout Korea. Moreover, we examined person-centered care environment and other factors related to job satisfaction and turnover intention using data from all care staff who were involved in direct resident care, including RNs, CNAs, and PCWs. Although CNAs are considered nursing staff in Korean long-term care facilities, CNAs and PCWs are usually considered paraprofessional nursing personnel and are likely to provide most direct resident care under the supervision of RNs (Choi & Johantgen, 2012; McGilton et al., 2016). Some studies have found that supportive supervision is one of the most significant factors related to turnover intention among PCWs (Bethell et al., 2018; Radford et al., 2015). Perceptions of person-centered care environments as well as factors influencing job satisfaction and turnover intention among RNs may differ from CNAs and PCWs. Thus, more research is needed to better understand the influence of person-centered care environments and other factors on job satisfaction and turnover intention at each staffing level in long-term care facilities.

Conclusions

Despite the limitations, the findings of this study indicate that promoting a person-centered care environment in long-term care facilities is vital to increasing job satisfaction and decreasing turnover intention in care staff who work in these facilities. In the long-term care practice, closer relationships and improved communications between staff and residents may decrease staff burnout and work-related emotional exhaustion and increase job satisfaction. Furthermore, care staff who provide individualized care to residents based on person-centeredness are more likely to experience enhanced confidence, which may suggest a significant strategy for retaining competent care staff in long-term care settings. Thus, more efforts should be made to develop person-centered care environments that facilitate tailored care processes that address the unique value, dignity, and preferences of individuals through a therapeutic relationship between all care providers and residents. Related changes will benefit not only residents but also care staff, who are invaluable caregivers in long-term care facilities in Korea.

Acknowledgments

This research was supported by the Research Resettlement Fund for the new faculty of Seoul National University and also by the Basic Science Research Program through the National Research Foundation of Korea funded by the Ministry of Science, ICT & Future Planning (Grant No. 2017R1C1B1002872, PI: J. Y. Y.). The funding sources had no role in the study design, data collection and analysis, interpretation of the data, writing of the manuscript, or decision to submit the manuscript for publication.

Author Contributions

Study conception and design: All authors
Data collection: DEK, JYY
Data analysis and interpretation: All authors
Drafting of the article: All authors
Critical revision of the article: JSC, JYY

References

Bethell, J., Chu, C. H., Wodchis, W. P., Walker, K., Stewart, S. C., & McGilton, K. S. (2018). Supportive supervision and staff intent to turn over in long-term care homes. *Gerontologist, 58*(5), 953–959. https://doi.org/10.1093/geront/gnx008

Chamberlain, S. A., Hoben, M., Squires, J. E., & Estabrooks, C. A. (2016). Individual and organizational predictors of health care aide job satisfaction in long term care. *BMC Health Services Research, 16,* Article No. 577. https://doi.org/10.1186/s12913-016-1815-6

Choi, J., & Johantgen, M. (2012). The importance of supervision in retention of CNAs. *Research in Nursing & Health, 35*(2), 187–199. https://doi.org/10.1002/nur.21461

Donoghue, C. (2010). Nursing home staff turnover and retention: An analysis of national level data. *Journal of Applied Gerontology, 29*(1), 89–106. https://doi.org/10.1177/0733464809334899

Edvardsson, D., Sandman, P.-O., & Rasmussen, B. (2009). Construction and psychometric evaluation of the Swedish language Person-centred Climate Questionnaire–Staff version.

Journal of Nursing Management, 17(7), 790–795. https://doi.org/10.1111/j.1365-2834.2009.01005.x

Edvardsson, D., Sjögren, K., Lood, Q., Bergland, Å., Kirkevold, M., & Sandman, P.-O. (2017). A person-centred and thriving-promoting intervention in nursing homes—Study protocol for the U-Age nursing home multi-centre, non-equivalent controlled group before–after trial. *BMC Geriatrics, 17*(1), Article No. 22. https://doi.org/10.1186/s12877-016-0404-1

Gilster, S. D., Boltz, M., & Dalessandro, J. L. (2018). Long-term care workforce issues: Practice principles for quality dementia care. *Gerontologist, 58*(1, Suppl.), S103–S113. https://doi.org/10.1093/geront/gnx174

June, K. J., & Choi, E. S. (2013). Reliability and validity of the Korean version of the Copenhagen Psycho-social Questionnaire Scale. *Korean Journal of Occupational Health Nursing, 22*(1), 1–12. https://doi.org/10.5807/kjohn.2013.22.1.1 (Original work published in Korean)

Karantzas, G. C., Mellor, D., McCabe, M. P., Davison, T. E., Beaton, P., & Mrkic, D. (2012). Intentions to quit work among care staff working in the aged care sector. *The Gerontologist, 52*(4), 506–516. https://doi.org/10.1093/geront/gnr161

Koren, M. J. (2010). Person-centered care for nursing home residents: The culture-change movement. *Health Affairs (Millwood), 29*(2), 312–317. https://doi.org/10.1377/hlthaff.2009.0966

Kuo, H. T., Lin, K. C., & Li, I. C. (2014). The mediating effects of job satisfaction on turnover intention for long-term care nurses in Taiwan. *Journal of Nursing Management, 22,* 225–233. https://doi.org/10.1111/jonm.12044

Lee, B. R. (2016). *The temporal–spatial patterns of elderly long-term care facilities and regional comparison of their service qualities* [Unpublished master's thesis]. Seoul National University, Republic of Korea.

Lee, H. Y., Shin, J. H., & Harrington, C. (2015). Comparing the nurse staffing in Korean and US nursing homes. *Nursing Outlook, 63*(2), 137–143. https://doi.org/10.1016/j.outlook.2014.08.005

Lee, M., Choi, J.-S., Lim, J., & Kim, Y. S. (2013). Relationship between staff-reported culture change and occupancy rate and organizational commitment among nursing homes in South Korea. *The Gerontologist, 53*(2), 235–245. https://doi.org/10.1093/geront/gns106

Lerner, N. B., Johantgen, M., Trinkoff, A. M., Storr, C. L., & Han, K. (2014). Are nursing home survey deficiencies higher in facilities with greater staff turnover. *Journal of the American Medical Directors Association, 15,* 102–107. https://doi.org/10.1016/j.jamda.2013.09.003

McCormack, B., Dewing, J., Breslin, L., Coyne-Nevin, A., Kennedy, K., Manning, M., Peelo-Kilroe, L., Tobin, C., & Slater, P. (2010). Developing person-centred practice: Nursing outcomes arising from changes to the care environment in residential settings for older people. *International Journal of Older People Nursing, 5,* 93–107. https://doi.org/10.1111/j.1748-3743.2010.00216.x

McCormack, B., & McCance, T. V. (2006). Development of a framework for person-centred nursing. *Journal of Advanced Nursing, 56*(5), 472–479. https://doi.org/10.1111/j.1365-2648.2006.04042.x

McGilton, K. S., Bowers, B. J., Heath, H., Shannon, K., Dellefield, M. E., Prentice, D., Peelo-Kilroe, L., Tobin, C., Siegel, E. O., Meyer, J., Chu, C. H., Ploeg, J., Boscart, V. M., Corazzini, K. N., Anderson, R. A., & Muller, C. A. (2016). Recommendations from the international consortium on professional nursing practice in long-term care homes. *Journal of the American Medical Directors Association, 17,* 99–103. https://doi.org/10.1016/j.jamda.2015.11.001

Pejtersen, J. H., Kristensen, T. S., Borg, V., & Bjorner, J. B. (2010). The second version of the Copenhagen Psychosocial Questionnaire. *Scandinavian Journal of Public Health, 38*(3, Suppl.), 8–24. https://doi.org/10.1177/1403494809349858

Radford, K., Shacklock, K., & Bradley, G. (2015). Personal care workers in Australian aged care: Retention and turnover intentions. *Journal of Nursing Management, 23*(5), 557–566. https://doi.org/10.1111/jonm.12172

Rokstad, A. M. M., Vatne, S., Engedal, K., & Selbaek, G. (2015). The role of leadership in the implementation of person-centred care using dementia care mapping: A study in three nursing homes. *Journal of Nursing Management, 23*(1), 15–26. https://doi.org/10.1111/jonm.12072

Sagong, H., Kim, D. E., Bae, S., Lee, G. E., Edvardsson, D., & Yoon, J. Y. (2018). Testing reliability and validity of the Person-centered Climate Questionnaire-Staff version in Korean for long-term care facilities. *Journal of Korean Academy of Community Health Nursing, 29*(1), 11–20. https://doi.org/10.12799/jkachn.2018.29.1.11

Sagong, H., & Lee, G. E. (2016). Person-centered care and nursing service quality of nurses in long-term care hospitals. *Journal of Korean Academy of Community Health Nursing, 27*(4), 309–318. https://doi.org/10.12799/jkachn.2016.27.4.309

Snijders, T. A. B. (2005). *Power and sample size in multilevel linear models.* In B. S., Everitt & D. C., Howell (Eds.), *Encyclopedia of statistics in behavioral science* (pp. 1570–1573). Wiley.

Squires, J. E., Hoben, M., Linklater, S., Carleton, H. L., Graham, N., Estabrooks, C. A., & Estabrooks, C. A. (2015). Job satisfaction among care aides in residential long-term care: A systematic review of contributing factors, both individual and organizational. *Nursing Research and Practice, 2015,* Article ID 157924. https://doi.org/10.1155/2015/157924

Statistics Korea. (2018). *2018 elderly population statistics.* http://kosis.kr/publication/publicationThema.do (Original work published in Korean)

te Boekhorst, S., Willemse, B., Depla, M. F., Eefsting, J. A., & Pot, A. M. (2008). Working in group living homes for older people with dementia: The effects on job satisfaction and burnout and the role of job characteristics. *International Psychogeriatrics, 20*(5), 927–940. https://doi.org/10.1017/S1041610208007291

Trinkoff, A. M., Han, K., Storr, C. L., Lerner, N., Johantgen, M., & Gartrell, K. (2013). Turnover, staffing, skill mix, and resident outcomes in a national sample of US nursing homes. *The Journal of Nursing Administration, 43*(12), 630–636. https://doi.org/10.1097/NNA.0000000000000004

Wallin, A. O., Jakobsson, U., & Edberg, A.-K. (2012). Job satisfaction and associated variables among nurse assistants working in residential care. *International Psychogeriatrics, 24,* 1904–1918. https://doi.org/10.1017/S1041610212001159

Waltz, C. F., Strickland, O. L., & Lenz, E. R. (2017). *Measurement in nursing and health research* (5th ed.). Springer Publishing Company.

Zhang, Y., Punnett, L., & Gore, R. (2019). Predictors of nursing staff voluntary termination in nursing homes: A case–control study. *Journal of Applied Gerontology, 38*(11), 1518–1536. https://doi.org/10.1177/0733464817724043

3

The Mediation and Suppression Effect of Demoralization in Breast Cancer Patients After Primary Therapy: A Structural Equation Model

Hsiu-Ling PENG[1] • Hui-Wen HSUEH[2] • Yu-Hsing CHANG[3] • Ren-Hau LI[1]*

ABSTRACT

Background: Because of the increasing 5-year survival rate of breast cancer, adjustment to breast cancer survivorship is pertinent to the patient's life after diagnosis. Despite the psychological changes occurring during the transitional period (first 5 years after diagnosis) and after primary therapy having a known, critical effect on survivorship status, the data related to this topic are very limited.

Purpose: This study was designed to examine the relationships among demoralization, stress, sleep disturbance, and psychological well-being in women with breast cancer after primary therapy.

Methods: Two hundred eight women with breast cancer (mean age = 51.96 ± 8.27) participated in a cross-sectional study in central Taiwan. Recruitment was conducted using convenience snowball sampling at a local teaching hospital. All of the participants had completed primary therapy and were in the 5-year postdiagnosis period. The average duration of cancer was 28 months. The participants completed the Stress of Breast Cancer after Primary Therapy Scale, Demoralization Scale, Pittsburgh Sleep Quality Inventory, and Ryff's Psychological Well-Being Scale–Short Form. Data were analyzed using a structural equation model to find plausible path relationships among stress, demoralization, sleep disturbances, and psychological well-being.

Results: Demoralization was shown to completely mediate the effect of stress on sleep disturbances. In addition, the predictive effect of sleep disturbances on psychological well-being was overwhelmingly explained by demoralization when competing with sleep disturbances. Furthermore, a positive path was found between stress and psychological well-being because of the suppression effect of demoralization.

Conclusions/Implications for Practice: Demoralization was found to be a mediator that suppressed the relationships among stress, sleep disturbances, and psychological well-being in the adaptation process of patients with breast cancer after primary therapy. This article adds to the limited research on women with breast cancer after primary therapy who are in their initial 5 years of diagnosis. In addition, this study used structural equation model to find the plausible path relationships among the psychological factors involved in the well-being of women with breast cancer. Supporting patients with cancer and effectively reducing their perceived demoralization will be key to transforming stress into personal growth and a facilitator of long-term recovery.

KEY WORDS:
breast cancer, demoralization, psychological well-being, stress, sleep disturbances.

Introduction

Parallel with the increase in the morbidity rate of breast cancer in recent years, the 5-year survival rate for breast cancer has increased to more than 90% (Health Promotion Administration, 2019; Howlader et al., 2018). The levels of threat and chronic stress related to this disease are pertinent to the lives of survivors of breast cancer. Over the last two decades, research has confirmed the beneficial effects of psychosocial factors on women with breast cancer (Rodin, 2018). Although many of these studies focused on the experiences of newly diagnosed (Lauzier et al., 2010; T. Y. Lee et al., 2013) or chronic patients with breast cancer (Bloom et al., 2012; Pudrovska et al., 2013), limited data exist on the physiological and psychological health changes in women during the transitional period after primary therapy and in women in the initial 5 years after their breast cancer diagnosis. Primary therapy for breast cancer typically includes surgery, chemotherapy, radiation therapy, and/or targeted therapy. The period after the completion of all primary therapy interventions with the exception of hormone therapy is a critical period during which patients should move beyond their cancer experiences and reestablish a normal daily routine. Pinpointing key psychological factors that may improve the quality of life of patients with breast cancer after primary therapy will help healthcare providers develop effective strategies to facilitate the adjustment of these patients.

[1]*PhD, Associate Professor, Department of Psychology, Chung-Shan Medical University, and Adjunct Consultant, Department of Psychiatry, Chung-Shan Medical University Hospital, Taichung, Taiwan, Republic of China* • [2]*MS, Psychologist, Department of Clinical Psychology, National Cheng Kung University Hospital, Dou-Liou Branch, Yunlin, Taiwan, Republic of China* • [3]*MS, Research Assistant, Department of Anesthesiology and Pain Medicine, Boston Children's Hospital, Boston, MA, USA.*

Breast cancer is a cause of life-threatening stress that may induce posttraumatic stress disorder or posttraumatic growth (Arnaboldi et al., 2017; Costanzo et al., 2012). Folkman's (2012) stress–coping model has shown that stress may produce not only negative emotions such as depression and demoralization but also negative reactions such as sleep disturbances, leading to poor psychological well-being. Moreover, depression and sleep disturbance are common factors in breast-cancer-related stress reactions (Rowland & Massie, 2010; Yue & Dimsdale, 2010).

Depression may take many forms in patients with breast cancer both after diagnosis and in daily life, significantly increasing functional disability in these patients (Tang et al., 2015). Kissane and Doolittle (2013) highlighted the divergence between depression and demoralization in patients with cancer, as anhedonic traits are not present in demoralization. "Demoralization" was defined in their study as an expression of existential distress, hopelessness, helplessness, and loss of meaning and purpose in life. Although demoralization is common in patients with cancer, some patients may experience demoralization without experiencing depression (Robinson et al., 2015). Therefore, using depression exclusively to evaluate patients with cancer may neglect as much as 25% of those patients who experience high levels of demoralization but do not present with major depressive disorders (C. Y. Lee et al., 2012; Robinson et al., 2015). In some studies, demoralization was identified as a better construct than depression to predict quality of life in survivorship (Robinson et al., 2015; Tecuta et al., 2015). Hence, demoralization may be described as the experience of hopelessness or helplessness that leads an individual to exhaustion and poor adjustment.

Sleep disturbance is another common stress reaction in breast cancer adaptation (Palesh et al., 2013). The highest prevalence of insomnia among patients with cancer has been reported in those with breast cancer, both during the primary therapy period (Sanford et al., 2013) and afterward (Otte et al., 2010). Furthermore, the findings of studies have indicated that psychological stress may be a precipitating factor of sleep disturbance and that these sleep disturbances may impact negatively on quality of life. Other studies have shown that sleep disturbances may be the cause or consequence of depression, which, in turn, worsens the adaptation of patients with breast cancer (Palesh et al., 2013). In light of the complex, contradictory relationships among stress, depression, and sleep disturbances, this study was developed to establish a model to better depict the path relationships among the above factors.

In their review of the literature on psychological well-being over the past 30 years, Ryff (2014) noted that a multitude of physical illnesses have been implicated as factors that impair psychological well-being. Accordingly, in this study, psychological well-being was used to measure quality of life in patients with breast cancer.

The purpose of this study was to explore the relationships among stress, sleep disturbance, demoralization, and psychological well-being in women with breast cancer after primary therapy. On the basis of the stress–coping model (Folkman, 2012) and the related literature on the plausible relationships among these factors, it was hypothesized in this study that experiencing stress, demoralization, and sleep disturbances may impact the psychological well-being of patients. Furthermore, this study aimed to investigate the role of demoralization and sleep disturbances in the stress–coping process. In the hypothesized relationship model, stress serves as an initial cause that affects other factors, whereas psychological well-being serves as an endpoint outcome. Moreover, in this model, demoralization plays an important, core role in terms of determining the extent of the impact on sleep disturbance. The results are expected to identify a number of mediation effects and to improve scholarly understanding regarding the mechanism at work among these factors.

Methods

Design

This cross-sectional study was conducted at a local teaching hospital in central Taiwan. Participants were recruited using a convenience snowball sampling technique. After receiving informed consent, a demographic datasheet and four psychological testing instruments were used to collect the data.

Participants

Two hundred seventeen participants were initially recruited for the study. Patients were included if they were female, diagnosed with breast cancer during the past 5 years, and had completed primary therapy. Exclusion criteria included diagnosis of psychotic or neurocognitive disorders, presenting with any acute or chronic condition that would limit the ability of the patient to participate in the study, being unable to communicate in Chinese, and refusal to give informed consent. Of the recruited population, 4.15% ($n = 9$) were lost because of incomplete data. The valid response rate was thus 95.85%, with 208 participants.

Procedures

This cross-sectional study was conducted from December 2013 to September 2015. Approval from the Chung Shan Medical Hospital's institutional review board to collect and analyze data was obtained before conducting the study (No. CS13203). Once the patients were recruited and informed consent was obtained in person, the participants completed the questionnaires, providing information on their demographics, medical history, stress, demoralization, sleep quality, and psychological well-being.

Instruments

The stress of breast cancer after primary therapy scale

The 13-item Stress of Breast Cancer after Primary Therapy Scale (Stress-BCAPTS) was partly adopted from the Mandarin version

Table 1

Participant Demographic Information (N = 208)

Variable	*n*	%
Educational level		
Illiterate	3	1.4
Elementary/junior high school	47	22.6
Senior high school/vocational school	129	62.0
University and above	29	14.0
Marital status		
Unmarried	17	8.2
Married	171	82.2
Separated	12	5.8
Widowed	8	3.8
Monthly income (NT$)		
No income	65	31.3
Below 20,000	40	19.2
20,000–50,000	78	37.5
51,000–80,000	19	9.1
Over 80,000	6	2.9
Comorbidities		
No	144	69.2
Yes	64	30.8

Note. NT$ = New Taiwan dollar.

of the Newly Diagnosed Breast Cancer Stress Scale (NDBCSS; T. Y. Lee et al., 2013). Each item of the scale is measured on a 4-point Likert scale, ranging from 0 (*strongly disagree*) to 3 (*strongly agree*), with higher scores indicating higher experienced stress. The Stress-BCAPTS has good criterion-related validity with the Perceived Stress Scale ($r = .46$, $p < .001$) and the anxiety ($r = .57$, $p < .001$) and depression ($r = .35$, $p < .001$) subscales of the Hospital Anxiety and Depression Scale. The NDBCSS has four subscales: perceptions of unpredictability, perceptions of uncontrollability, perceptions of a heavy psychological load, and perceptions of facing challenge. The perceptions of facing challenge subscale was excluded from the Stress-BCAPTS, whereas the other three were retained. The Cronbach's α is .89 for the Stress-BCAPTS and .62–.77 for its three subscales. Confirmatory factor analysis showed that each item had a factor loading of .41–.83, indicating acceptable construct validity.

Demoralization scale

The Demoralization Scale (Kissane et al., 2004) consists of 24 questions and has been translated into Mandarin (Hung et al., 2010). Each item is measured on a 5-point Likert scale ranging from 0 (*strongly disagree*) to 4 (*strongly agree*), with higher scores associated with higher demoralization. The Demoralization Scale has good criterion-related validity and divergent validity (Kissane et al., 2004), earning a Cronbach's α of .93 for the full scale and α of .60–.86 for its five facets, including loss of meaning and purpose, dysphoria, disheartenment, helplessness, and sense of failure. The translated Mandarin version maintained the same validity and may thus be effectively applied to Mandarin-speaking patients with cancer (Hung et al., 2010). Furthermore, confirmatory factor analysis indicated the factor loading for each item as between .49 and .87, showing acceptable construct validity.

Pittsburgh sleep quality inventory

The Pittsburgh Sleep Quality Inventory (PSQI; Buysse et al., 1989) has been translated into Mandarin (Fu, 2007). The PSQI is a self-report questionnaire consisting of 19 items that are designed to assess the respondent's quality of sleep during the past month. The PQSI investigates seven indicators of sleep quality, including (a) subjective sleep quality, (b) sleep latency, (c) sleep duration, (d) habitual sleep efficiency, (e) sleep disturbances, (f) use of sleeping medication, and (g) daytime dysfunction, with higher scores indicating worse quality of sleep. The questionnaire has good reliability and validity and has been the most effective and most widely used self-report scale in sleep research for cancer (Palesh et al., 2010). The Cronbach's α of this scale is .77, and the results of confirmatory factor analysis indicate that each factor loading ranges from .41 to .86, showing acceptable construct validity.

Ryff's psychological well-being scale–short form

Ryff's Psychological Well-Being Scale (Ryff, 1989) has been translated into Mandarin and condensed from the original

Table 2

Descriptive Statistics and Correlation Matrix Between Variables

Variable	Descriptive Statistics		Pearson's Correlation Coefficients			
	Mean	*SD*	1	2	3	4
1. Stress	11.53	7.55	–	(.49***)	(.22**)	(–.05)
2. Demoralization	25.96	13.75	.42***	–	(.49***)	(–.67***)
3. Sleep disturbances	8.26	3.95	.18**	.40***	–	(–.36***)
4. Psychological well-being	83.62	12.37	–.09	–.58***	–.26***	–

Note. Data in the parentheses represent correlation coefficients among latent variables.
$^{**}p < .01$. $^{***}p < .001$ (two-tailed).

Table 3

Descriptive Statistics and Correlation Matrix Between Each Subscale of All Variables

Subscale	Descriptive Statistics		Pearson's Correlation Coefficients								
	M	*SD*	Sp1	Sp2	Sp3	Sp4	Sp5	Sp6	Sp7	D1	D2
Sp1	1.51	0.87	1.0								
Sp2	1.67	0.87	.55**	1.0							
Sp3	1.16	0.91	.37**	.24**	1.0						
Sp4	0.75	0.96	.42**	.40**	.53**	1.0					
Sp5	1.65	0.63	.45**	.33**	.23**	.22**	1.0				
Sp6	0.58	1.05	.44**	.38**	.19**	.20**	.27**	1.0			
Sp7	0.94	0.80	.46**	.27**	.15*	.14*	.41**	.21**	1.0		
D1	3.87	3.03	.34**	.30**	.10	.09	.29**	.21**	.27**	1.0	
D2	6.83	3.81	.37**	.21**	.10	.17*	.32**	.11	.44**	.58**	1.0
D3	6.76	4.31	.35**	.21**	.03	.10	.32**	.16*	.39**	.67**	.80**
D4	4.05	2.95	.36**	.31**	.10	.19**	.27**	.16*	.32**	.71**	.70**
D5	4.46	2.14	.28**	.23**	.05	.15*	.28**	.13	.21**	.58**	.41**
St1	3.73	2.91	.08	−.01	−.08	−.12	.16*	.06	.22**	.23**	.32**
St2	3.68	2.71	.26**	.06	.04	−.04	.29**	.15*	.29**	.24**	.36**
St3	4.13	3.06	.18*	.14*	.05	−.04	.26**	.14*	.25**	.30**	.38**
P1	14.84	2.77	−.19**	−.17*	−.08	−.13	−.16*	.01	−.07	−.37**	−.27**
P2	13.75	3.02	−.19**	−.16*	−.05	−.06	−.14*	−.07	−.10	−.44**	.29**
P3	14.25	2.48	−.19**	−.22**	−.06	−.15*	−.23**	−.01	−.19**	−.33**	−.23**
P4	12.80	2.72	−.22**	−.18**	−.00	−.08	−.15*	−.07	−.10	−.22**	−.28**
P5	14.66	2.59	−.21**	−.21**	.00	−.08	−.19**	−.02	−.21**	−.45**	−.40**
P6	13.31	2.69	−.26**	−.28**	−.12	−.16*	−.28**	−.08	−.31**	−.44**	−.47**

Note. Sp1–Sp7 indicate subscale scores, respectively, as subjective sleep quality, sleep latency, sleep duration, habitual sleep efficiency, sleep disturbances, use of sleeping medication, and daytime dysfunction in Pittsburgh Sleep Quality Inventory; D1–D5 indicate subscale scores, respectively, as loss of meaning and purpose, dysphoria, disheartenment, helplessness, and sense of failure in the Demoralization Scale; St1–St3 indicate subscale scores, respectively, as perceptions of unpredictability, perceptions of uncontrollability, and perceptions of a heavy psychological load in the Stress of Breast Cancer after Primary Therapy Scale; and P1–P6 indicate subscale scores, respectively, as Ryff's personal growth, purpose of life, positive relationships with others, autonomy, environmental mastery, and self-acceptance in the Psychological Well-Being Scale–Short Form.

$^{*}p < .05$. $^{**}p < .01$ (two-tailed).

84 items to an 18-item version with good reliability and validity (Li, 2014). Three items were selected from six indexes that respectively measure (a) self-acceptance, (b) positive relations with others, (c) autonomy, (d) environmental mastery, (e) purpose in life, and (f) personal growth. Each item is measured on a 6-point Likert scale ranging from 1 (*strongly disagree*) to 6 (*strongly agree*), with higher scores indicating better psychological well-being. The Psychological Well-Being Scale–Short Form has a Cronbach's α of .93, and the subscales have α values of .79–.91. Confirmatory factor analysis has shown factor loadings between .67 and .94, indicating acceptable construct validity.

Analyses

Statistical analyses were conducted using IMB SPSS Statistics Version 23 (IBM, Inc., Armonk, NY, USA) for both descriptive and correlational analyses. Structural equation modeling (SEM) was determined using LISREL 8.8 to explore and understand the path relationships among the constructs of interest in the sample. The sample size was expected to be over 200 for SEM models containing five or fewer constructs, each with more than three observed variables, and modest communalities of the observed variables (Hair et al., 2006). In this research, the absolute values of skewness of the 21 variables (subscales) ranged from 0.03 to 1.56 (standard error = 0.17), whereas the absolute values of kurtosis ranged from .05 to .93 (standard error = .34). These values are generally in line with the normal distribution assumed in the hypothesis. According to the recommendation of Hooper et al. (2008), indices such as chi-square statistic (χ^2), degrees of freedom (*df*), *p* value, χ^2/df, root mean square error of approximation (RMSEA) and its confidence interval, standardized root mean square residual (SRMR), comparative fit index (CFI), and parsimony goodness-of-fit index (PGFI) should be reported. In addition, goodness-of-fit index

D3	D4	D5	St1	St2	St3	P1	P2	P3	P4	P5	P6
1.0											
.67**	1.0										
.55**	.54**	1.0									
.36**	.28**	.13	1.0								
.36**	.33**	.16*	.67**	1.0							
.43**	.28**	.15*	.63**	.60**	1.0						
−.38**	−.37**	−.46**	.08	−.01	.05	1.0					
−.35**	−.36**	−.48**	−.04	−.04	.00	.71**	1.0				
−.37**	−.27**	−.49**	.00	.01	−.02	.54**	.43**	1.0			
−.28**	−.23**	−.41**	−.06	−.02	−.09	.41**	.37**	.42**	1.0		
−.38**	−.45**	−.46**	−.14*	−.11	−.20**	.43**	.44**	.42**	.53**	1.0	
−.54**	−.49**	−.57**	−.13	−.17*	−.18**	.55**	.61**	.47**	.48**	.54**	1.0

(GFI) may also be presented for reference. Specifically, p value > .05, χ^2/df < 2 or 3, CFI > .95, GFI > .95, PGFI > .50, SRMR < .08, and RMSEA < .07 with an upper confidence interval limit of < .08 are preferred.

Results

Descriptive Statistics

The average age of the 208 participants was 51.96 years, with a standard deviation of 8.27 and a range of 29–76 years. Most (89.9%) of the participants were postmenopausal, whereas 95.2% had received surgery, 77.4% had received chemotherapy, 67.8% had received radiation therapy, and 60.6% had received hormone therapy during primary therapy. The average period of remission was 28 months, whereas 42.3% had been diagnosed with Stage 2 breast cancer and 37.5% had been diagnosed with Stage 1. These percentage distributions are largely similar to official government statistics for Taiwan (Health Promotion Administration, 2019). Other sociodemographic characteristics of the sample are shown in Table 1.

Table 2 shows the average level of each scale score and correlation coefficient among their observed scores and among their latent variables for patients with breast cancer after primary therapy. The correlation coefficients among the scale scores were all significant, with the exception of the correlation between stress and psychological well-being. In addition to the SEM, statistics such as means, standard deviations, and correlation coefficients among each subscale scores of all variables are presented in Table 3. In summary, most of the subscales correlated significantly with each other. However, sleep duration did not correlate significantly with all of the subscales of the other three variables, habitual sleep efficiency did not correlate significantly with all of the subscales of stress, use of sleeping medication did not correlate significantly with all of the subscales of

Figure 1

Confirmatory Factor Analysis Model for Stress, Demoralization, Sleep Disturbance, and Psychological Well-Being (Completely Standardized Solution)

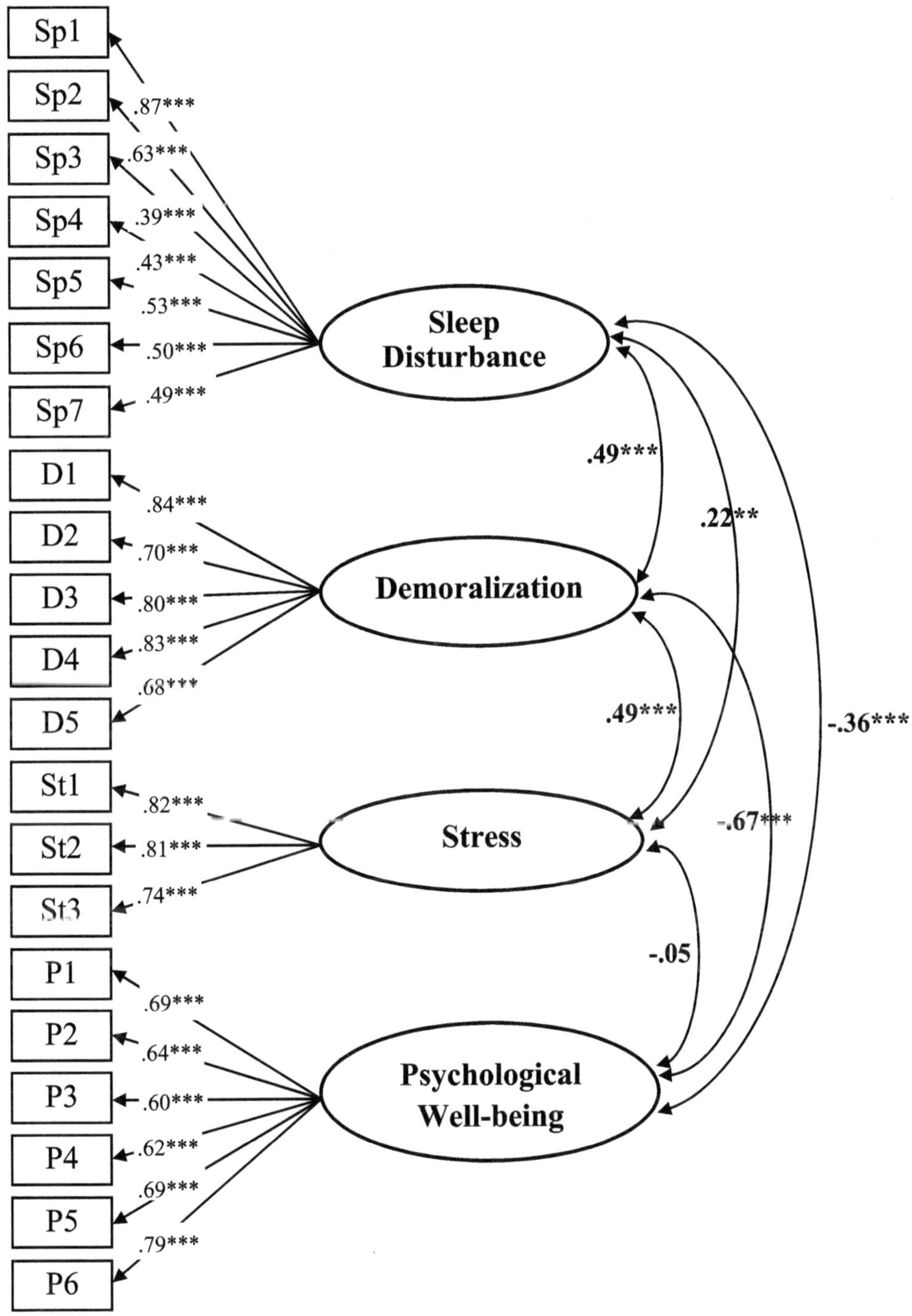

Note. Sp1–Sp7 indicate subscale scores, respectively, as subjective sleep quality, sleep latency, sleep duration, habitual sleep efficiency, sleep disturbances, use of sleeping medication, and daytime dysfunction in the Pittsburgh Sleep Quality Inventory; D1–D5 indicate subscale scores, respectively, as loss of meaning and purpose, dysphoria, disheartenment, helplessness, and sense of failure in the Demoralization Scale; St1–St3 indicate subscale scores, respectively, as perceptions of unpredictability, perceptions of uncontrollability, and perceptions of a heavy psychological load in the Stress of Breast Cancer after Primary Therapy Scale; and P1–P6 indicate subscale scores, respectively, as Ryff's personal growth, purpose of life, positive relationships with others, autonomy, environmental mastery, and self-acceptance in the Psychological Well-Being Scale–Short Form. χ^2 = 123.14 (df = 128, p = .60), comparative fit index = 1.00, goodness-of-fit index = .95, parsimony goodness-of-fit index = .52, standardized root mean square residual = .054, and root mean square error of approximation < .001. $^{**}p < .01$, $^{***}p < .001$ (two-tailed).

Figure 2

Structural Equation Modeling for Relationships Among Stress, Demoralization, Sleep Disturbances, and Psychological Well-Being (Completely Standardized Solution)

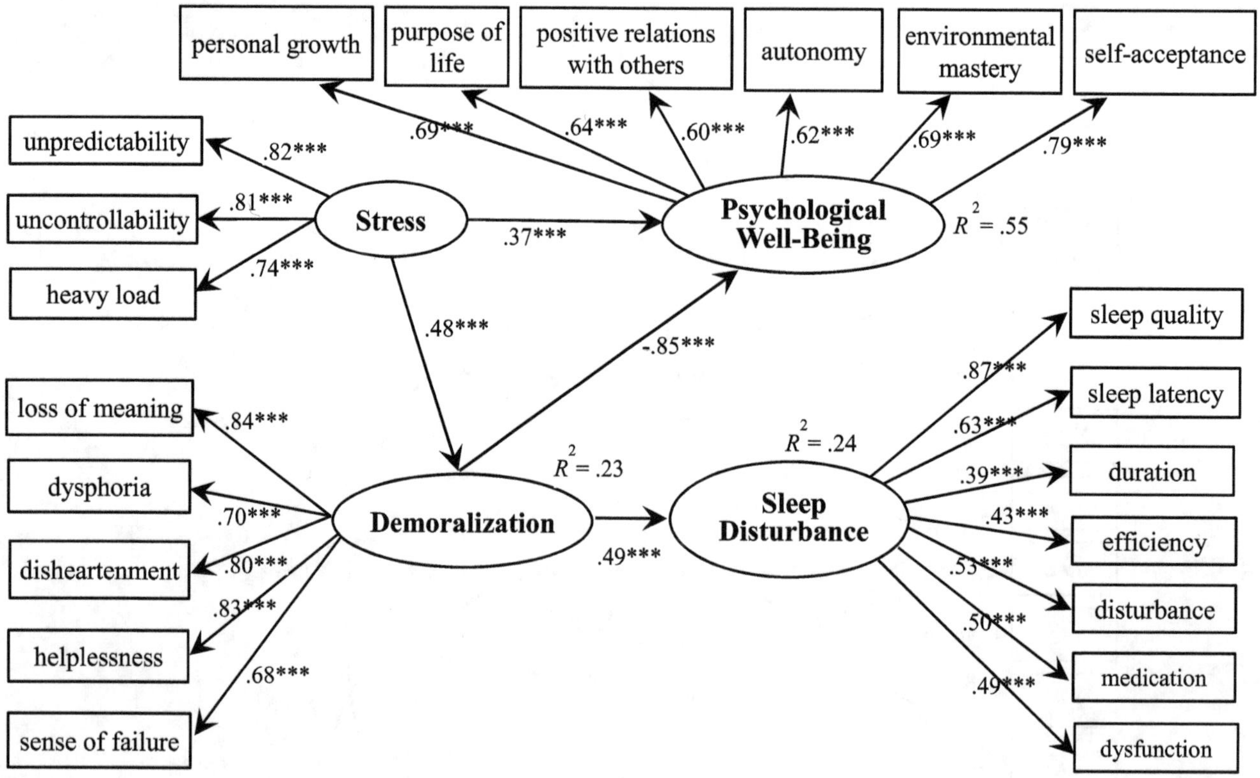

Note. χ^2 = 123.54 (df = 130, p = .64). CFI = 1.00, GFI = .95, PGFI = .53, SRMR = .054, RMSEA < .001. ***p < .001 (two tailed).

psychological well-being, and none of the subscales of stress correlated significantly with the first four subscales of psychological well-being.

The Mediation and Suppression Role of Demoralization

The confirmatory factor analysis of all of the factors, which had been modified by adding correlation coefficients between errors, is shown in Figure 1, with results showing that χ^2 = 123.14, df = 128, p = .60, χ^2/df = .96, CFI = 1.00, GFI = .95, PGFI = .52, SRMR = .054, and RMSEA < .001 with a 90% confidence interval of .00 < RMSEA < .031. The SEM with the same modification is shown in Figure 2. The model fit showed χ^2 = 123.54, df = 130, p = .64, χ^2/df = .95, CFI = 1.00, GFI = .95, PGFI = .53, SRMR = .054, and RMSEA < .001 with a 90% confidence interval of .00 < RMSEA < .029, indicating an acceptable model fit. In addition, all of the structural coefficients (β) of the SEM were significant (ps < .001). Specifically, the direct effects of stress were .48 for demoralization and .37 for psychological well-being. Moreover, demoralization was found to have a direct effect on sleep disturbances (β = .49) and psychological well-being (β = –.85). Besides, the indirect effects of stress on psychological well-being and sleep disturbances, respectively, were –.41 and .24. In particular, there were two paths in the model, from stress to sleep disturbances and from sleep disturbances to psychological well-being, which were no longer significant as their corresponding bivariate correlation coefficients (refer to Table 2 for details on the correlation coefficients between the latent variables, r = .22 and r = –.36). In other words, the effect of stress on sleep disturbances were completely mediated by demoralization, and demoralization influenced psychological well-being more strongly than sleep disturbances, resulting in the invalidation of the effects of sleep disturbances on psychological well-being.

Furthermore, when the effect of stress on psychological well-being was mediated by demoralization, the path of the latent variables changed from the initial value of –.05 to a subsequent value of .37 (refer to Table 2 and Figure 2). Experienced stress appeared to not significantly correlate with psychological well-being (–.05) but had a significant effect (.37) under the mediation of demoralization. This phenomenon is known as the suppression effect (MacKinnon, 2008), in which the effect of demoralization on psychological well-being is reinforced (from −.67 to −.85; refer to Table 2 and Figure 2) and the effect of stress on psychological well-being changes in terms of both sign and size (from −.05 to .37).

Discussion

The results of this study indicate the presence of significant psychological stress in patients with breast cancer after primary therapy, although the measured stress levels (M = 11.53) were lower than in patients who had just received their diagnosis (M = 17.44; T. Y. Lee et al., 2013). The NDBCSS factor analysis, heavy perceived psychological load, unpredictability, and uncontrollability were found to effectively reflect degree of stress, whereas perceptions of facing challenges were found to have a very low factor loading on stress. This may be because certain items considered in the facing challenge perception factor refer to the period immediately after diagnosis rather than after primary therapy (T. Y. Lee et al., 2013). This was why the subscale was not included in the model. The transition to the role of a survivor of breast cancer after primary therapy commences after radical physical therapy has been completed and before the start of relatively easier hormone therapy procedures. From this, we inferred that the perceived challenges may influence postdiagnosis stress in terms of representing the shock of being threatened by the cancer and the physiological pain. Meanwhile, the subfactor of perceptions of unpredictability included some items related to the fear of recurrence. This fear was found to be an important factor affecting post-primary-therapy adjustment, earning the highest factor loading on stress (.82). Age and stress were found to have a statistically significant and negative correlation (r = −.25, p < .001). This is consistent with previous research findings that, on average, the younger a patient is, the higher the experienced stress (Helgeson et al., 2004). It may be that older women experience more life events and are less worried about facing uncontrolled and unpredictable relapse and death and thus are less overloaded. This is an important point in the development of intervention protocols and self-care programs for younger patients with breast cancer.

On the basis of the results of SEM, demoralization was found to exert mediation and suppression effects in the model. Demoralization had a stronger influence on psychological well-being than sleep disturbances, resulting in the invalidation of the effects of sleep disturbances on psychological well-being. We further found that stress, via demoralization, affected sleep disturbances (0.48 x 0.49 = 0.24; MacKinnon, 2008). In addition, stress was found to directly affect demoralization, which, in turn, influenced psychological well-being (0.48x(−0.85) = −0.41; MacKinnon, 2008). When patients cope adequately with demoralization, both the negative effect of stress on sleep disturbances and the negative effect of sleep disturbances on psychological well-being may be expected to decrease drastically, to the point at which stress should become a factor promoting wellness (β = .37). In contrast, when demoralization is coped with poorly, the stress may increase sleep disturbances and, in turn, lower wellness. Furthermore, we found that demoralization competed with sleep disturbances in explaining psychological well-being. Thus, demoralization cannot be taken lightly. Ultimately, paying attention to demoralization is crucial to promoting overall wellness in survivors of breast cancer.

Clinical Implications

This study found that demoralization plays mediating and suppressive roles in the model involving stress, sleep disturbances, and psychological well-being, which is an important finding for those patients with breast cancer who had completed primary therapy and have been struggling to adapt to their new lives as survivors. This finding echoes previous research that emphasized demoralization findings among women with breast cancer (Kissane & Doolittle, 2013; C. Y. Lee et al., 2012; Robinson et al., 2015). Successfully managing demoralization in survivors of breast cancer will help decrease stressful feelings and death anxiety and improve psychological well-being (Rodin et al., 2018). Kissane and Doolittle (2013) suggested dignity and meaning-centered therapies as models of psychotherapy that focus on alleviating demoralization and also suggested combining interpersonal psychotherapy, behavioral activation strategies, psychodynamic life review, and pharmacological treatment into an effective strategy. Some researchers productively proposed "Moving Beyond Cancer" (Ganz et al., 2004) and "Managing Cancer and Living Meaningfully" (Rodin et al., 2018) as psychological intervention trials to evaluate the physical and psychosocial functioning of patients with breast cancer after primary therapy. These protocols indeed significantly improved the participants' adjustment efficacy. With respect to the Managing Cancer and Living Meaningfully therapy, the authors showed that demoralization is a good predictor of the effects of the intervention in patients with breast cancer with moderate death anxiety. This anxiety improved 3 months after primary therapy as compared with initial diagnosis and with the end of primary therapy (Rodin et al., 2018). Demoralization should be cautiously evaluated in psychoeducation, individual counseling, and group counseling settings. According to the model in this study, the beneficial effects of stress increase psychological well-being when the patient is coping with demoralization.

This study contributes to the care of patients with breast cancer, especially during the period of adaptation after primary therapy. Patients who have completed primary therapy and are within 5 years of diagnosis have been the least-discussed target group in breast cancer research to date. However, the adaptation process is fluid and chronic and should not be treated the same way as treating post-traumatic stress disorder or in an urgent manner. During surgery, chemotherapy, radiation therapy, and other forms of primary therapy, the physical pain and discomfort are usually the main responses that a patient with breast cancer experiences. Negative moods and other psychological responses during primary therapy are often masked by the physiological pain, making these often not visible and difficult to address. When the primary therapy has ended, along with diminishing physiological responses, the real psychological adaptation process for patients with breast cancer begins. Therefore, demoralization as a treatable psychological factor should be emphasized in related therapeutic interventions (Robinson et al., 2015).

Study Limitations

Despite the benefits of this unique data set and the value of being able to obtain data from SEM, several limitations to this study must be acknowledged. Although the sample comprised a population with characteristics that approximated the average national characteristics in published government statistics, the small sample size and convenient sampling approach may have biased this sample and affected the generalizability of the findings. The evidence reported here suggests that benefit finding associated with having breast cancer and undergoing treatment may have the potential to promote greater psychological well-being over time. It is important to keep in mind that not all patients with breast cancer fit the scenario described in this study. In addition, this study did not include a control group or conduct random sampling. Both should be considered when planning future research. Furthermore, variables such as fear of recurrence are suggested in studies of stress in patients with breast cancer to explore their adaptation. This research used a cross-sectional design, and although the SEM analysis showed that the overall model fitness was acceptable for the relationships among stress, demoralization, sleep disturbances, and psychological well-being, any conclusions regarding causal relationships should be carefully considered. Future research should test the fitness of the model using a longitudinal design or a treatment-intervention design.

Author Contributions

Study conception and design: HLP, RHL
Data collection: HLP, HWH
Data analysis and interpretation: HLP, RHL
Drafting of the article: All authors
Critical revision of the article: HLP, RHL

References

Arnaboldi, P., Riva, S., Crico, C., & Pravettoni, G. (2017). A systematic literature review exploring the prevalence of post-traumatic stress disorder and the role played by stress and traumatic stress in breast cancer diagnosis and trajectory. *Breast Cancer (Dove Medical Press), 9*, 473–485. https://doi.org/10.2147/BCTT.S111101

Bloom, J. R., Stewart, S. L., Oakley-Girvan, I., Banks, P. J., & Shema, S. (2012). Quality of life of younger breast cancer survivors: Persistence of problems and sense of well-being. *Psycho-Oncology, 21*(6), 655–665. https://doi.org/10.1002/pon.1965

Buysse, D. J., Reynolds, C. F., Monk, T. H., Berman, S. R., & Kupfer, D. J. (1989). The Pittsburgh Sleep Quality Index: A new instrument for psychiatric practice and research. *Psychiatry Research, 28*(2), 193–213. https://doi.org/10.1016/0165-1781(89)90047-4

Costanzo, E. S., Stawski, R., Ryff, C., Coe, C., & Almeida, D. (2012). Cancer survivors' responses to daily stressors: Implications for quality of life. *Health Psychology, 31*(3), 360–370. https://doi.org/10.1037/a0027018

Folkman, S. (2012). *The Oxford handbook of stress, health, and coping*. Oxford University Press.

Fu, Y. W. (2007). *Psychometric evaluation of the Pittsburgh Sleep Quality Index in Taiwanese cancer patients* [Unpublished master's thesis]. Taipei Medical University, Taiwan, ROC.

Ganz, P. A., Kwan, L., Stanton, A. L., Krupnick, J. L., Rowland, J. H., Meyerowitz, B. E., Bower, J. E., & Belin, T. R. (2004). Quality of life at the end of primary treatment of breast cancer: First results from the moving beyond cancer randomized trial. *Journal of the National Cancer Institute, 96*(5), 376–387. https://doi.org/10.1093/jnci/djh060

Hair, J. F., Black, W. C., Babin, B. J., Anderson, R. E., & Tatham, R. L. (2006). *Multivariate data analysis* (6th ed.). Prentice Hall.

Health Promotion Administration. (2019). *Cancer registry annual report*. Ministry of Health and Welfare, Taiwan, ROC.

Helgeson, V. S., Snyder, P., & Seltman, H. (2004). Psychological and physical adjustment to breast cancer over 4 years: Identifying distinct trajectories of change. *Health Psychology, 23*(1), 3–15. https://doi.org/10.1037/0278-6133.23.1.3

Hooper, D., Coughlan, J., & Mullen, M. (2008). Structural equation modelling: Guidelines for determining model fit. *Electronic Journal of Business Research Methods, 6*(1), 53–60. https://doi.org/10.21427/D7CF7R

Howlader, N., Noone, A. M., Krapcho, M., Miller, D., Bishop, K., Kosary, C. L., Yu, M., Ruhl, J., Tatalovich, Z., Mariotto, A., Lewis, D. R., Chen, H. S., Feuer, E. J., & Cronin, K. A. (2018). *SEER cancer statistics review, 1975–2014*. National Cancer Institute. https://seer.cancer.gov/csr/1975_2014/

Hung, H.-C., Chen, H.-W., Chang, Y.-F., Yang, Y.-C., Liu, C.-L., Hsieh, R.-K., Leu, Y.-S., Chen, Y.-J., Wang, T.-E., Tsai, L.-Y., Liu, S.-I., & Fang, C. K. (2010). Evaluation of the reliability and validity of the Mandarin version of demoralization scale for cancer patients. *Journal of Internal Medical of Taiwan, 21*(6), 427–435. https://doi.org/10.6314/JIMT.2010.21(6).06

Kissane, D. W., & Doolittle, M. (2013). Demoralization and depression in cancer. In T. N. Wise, M. Biondi, & A. Costantini (Eds.), *Psychooncology* (pp. 91–115). American Psychiatric Association.

Kissane, D. W., Wein, S., Love, A., Lee, X. Q., Kee, P. L., & Clarke, D. M. (2004). The demoralization scale: A report of its development and preliminary validation. *Journal of Palliative Care, 20*(4), 269–276. https://doi.org/10.1177/082585970402000402

Lauzier, S., Maunsell, E., Levesque, P., Mondor, M., Robert, J., Robidoux, A., & Provencher, L. (2010). Psychological distress and physical health in the year after diagnosis of DCIS or invasive breast cancer. *Breast Cancer Research and Treatment, 120*(3), 685–691. https://doi.org/10.1007/s10549-009-0477-z

Lee, C.-Y., Fang, C.-K., Yang, Y.-C., Liu, C.-L., Leu, Y.-S., Wang, T.-E., Chang, Y.-F., Hsieh, R. K., Chen, Y.-J., Tsai, L.-Y., Liu, S.-I., & Chen,

H. W. (2012). Demoralization syndrome among cancer outpatients in Taiwan. *Supportive Care in Cancer, 20*(10), 2259–2267. https://doi.org/10.1007/s00520-011-1332-4

Lee, T.-Y., Chen, H.-H., Yeh, M.-L., Li, H.-L., & Chou, K.-R. (2013). Measuring reliability and validity of a newly developed stress instrument: Newly diagnosed breast cancer stress scale. *Journal of Clinical Nursing, 22*(17–18), 2417–2425. https://doi.org/10.1111/jocn.12107

Li, R.-H. (2014). Reliability and validity of a shorter Chinese version for Ryff's psychological well-being scale. *Health Education Journal, 73*(4), 446–452. https://doi.org/10.1177/0017896913485743

MacKinnon, D. P. (2008). *Multivariate applications series. Introduction to statistical mediation analysis.* Lawrence Erlbaum Associates.

Otte, J. L., Carpenter, J. S., Russell, K. M., Bigatti, S., & Champion, V. L. (2010). Prevalence, severity, and correlates of sleep–wake disturbances in long-term breast cancer survivors. *Journal of Pain and Symptom Management, 39*(3), 535–547. https://doi.org/10.1016/j.jpainsymman.2009.07.004

Palesh, O. G., Aldridge-Gerry, A., Ortiz-Tudela, E., & Capuron, L. (2013). Sleep disruption in breast cancer patients and survivors. *Journal of the National Comprehensive Cancer Network, 11*(12), 1523–1530.

Palesh, O. G., Roscoe, J. A., Mustian, K. M., Roth, T., Savard, J., Ancoli-Israel, S., Heckler, C., Purnell, J. Q., Janelsins, M. C., & Morrow, G. R. (2010). Prevalence, demographics, and psychological associations of sleep disruption in patients with cancer: University of Rochester Cancer Center-Community Clinical Oncology Program. *Journal of Clinical Oncology, 28*(2), 292–298. https://doi.org/10.1200/JCO.2009.22.5011

Pudrovska, T., Carr, D., McFarland, M., & Collins, C. (2013). Higher-status occupations and breast cancer: A life-course stress approach. *Social Science & Medicine, 89*, 53–61. https://doi.org/10.1016/j.socscimed.2013.04.013

Robinson, S., Kissane, D. W., Brooker, J., & Burney, S. (2015). A systematic review of the demoralization syndrome in individuals with progressive disease and cancer: A decade of research. *Journal of Pain and Symptom Management, 49*(3), 595–610. https://doi.org/10.1016/j.jpainsymman.2014.07.008

Rodin, G. (2018). From evidence to implementation: The global challenge for psychosocial oncology. *Psycho-Oncology, 27*(10), 2310–2316. https://doi.org/10.1002/pon.4837

Rodin, G., Lo, C., Rydall, A., Shnall, J., Malfitano, C., Chiu, A., Panday, T., Watt, S., An, E., Nissim, R., Li, M., Zimmermann, C., & Hales, S. (2018). Managing cancer and living meaningfully (CALM): A randomized controlled trial of a psychological intervention for patients with advanced cancer. *Journal of Clinical Oncology, 36*(23), 2422–2432. https://doi.org/10.1200/JCO.2017.77.1097

Rowland, J. H., & Massie, M. J. (2010). Breast cancer. In J. C. Holland, W. S. Breitbart, P. B. Jacobsen, M. S. Lederberg, M. J. Loscalzo, & R. McCorkle (Eds.), *Psychooncology* (2nd ed., pp. 177–186). Oxford University Press.

Ryff, C. D. (1989). Happiness is everything, or is it? Explorations on the meaning of psychological well-being. *Journal of Personality and Social Psychology, 57*(6), 1069–1081. https://doi.org/10.1037/0022-3514.57.6.1069

Ryff, C. D. (2014). Psychological well-being revisited: Advances in the science and practice of eudaimonia. *Psychotherapy and Psychosomatics, 83*(1), 10–28. https://doi.org/10.1159/000353263

Sanford, S., Wagner, L., Beaumont, J., Butt, Z., Sweet, J., & Cella, D. (2013). Longitudinal prospective assessment of sleep quality: Before, during, and after adjuvant chemotherapy for breast cancer. *Supportive Care in Cancer, 21*(4), 959–967. https://doi.org/10.1007/s00520-012-1612-7

Tang, P.-L., Wang, H.-H., & Chou, F.-H. (2015). A systematic review and meta-analysis of demoralization and depression in patients with cancer. *Psychosomatics, 56*(6), 634–643. https://doi.org/10.1016/j.psym.2015.06.005

Tecuta, L., Tomba, E., Grandi, S., & Fava, G. A. (2015). Demoralization: A systematic review on its clinical characterization. *Psychological Medicine, 45*(4), 673–691. https://doi.org/10.1017/S0033291714001597

Yue, H. J., & Dimsdale, J. E. (2010). Sleep and cancer. In J. C. Holland, W. S. Breitbart, P. B. Jacobsen, M. S. Lederberg, M. J. Loscalzo, & R. McCorkle (Eds.), *Psychooncology* (2nd ed., pp. 258–269). Oxford University Press.

4

Utility of Equivalence and Cognition Models in Enhancing Validity of Translated Questionnaires: A Methodological Example Using the Heart Quality-of-Life Questionnaire

Wan Ling LEE[1]* • Khatijah LIM ABDULLAH[2] • Karuthan CHINNA[3] • Imran Z. ABIDIN[4]

ABSTRACT

Background: The cross-cultural adaptation of questionnaires has tenuous theoretical underpinnings that limit the rigor of data collection and the meaningful analysis of cognitive interview data. An adaptation of existing models of equivalence and cognition provides structure to the comprehensive investigation of various equivalence types in enhancing the validity of translated questionnaires.

Purpose: In this study, a framework comprising equivalence and cognition models was used to assess and finalize the Heart Quality-of-Life (HeartQoL)-Bahasa Malaysia (BM) questionnaire, which was derived from both forward–backward (FB) and dual-panel (DP) translation methods.

Methods: Investigation and finalization of two initial versions of the questionnaire were conducted based on findings from an expert assessment (n = 3 sociolinguists blinded to translation methods) and cognitive interviews with purposively sampled patients (FB: n = 11; DP: n = 11). The equivalence model of Herdman et al. and the question-and-answer model of Collins were adapted to form a "cognition-and-equivalence" model to guide data collection and analysis through modified cognitive interviews. The final HeartQoL-BM was completed by 373 patients with ischemic heart disease from two medical centers, and the data were analyzed using confirmatory factor analysis to assess the evidence of equivalence.

Results: Findings from the expert assessment and cognitive interview showed the existence of semantic and item equivalence on almost all of the FB and DP items, identified some subtle potential equivalence gaps, and guided the process of item finalization. Confirmatory factor analysis, including tests of factorial invariance on the final two-factor model of HeartQoL-BM, confirmed conceptual, item, measurement, and operational equivalence, which supports functional equivalence.

Conclusions: The potential use of the cognition-and-equivalence model for modified cognitive interviewing and the application of the six equivalence types of Herdman et al. were supported by the HeartQoL-BM showing functional equivalence with its source. HeartQoL-BM is a potentially valid measure of health-related quality of life for patients with ischemic heart disease independent of conditions such as angina, myocardial infarction, and heart failure.

KEY WORDS:
coronary nursing, translations, health-related quality of life, patient-reported outcome measures, cognitive interviewing.

Introduction

An adapted questionnaire (also known as a target or translated version) is assumed to be comparable with the original (or source) questionnaire after equivalence between the two versions has been established. Findings based on the equivalent target version are taken as valid, which allows data pooling and interstudy comparisons to be made across cultures. The methods used to test equivalence vary, and current empirical evidence is not adequate to pool consensus. Moreover, no gold standard exists to define the degree of acceptable similarities or tolerable variance to conclude equivalence between target and source versions. Experts, in general, agree on a multistep process for the cross-cultural adaptation of questionnaires (Fremenco et al., 2017). Most experts support using cognitive interviews to examine comparability between versions by exploring respondents' thought processes, especially with regard to their interpretation of item meanings and relevance. The wide-ranging, cross-cultural application of questionnaires with no consensus on analysis approach is the Achilles' heel of cognitive interviewing (Willis, 2015a). Thus, research advancing an appropriate analysis model is warranted. Research on the theoretical basis and the methodology necessary to establish equivalence is lacking, and the number of studies examining issues surrounding the cross-cultural adaptation of questionnaires has declined in recent years. Researchers are more explicit in reporting psychometrics properties (i.e., measurement equivalence) than other types of

[1]PhD, RN, Senior Lecturer, Faculty of Medicine, Department of Nursing Science, University of Malaya, Kuala Lumpur, Malaysia • [2]DClinP, RN, Professor, Department of Nursing, School of Healthcare and Medical Sciences, Sunway University, Kuala Lumpur, Malaysia • [3]PhD, Associate Professor, Faculty of Health and Medical Sciences, School of Medicine, Taylor's University, Malaysia • [4]MMed, MBBS, Professor, Faculty of Medicine, Department of Medicine, University of Malaya, Kuala Lumpur, Malaysia.

equivalence. To establish the many types of equivalence, both qualitative and quantitative approaches are needed, as no single method is able to address all equivalence types.

Background

This study sought to adapt the equivalence model of Herdman et al. (1998) and the "question-and-answer" cognition model of Collins (2003) as part of a larger study that was designed to establish six types of equivalence (conceptual, item, semantic, operational, measurement, and functional) in the Malay version of the Heart Quality-of-Life (HeartQoL) scale. According to Herdman et al., "conceptual equivalence" exists if the adapted questionnaire has the same relationship to the underlying concept (i.e., factors) between source and target culture. "Item equivalence" is the extent to which items are relevant and acceptable across cultures. This term also refers to the extent to which items estimate the same parameters of factor structures. "Semantic equivalence" refers to the transfer of item meaning to achieve a similar effect on respondents in different languages. "Operational equivalence" exists when a similar format, instructions, mode of administration, and measurement methods produce comparable results between adapted and source questionnaires. "Measurement equivalence" is the extent to which the properties of the measurements in the adapted questionnaire approximate its source. "Functional equivalence" (aka the summary of equivalence), which refers to the extent to which an instrument performs equally well across cultures, may be established only after the other five equivalence types have been substantiated. A framework mapping the six equivalence types to the complete process of cross-cultural adaptation of questionnaire has been proposed (W. L. Lee et al., 2019). However, the concepts of equivalence and how they link to the cognition processes underpinning cognitive interview remain underexplored in the literature. Thus, this study was designed to integrate equivalence into a cognition model to propose a structured guide for data collection and analysis of cognitive interviews employed in pretesting of translated questionnaires.

The methodologies used to translate questionnaire are still largely opinion based, with existing evidence insufficient to verify conclusively the value of back-translation, which currently dominates the field (Colina et al., 2017; Epstein et al., 2015). Therefore, in this study, the HeartQoL scale was translated into Malay (Bahasa Malaysia or BM) using two popular translation methods, the forward–backward (FB) method and the dual-panel (DP) method, as described respectively by Beaton et al. (2000) and Swaine-Verdier et al. (2004). The methodology used to finalize and validate the synthesized HeartQoL-BM to establish the six types of equivalence is described in this article.

Heart Quality-of-Life Questionnaire

The copyrighted, 14-item HeartQoL is a core measure of health-related quality of life (HRQoL) for patients with ischemic heart disease (IHD) that is independent of myocardial infarction, angina, and heart failure conditions. The participants were asked to rate on a scale of 0 (*none*) to 3 (*a lot*) regarding how much they felt bothered when in specific situations or while doing specific tasks. The detailed content of the HeartQoL is available elsewhere (Oldridge et al., 2014). Although the test–retest reliability of this scale has been verified in Malaysia (W. L. Lee et al., 2016), its construct validity has been established predominantly in Western populations (De Smedt et al., 2016; Oldridge et al., 2014). Thus, qualitative inquiry is deemed necessary to assess HeartQoL equivalence from an East Asian perspective.

Methods

Ethics clearance to conduct this study at two medical centers in Kuala Lumpur (reference: No 996.45 and RD5/25/14) and permission to translate the HeartQoL into BM were obtained. The preliminary conceptual and item equivalences of the original HeartQoL were verified by two local cardiologists and five English-speaking patients as recommended in Herdman et al. (1998). Because of the high level of semantic similarity between the FB and DP versions (W. L. Lee et al., 2019), further examination was conducted to assess the equivalence of each version with the source questionnaire using expert assessment and cognitive interviews to aid decision making in item finalization for a synthesized HeartQoL-BM. Afterward, the finalized HeartQoL-BM was validated using a cross-sectional survey.

Details on the original model of equivalence (Herdman et al., 1998) and the question-and-answer model (Collins, 2003) are provided elsewhere. This article was designed to affirm the semantic and item equivalences by analyzing cognitive interviews using the proposed cognition-and-equivalence model. Evidence of conceptual, item, operational, and measurement equivalences were verified using a confirmatory factor analysis of the HeartQoL-BM, which was administered in a survey. Functional equivalence was confirmed when the five equivalence types were substantiated, which, in turn, supported the workability of the proposed framework.

The following sections describe the data collection and analysis approaches used in the expert assessment, cognitive interviews, and survey, which were conducted between December 2015 and April 2016. Expert assessment was performed by sociolinguists from three different universities. All of these individuals were native BM speakers, proficient in English, and experienced translators. The patients who participated in the cognitive interview and survey proceedings were recruited from cardiac wards if they had an indexed diagnosis of IHD, were > 18 years old, and spoke BM as a first or second language. Patients who were cognitively unfit or hemodynamically unstable were excluded.

Expert Assessment

This method produced grand means and corresponding comments on semantic equivalence. The findings were triangulated with the cognitive interviews to aid item finalization.

Three bilingual sociolinguists who were blinded to the translation process performed independent assessments of the FB and DP versions. Detailed ratings across three aspects of semantic equivalence are available elsewhere (W. L. Lee et al., 2019). In this study, ratings were averaged to compute a grand mean (X_{GM}) value ranging from 0 (*very poor*) to 6 (*excellent*). An X_{GM} of 4.0–6.0 was taken as an indicator of good-to-excellent overall semantic equivalence (Keller et al., 1998), with a higher X_{GM} value indicating closer semantic equivalence of the item version to its source.

Cognitive Interview

In assessing semantic and item equivalences in terms of item content relevance, the proposed cognition-and-equivalence model was applied to guide the data collection and analysis of the cognitive interview process. Eligible patients were selected using purposive parallel quota sampling (Collins & Gray, 2015) to acquire a sample that was representative across the following demographics: (a) male and female gender; (b) primary, secondary, and tertiary levels of education; (c) Malay and non-Malay ethnicity; and (d) age groups (< 50, 50–60, and > 60 years). Sampling ceased at data saturation, and sample sizes were equal for both FB and DP versions. As the copyright use agreement prohibited the modification or deletion of items, it was pragmatic to employ a modified cognitive interview process that focused on examining items primarily for semantic and item equivalence.

Collins' (2003) question-and-answer model, which underpins Tourangeau's four-stage cognition, was adapted in this study to guide the equivalence investigation (via the cognition-and-equivalence model). In Figure 1, the two-headed arrow linking the "comprehension" and "decision-making" components of cognition represents the interdependency and iterative interaction of these two components. The "decision-making" component represents the complex, intertwined interactions between the retrieval, judgment, and response processes of cognition, which help respondents determine their answer.

Assumptions of the cognition-and-equivalence model

The evidence for "semantic equivalence" and "item equivalence" were extracted by exploring

(a) patients' comprehension, that is, whether each item was understood or interpreted as intended by the original item using questions such as "Can you explain the meaning of this sentence (or this term 'X')?" and "Please give examples to explain its meaning"; and

(b) patients' decision making, that is, whether the item was perceived as relevant and appropriate to their setting by eliciting the reasoning used by the participants to determine their answers. Example questions include "Why did you choose that particular answer?", "Is it suitable to ask this question? Why?", and "Why is the question difficult or easy to answer?"

Figure 1

The "cognition-and-equivalence" model used to guide the cognitive interviews was adapted from the question-and-answer model (Collins, 2003) and the equivalence model (Herdman et al., 1998)

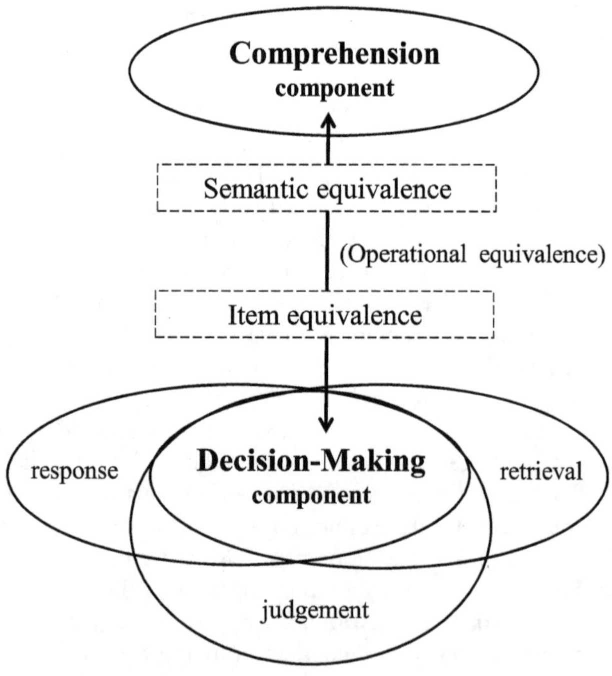

In addition, participant feedback was solicited regarding the clarity of instructions and response options, the practicality of the format layout, and the 4-week recall period using questions such as "Give an example of the timeframe you are thinking of when answering?" (referring to a 4-week recall), "What do you think of the wording size and layout?", and "Which part of the questionnaire do you not like?" However, this approach is adequate only to support "preliminary operational equivalence." According to Herdman et al. (1998), full operational equivalence should be established based on findings related to measurement properties during questionnaire validation.

The participants were interviewed after self-administering either the FB or DP version. The interview sessions were kept within 30 minutes, as the participants get tired easily. The interviews were generally audio-recorded. Alternatively, interviewer notes were used when participants declined permission to be audio-recorded. About two interviews were conducted per day, and the data were analyzed on the same day. Scripted probes were revised accordingly to suit Malaysian patients, especially those with less education, with lower survey literacy, and of higher ages, who were likely to be relatively reticent, less accustomed to research culture, and less articulate than their peers in other cultural settings (Park et al., 2016). To ensure consistency, the same interviewer and coresearch team analyzed the data and performed peer-checking. Descriptive analyses of the data were performed using a text-summary approach (Willis, 2015a) to confirm semantic, item, and preliminary operational equivalences and identify significant problems in drawing conclusions. The findings were summarized in a matrix framework based on the primary objectives of the modified cognitive interview process. According to Willis (2015b), the detection of flaws and resultant decisions depend on the judgment of researchers instead of the opinions of participants, as the latter are not generally regarded as "experts" in cognitive interview proceedings. Findings on the corresponding FB and DP items were compared to aid decision making in finalizing the HeartQoL-BM.

Survey

A survey was used to generate the responses for the confirmatory factor analysis (CFA), which assessed the HeartQoL-BM in terms of conceptual, item, operational, and measurement equivalences. To assess HeartQoL-BM across the three IHD conditions, eligible patients were consecutively sampled to recruit a minimum of 100 participants from each one of the three subgroups (Kline, 2005): patients with a myocardial infarction between 1 and 6 months, patients treated mainly for angina, and patients who had ischaemic heart failure. Data from the 4-point HeartQoL were treated as ordered categorical data to generate polychoric correlation matrices for CFA using EQS Version 6.3 (Multivariate Software, Inc., Temple, CA, USA). The nonnormal data were analyzed using a robust (or corrected) maximum likelihood estimator to provide adjusted standard errors and Satorra–Bentler scaled chi-square statistics. The acceptability of overall model fit was based on Hu and Bentler's (1999) recommendations, whereas the Fornell and Larcker (1981) model was used to test the discriminant validity of the model-based factors. The HeartQoL-BM was tested equivalently across the subgroups for measurement invariance. Goodness-of-fit may be confirmed only when the p value of the corrected Satorra–Bentler's χ^2 difference is > .05 (Satorra & Bentler, 2010) and the comparative fit index–robust difference is $\leq$ 0.01 (Byrne, 2006).

Ethical Considerations

Informed consent was obtained from all of the participants, and all procedures were undertaken in accordance with the ethical principles outlined in the Declaration of Helsinki.

Results

In comparing the corresponding items in the FB and DP versions, four item pairs (HQ [HeartQoL item] 1, HQ2, HQ6, and HQ14) were found to be nonidentical (28.6%), whereas the remaining items were identical or almost identical in wording. All item versions had good overall semantic equivalence ($X_{GM} \geq 4.0$) with the exception of $HQ6_{FBversion}$, $HQ9_{FBversion}$, $HQ9_{DPversion}$, and $HQ14_{DPversion}$ (X_{GM} = 2.55–3.83). The final HeartQoL-BM included the item versions that earned the highest grand mean scores, while taking into consideration the findings of cognitive interviews. The resultant HeartQoL-BM was composed of six DP items ($HQ_{DPversion}$ 1, 2, 4, 6, 10, and 13), four FB items ($HQ_{FBversion}$ 3, 8, 9, and 14), and four identical items. A sample detailing the findings of the expert assessment and cognitive interviews that guided item finalization in HeartQoL-BM is shown in Table 1.

Cognitive Interviews and Expert Assessment

The patient subgroups (N = 22) included in the cognitive interview process were, by FB–DP ratio, (a) male (8:7) and female (3:4); (b) Malays (6:7), Chinese (2:1), and Indians (3:3); (c) 25–49 years old (4:2), 50–59 years old (4:5), and 60–77 years old (3:4); and (d) primary (3:1), secondary (5:7), and tertiary (3:3) education. The expert feedback was congruent with the findings from the cognitive interviews. Selected examples of flagged items with potential gaps of semantic and item equivalences are shown in Table 1. In the final version, item versions with relatively higher grand means were selected over their equivalent, lower-grand-mean versions unless shortcomings were identified during the cognitive interview process.

All of the participants were able to read out the texts and mark their responses on paper. Similar findings were identified across FB and DP subgroups. Some participants (e.g., Patients H and k) described their mental retrieval of memory on a whole-month rather than week-to-week basis in recalling a 4-week event or experience. Some participants (e.g., Patients F, G, and g) preferred to estimate their degree of bother by recalling the frequency rather than the intensity of symptoms unless these symptoms were severe. Moreover, both participants and experts expressed difficulty in quantifying the response option "somewhat bothered," as there is no equivalent expression in BM. As some participants (e.g., Participant B) commented on having a natural inclination to associate "none" with a score of 0, the final HeartQoL-BM scale was scored in ascending order, with 0 = *not bothered at all* and 3 = *greatly bothered*. These responses were reverse coded before computing scores. These observations shed light on the value of cognitive methods in creating awareness of the complexity surrounding the cross-cultural adaptation of questionnaires. However, it is beyond the scope of this article to elaborate on this issue.

Factor Structure of the Final Heart Quality-of-Life–Bahasa Malaysia

Responses from 373 patients were used in factor structure testing. As shown in Table 2, no significant difference in the distribution of patients' characteristics across the three IHD conditions was found. Moreover, the ceiling effect was evident in the emotional subscale for patients with angina and those with myocardial infarction. Table 3 illustrates a summary of the assessments of various models of HeartQoL-BM. The three-factor model (Model C) lacked discriminant validity, as F2 (physical functioning) was highly correlated with

Table 1

Selected Examples of Findings—Summary of Flagged Items of HeartQoL-BM and Its Corresponding Item Finalization

Expert Assessment ($n = 3$)	Cognitive Interview (FB: $n = 11$; DP: $n = 11$)	Item Finalization
Items with potential gaps in semantic equivalence		
HQ7 (being physically restricted): $X_{GM} = 5.06$ (FB = DP) Experts A and C commented the term "fizikal" (physical) sounded technical.	Two patients with low education could not define the term "fizikal" (e.g., Patients d and i).	Although HQ7 was identical between the FB and DP versions, the semantic equivalence of item was enhanced with "anggota badan" added to cue the meaning of "fizikal."
HQ10 (feeling depressed): $X_{GM} = 4.22_{FB}$ vs. 5.22_{DP} All experts suggested the use of "depress" rather than "murung."	Nonnative Bahasa-Malaysia-speaking patients were not familiar with "murung" (e.g., Patients B and d).	$HQ10_{DPversion}$ with added synonyms, i.e., "murung (depression/sangat sedih/hilang semangat hidup)" was accepted as it had higher scores.
Items with potential gaps in item equivalence		
HQ2 (gardening/vacuum/carry groceries): $X_{GM} = 4.95_{FB}$ vs. 4.28_{DP} Experts B and C preferred "barangan dapur" than "barangan runcit" to describe groceries.	Tasks in HQ2 were valued differently because of patriarchal gender-role, e.g., womenfolk doing household chores most of the times.	Although $HQ2_{DPversion}$ had a slightly lower X_{GM}, it was selected for its culturally relevant examples. The final HQ2 had sweeping/mopping added to the original item.
All experts commented that sweeping and mopping were more common than vacuuming as a cleaning chore in typical Malaysian households.	Sixteen of 22 patients swept and mopped the floor more frequently than vacuuming.	

Note. Bahasa Malaysia is also known as the Malay language; words in quotation marks are of Malay language. HeartQoL-BM = Heart Quality-of-Life-Bahasa Malaysia questionnair; HQ = HeartQoL item; FB = forward–backward; DP = dual-panel; X_{GM} = mean of ratings from three experts.

F3 (physical symptoms) at r of .93. Hence, the popular Wilson–Cleary's HRQoL model was not supported. The two-factor model (Model B) showed acceptable fit indices with sufficient discriminant validity, with all factor loadings > .80. The second-order factor structure model (Model B.1) showed good model fit, with factor loadings ranging from .64 to .98. As shown in Table 4, Model B had sufficient factorial invariance across the subgroups of myocardial infarction, angina, and heart failure as well as across native and nonnative BM speakers.

Discussion

The perspectives of participants, which were gathered via cognitive interviews, were congruent with the assessments of the sociolinguists, suggesting that the two methods are mutually complementary. Noteworthy findings are elaborated in this section to show the value of qualitative inquiry to eliciting insights and identifying potential gaps. In addition, how the resultant version achieved the six types of equivalence is discussed to support the efficacy of applying the cognition-and-equivalence model, using cognitive interviews with or without expert assessment, to pretest translated questionnaires.

Noteworthy Observations From the Cognitive Interviews and Expert Assessments

In this study, by translation alone, neither the FB nor DP method achieved optimal equivalence. Moreover, qualitative pretesting methods such as modified cognitive interviewing may offer additional insight. Although most items exhibited good semantic equivalence ($X_{GM} > 4.0$), the findings from the experts and the cognitive interviews suggest that minor revisions should be made to enhance equivalence. For example, adding alternative wordings to items (e.g., HQ7, HQ10, HQ12) may promote comprehension of item meanings among respondents (Weeks et al., 2007). The cognitive interviews highlighted potential gaps of equivalence, including gaps overlooked by translators. For example, the technical term "physical" ("fizikal") in both the FB and DP versions of HQ7 was found to be potentially problematic for respondents with lower levels of education. Conversely, the cognitive interviews tended to affirm the suggestions of the translators. For example, adding an example of a football field to item $HQ4_{DP}$ helped respondents better comprehend the distance covered by 100 yards. However, as this example was not included in the original item, $HQ4_{DP}$ earned a lower equivalence rating from the experts ($HQ4_{DP} = X_{GM}$ of 4.05 vs. $HQ4_{FB} = X_{GM}$

Table 2

Distribution of Patient Characteristics and Floor Ceiling Effects, by Total Group and Subgroups in the Survey

Patient Subgroup and Characteristic[a]	Myocardial Infarction (*n* = 123)		Angina (*n* = 139)		Heart Failure (*n* = 111)		Total Group (*N* = 373)	
	n	%	*n*	%	*n*	%	*n*	%
Male gender	104	84.6	113	81.3	98	88.3	315	84.5
Married	116	94.3	134	96.4	100	90.1	350	93.8
Ethnicity[b]								
Malay	73	59.3	62	44.6	55	49.5	190	50.9
Chinese	12	9.8	30	21.6	23	20.7	65	17.5
Indian	36	29.3	43	30.9	31	27.9	110	29.5
Others	2	1.6	4	2.9	2	1.8	8	2.1
Educational level								
Tertiary	30	24.4	47	33.8	25	22.5	102	27.3
Secondary	78	63.4	79	56.8	76	68.5	233	62.5
Primary	15	12.2	13	9.4	10	9.0	38	10.2
Employment status								
Employment	51	41.5	51	36.7	27	24.6	129	34.6
Retiree	47	38.2	57	41.0	46	41.8	150	40.2
Others	25	20.3	31	22.3	38	34.6	94	25.2
Diabetes mellitus	65	52.8	78	56.1	73	66.4	225	60.3
Hypertension	95	77.2	110	79.1	83	75.5	288	77.2
BMI > 30	2	1.6	12	8.6	6	5.5	20	5.4
Active smokers	32	26.0	17	12.2	13	11.8	63	16.9
Age (years; mean)	59.5	*SD* = 10.6	61	IQR = 12.0	58.9	*SD* = 13.4	60.0	IQR = 14.0
HeartQoL-BM version (score range: 0–3)								
Physical subscale (mean scoring of Items HQ1–HQ8, HQ13, and HQ14)								
Ceiling effect[c]	1	0.8	3	2.2	1	0.9	5	1.3
Floor effect[d]	0	0.0	0	0.0	2	1.8	2	0.5
Emotion subscale (mean of scoring Items HQ9–HQ12)								
Ceiling effect[c]	33	26.8	45	32.4	3	2.7	106	28.4
Floor effect[d]	2	1.6	0	0.0	6	5.5	8	2.1
Global subscale (mean of scoring all items HQ1–HQ14)								
Ceiling effect[c]	0	0.0	2	1.4	0	0.0	2	0.5
Floor effect[d]	0	0.0	0	0.0	1	0.9	1	0.3

Note. BMI = body mass index; IQR = interquartile range; HeartQOL-BM = Heart Quality-of-Life-Bahasa Malaysia questionnaire; HQ = HeartQoL item.
[a] No significant difference ($p > .05$) in age, gender, marital status, ethnicity, educational level, diabetes, and hypertension status across subgroups. [b] Patients of Malay ethnicity are native BM speakers, whereas the rest of ethnic groups are nonnative BM speakers. [c] Number of patients with a maximum mean score of 3.
[d] Number of patients with a minimum mean score of 0.

of 4.78). The neutrality of sociolinguistic experts enhanced objectivity in the translation assessments and played a supplementary role in cognitive interviews by aiding healthcare researchers who often lack expertise regarding addressing cross-cultural issues, item structural problems, and culture-related linguistic stylings (Conway et al., 2014).

Furthermore, in this study, a potential drawback in terms of overemphasizing back-translation was observed in $HQ6_{FB}$. This overemphasis was rectified to address a concern raised on the nonalike wording between back-translated and source versions, although these words were equivalent in meaning. To produce an exact back-translated wording for the term "short of breath," the revision of $HQ6_{FB}$ resulted in the unnatural sounding term "nafas pendek," which was rated poorly ($X_{GM} = 3.11$). This example illustrates the limits of back-translation, especially when words do not have equivalent expressions in other languages and when grammatical structures differ between languages, which may convey an equivalent meaning but use different wordings in the back-translated and source texts (Tsai et al., 2018). Therefore, back-translation should be used to promote discussion rather than provide an absolute indicator of quality. A competent bilingual committee that is carefully selected should be able to derive and assess semantic equivalence in translation (Epstein et al., 2015) and to identify item content that differs by culture. In this study, the suggestion made by the better-educated respondents to add

Table 3

Structure of the HeartQoL-BM: Summary of Model Assessment in Total or Single-Group Analyses (N = 373)

Model		Goodness of Fit						Factor-Based Reliability and Validity				
No.	Descriptions	*df* (Cutoff criteria)	$SB\chi^2$	TLI_{robust} (≥ .95 = good fit [a])	CFI_{robust}	$RMSEA_{robust}$/ 90% CI (< .06 = good fit [a]; > .10 = poor fit [b])	$CAIC_{robust}$		CR (> .7)	AVE (> .5)	MSV (< AVE)	ASV (< AVE)
First-order, one-factor Model A									–	–	–	–
A	F: HQ1–HQ14	77	757.17	.956	.962	.154 [.144, .164]	224.21					
First-order, two-factor Model B [c]												
B	F1 (emotion): HQ9–HQ12	76	150.82	.995	.996	.051 [.039, .063]	−375.22	F1	.843	.826	.407	.407
	F2 (physical): HQ1–HQ8, HQ13–HQ14							F2	.938	.722	.407	.407
	Source results [d]			.94	.95	.117						
First-order, three-factor Model C—based on Wilson and Cleary's conceptual model and exploratory confirmatory factory analysis												
C	F1 (emotion): HQ9–HQ12	73	99.3	.998	.999	.031 [.012, .046]	−405.97	F1	.843	.827	.473	.404
	F2 (physical functioning): HQ1–HQ5, HQ13							F2	.881	.661	.859 [e]	.597
	F3 (physical symptoms): HQ6–HQ8, HQ14, HQ13							F3	.860	.631	.859 [e]	.666
Second-order, two-factor Model B.1 [f]												
B.1	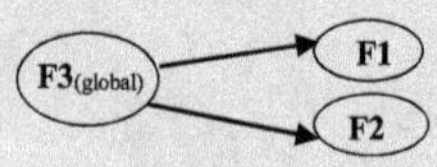	75	148.70	.995	.996	.051 [.039, .063]	−370.42		–	–	–	–

Note. HeartQOL-BM= Heart Quality-of-Life-Bahasa Malaysia questionnaire; HQ = HeartQoL item; *df* = degrees of freedom; $SB\chi^2$ = Satorra–Bentler corrected maximum likelihood chi-square; TLI_{robust} = corrected Tucker–Lewis Index; CFI_{robust} = corrected comparative fit index; $CAIC_{robust}$ = corrected, consistent Akaike information criterion; $RMSEA_{robust}$ = corrected root mean square error of approximation; CR = composite reliability; AVE = average variance extracted; MSV = maximum shared squared variance; ASV = average shared squared variance.

[a] Hu & Bentler (1999). [b] MacCallum et al. (1996). [c] Factor loadings at ≥ .80 with an F1–F2 correlation of .64. [d] De Smedt et al. (2016). [e] Values did not meet criteria as F2 was highly correlated with F3 at .93. [f] First-order factor loadings at ≥ .64 with F1 and F2 loadings at .69 and .60, respectively.

local household chores (sweeping and mopping) to item $HQ2_{DP}$ in the DP method resulted in better item equivalence during cognitive interviews and expert assessments. In addition to affirming the relevance of local chores, the cognitive interviews revealed the different values held among the participants, with some viewing household chores as "a woman's job," which is common in cultures with patriarchal family systems. This should be a point of consideration for those working to develop or cross-culturally adapt questionnaire items in the future.

According to Herdman et al. (1998), translation should consider using appropriate language levels, including the lingo and syntax of common language, to meet the needs of the target population. Hence, the process of translating the HeartQoL-BM version considered the variance in BM proficiency within Malaysia's multiethnic society and the country's unique linguistic landscape in which code-switching and code-mixing between English and BM are practiced commonly in social conversation (Y. L. Lee et al., 2012). Findings from the cognitive interviews and experts supported using lay lingo such as "tension," "frust," and "susah hati" for respective items HQ9, HQ11, and HQ12 to clarify meaning and more accurately reflect the original texts (Herdman et al., 1998). One final, notable encounter in this study was the initial misunderstanding of researchers regarding the original developer's intent for $HQ14_{DP}$. Hence, a document or manual that explicitly explains the conceptual basis of each item would be useful to facilitate the interpretation of item intent by translators (Wild et al., 2005).

The Six Equivalence Types of the Final Heart Quality-of-Life–Bahasa Malaysia

The semantic and item equivalences of the HeartQoL-BM were substantiated in the analysis of cognitive interview data using the cognition-and-equivalence model. In addition, areas of potential gaps because of differences in sociocultural factors, educational level, and linguistic expression were also identified. These findings, together with the opinions of the experts, offer valuable insights that may be used to enhance semantic and item equivalence in the final version of the HeartQoL-BM.

The conceptual, item, measurement, and operational equivalences of HeartQoL-BM were substantiated in the CFA. The two-factor Model B (Table 3) confirmed that HeartQoL-BM had adequate conceptual and item equivalences because the

Table 4

Tests for Invariance of the HeartQoL-BM Model Across Subgroups: Summary of Goodness-of-Fit Statistics in Multiple-Group Analyses

Index	$ML\chi^2$	$SB\chi^2$	*df*	CFI_{robust} (≥ .95 = good fit [a])	$RMSEA_{robust}$ [90% CI] (< .06 = good fit [a]; > .10 = poor fit [b])	Model Comparison	$\Delta SB\chi^2$	Δdf	*p* (> .05)	ΔCFI_{robust} (≤ .01)
	(Criteria of good fit)						(Criteria of invariance)			
Native BM speakers (n = 190) vs. nonnative BM speakers (n = 183)										
Model 1: configural model (no parameter constraints between groups)										
	639.34	237.15	152	.995	.055 [.041, .068]	–	–	–	–	–
Model 2: measurement model invariant (factor loadings between groups equally constrained)										
	645.03	242.50	164	.995	.051 [.036, .064]	2 vs. 1	2.582	12	> .1	< .001
Model 3: structural model invariant (all factor loadings and factor covariances between groups equally constrained)										
	651.66	245.24	165	.995	.051 [.037, .064]	3 vs. 1	5.587	13	> .1	< .001
Myocardial infarction (n = 123) vs. angina (n = 139) vs. heart failure (n = 111)										
Model 4: configural model (no parameter constraints between groups)										
	722.85	321.95	228	.993	.058 [.042, .072]	–	–	–	–	–
Model 5: measurement model invariant (factor loadings between groups equally constrained)										
	760.13	341.52	252	.993	.054 [.038, .067]	5 vs. 4	18.272	24	> .1	< .001
Model 6: Structural model invariant (all factor loadings and factor covariances between groups equally constrained)										
	771.41	340.23	254	.993	.052 [.037, .066]	6 vs. 4	19.733	26	> .1	< .001

Note. HeartQOL-BM = Heart Quality-of-Life (HeartQoL)-Bahasa Malaysia questionnaire; $ML\chi^2$ = maximum likelihood chi-square; $SB\chi^2$ = Satorra–Bentler scaled chi-square; *df* = degrees of freedom; Δ = difference; CFI_{robust} = corrected comparative fit index; $RMSEA_{robust}$ = corrected root mean square error of approximation.
[a] Hu & Bentler (1999). [b] MacCallum et al. (1996).

four items in the emotional dimension and the 10 items in the physical dimension respectively formed the single, underlying structures of F1 and F2, as discussed in the source study of De Smedt et al. (2016). Model B was shown to have good fit (i.e., a Tucker–Lewis index of .995, a comparative fit index of .996, and a root mean square error of approximation of .051). Moreover, adequate convergent validity among items was found in the physical and emotional subscales, with respective composite reliability scores of .94 and .84 and respective average variance extractions of .83 and .72. Findings for the model fit and internal consistency reliability of the HeartQoL-BM were comparable with the source (De Smedt et al., 2016; Oldridge et al., 2014), supporting measurement equivalence. Using a method of administration similar to source studies (De Smedt et al., 2016; Oldridge et al., 2014), the HeartQoL-BM elicited a comparable scoring distribution that confirmed operational equivalence. As shown in Table 2, all ceiling and floor effects were considered negligible, except for the emotional subscale, which showed a high ceiling effect > 15% among patients with angina and myocardial infarction.

The functional equivalence of HeartQoL-BM was confirmed in this study, with cognitive interviews findings supportive of semantic and item equivalence and confirmation of conceptual, item, measurement, and operational equivalences in the CFA. Therefore, studies that use HeartQoL-BM may be expected to yield comparable results with studies that use the original HeartQoL. Moreover, in this study, CFAs of the second-order model and factorial invariance testing were conducted to provide information that were precluded in the source study (De Smedt et al., 2016). As shown in Table 3, the fit indices for Model B.1 were good, thus supporting the validity of global scale scores in representing overall HRQoL level. The tests of invariance shown in Table 4 support the use of HeartQoL-BM for both native and nonnative BM speakers and using HeartQoL-BM to measure HRQoL in patients with IHD experiencing angina, myocardial infarction, or heart failure.

Study Limitations

Although more DP items than FB items constitute the final HeartQoL-BM, the DP method is not necessarily a better translation approach, as the sample of experts used in this study was small. Moreover, the qualitative nature of cognitive interviewing and the decision making in item finalization are inherently subjective. However, the feedback from experts and cognitive interviews provided important insights that were used to adapt the questionnaire to the needs and cultural expectations of the targeted patient population, while adhering to copyright and licensing agreement requirements. Invariances across gender and educational level were not tested, as the female–male gender ratio was ≈1:5 and the tertiary–secondary educational level ratio was ≈1:3. These unbalanced ratios within the sample group had different impacts on the χ^2 of the configural model, which may lead to invalid results.

Conclusions

The complementary and congruent findings of the expert assessment and cognitive interviews confirmed semantic and item equivalences, highlighted potential gaps to be addressed/rectified, and aided decision making with regard to item finalization. Findings from the CFA of the HeartQoL-BM confirmed its conceptual, item, measurement, and operational equivalences to the original instrument. Confirmation of these five equivalence types adequately shows the functional equivalence of the HeartQoL-BM to the source instrument. Therefore, the HeartQoL-BM is a potentially valid and acceptable core IHD-specific HRQoL instrument that functions equivalently across Malaysia's multiethnic culture and across those who speak Malay as a mother tongue and those who speak Malay as a second language. These findings lend support to adapting Herdman et al.'s and Collins' models (e.g., cognition-and-equivalence model) to the cross-cultural adaptation and translation of questionnaires.

Acknowledgments

This research was supported by a university grant (RF009C-2018). We would like to acknowledge Dr. Mahmoud Danaee for earlier statistical advice and Dr. Choo W. Y. for reviewing the quantitative results.

Author Contributions

Study conception and design: All authors.
Data collection: WLL, IZA
Data analysis and interpretation: WLL, KLA, KC
Drafting of the article: WLL
Critical revision of the article: WLL, KLA

References

Beaton, D. E., Bombardier, C., Guillemin, F., & Ferraz, M. B. (2000). Guidelines for the process of cross-cultural adaptation of self-report measures. *Spine, 25*(24), 3186–3191.

Byrne, B. M. (2006). *Structural equation modeling with EQS—Basic concepts, applications, and programming* (2nd ed.). Lawrence Erlbaum Associates.

Colina, S., Marrone, N., Ingram, M., & Sánchez, D. (2017). Translation quality assessment in health research: A functionalist alternative to back-translation. *Evaluation & the Health Professions, 40*(3), 267–293. https://doi.org/10.1177/0163278716648191

Collins, D. (2003). Pretesting survey instruments: An overview of cognitive methods. *Quality of Life Research, 12*(3), 229–238. https://doi.org/10.1023/a:1023254226592

Collins, D., & Gray, M. (2015). Sampling and recruitment. In D. Collins (Ed.), *Cognitive interviewing practice*. Sage Publication.

Conway, K., Acquadro, C., & Patrick, D. L. (2014). Usefulness of translatability assessment: Results from a retrospective study. *Quality of Life Research, 23*(4), 1199–1210. https://doi.org/10.1007/s11136-013-0572-9

De Smedt, D., Clays, E., Höfer, S., Oldridge, N., Kotseva, K., Maggioni, A. P., Janssen, B., De Bacquer, D., & EUROASPIRE Investigators (2016). Validity and reliability of the HeartQoL questionnaire in a large sample of stable coronary patients: The EUROASPIRE IV study of the European Society of Cardiology. *European Journal of Preventive Cardiology, 23*(7), 714–721. https://doi.org/10.1177/2047487315604837

Epstein, J., Osborne, R. H., Elsworth, G. R., Beaton, D. E., & Guillemin, F. (2015). Cross-cultural adaptation of the Health Education Impact Questionnaire: Experimental study showed expert committee, not back-translation, added, value. *Journal of Clinical Epidemiology, 68*(4), 360–369. https://doi.org/10.1016/j.jclinepi.2013.07.013

Eremenco, S., Pease, S., Mann, S., Berry, P., & PRO Consortium's Process Subcommittee. (2017). Patient-reported outcome (PRO) consortium translation process: Consensus development of updated best practices. *Journal of Patient-Reported Outcomes, 2*(1), Article No. 12. https://doi.org/10.1186/s41687-018-0037-6

Fornell, C., & Larcker, D. F. (1981). Evaluating structural equation models with unobservable variables and measurement error. *Journal of Marketing Research, 18*(1), 39–50. https://doi.org/10.1177/002224378101800104

Herdman, M., Fox-Rushby, J., & Badia, X. (1998). A model of equivalence in the cultural adaptation of HRQoL instruments: The universalist approach. *Quality of Life Research, 7*(4), 323–335. https://doi.org/10.1023/a:1024985930536

Hu, L.-t., & Bentler, P. M. (1999). Cutoff criteria for fit indexes in covariance structure analysis: Conventional criteria versus new alternatives. *Structural Equation Modeling: A Multidisciplinary Journal, 6*(1), 1–55. https://doi.org/10.1080/10705519909540118

Keller, S. D., Ware, J. E. Jr., Gandek, B., Aaronson, N. K., Alonso, J., Apolone, G., Bjorner, J. B., Brazier, J., Bullinger, M., Fukuhara, S., Kaasa, S., Leplège, A., Sanson-Fisher, R. W., Sullivan, M., & Wood-Dauphinee, S. (1998). Testing the equivalence of translations of widely used response choice labels: Results from the IQOLA project. International Quality of Life Assessment. *Journal of Clinical Epidemiology, 51*(11), 933–944. https://doi.org/10.1016/s0895-4356(98)00084-5

Kline, R. B. (2005). *Principles and practice of structural equation modeling* (2nd ed.). Guilford Press.

Lee, W. L., Chinna, K., Lim Abdullah, K., & Zainal Abidin, I. (2019). The forward–backward and dual-panel translation methods are comparable in producing semantic equivalent versions of a heart quality of life questionnaire. *International Journal of Nursing Practice, 25*(1), Article e12715. https://doi.org/10.1111/ijn.12715

Lee, W. L., Chinna, K., Bulgiba, A., Abdullah, K. L., Abidin, I. Z., & Höfer, S. (2016). Test–retest reliability of HeartQoL and its comparability to the MacNew heart disease health-related quality of life questionnaire. *Quality of Life Research, 25*(2), 351–357. https://doi.org/10.1007/s11136-015-1097-1

Lee, Y. L., Ng, Y. J., Chong, S. T., & Mohd Ariff, A. T. (2012). Code switching in Sepet: Unveiling Malaysians' communicative styles. *British Journal of Arts and Social Sciences, 6*(2), 166–181.

MacCallum, R. C., Browne, M. W., & Sugawara, H. M. (1996). Power analysis and determination of sample size for covariance structure modeling. *Psychological Methods, 1*(2), 130–149. https://doi.org/10.1037/1082-989X.1.2.130

Oldridge, N., Höfer, S., McGee, H., Conroy, R., Doyle, F., Saner, H., & for the HeartQoL Project Investigators. (2014). The HeartQoL: Part II. validation of a new core health-related quality of life questionnaire for patients with ischemic heart disease. *European Journal of Preventive Cardiology, 21*(1), 98–106. https://doi.org/10.1177/2047487312450545

Park, H., Sha, M. M., & Olmsted, M. (2016). Research participant selection in non-English language questionnaire pretesting: Findings from Chinese and Korean cognitive interviews. *Quality & Quantity, 50*(3), 1385–1398. https://doi.org/10.1007/s11135-015-0211-3

Satorra, A., & Bentler, P. M. (2010). Ensuring positiveness of the scaled difference chi-square test statistic. *Psychometrika, 75*(2), 243–248. https://doi.org/10.1007/s11336-009-9135-y

Swaine-Verdier, A., Doward, L. C., Hagell, P., Thorsen, H., & McKenna, S. P. (2004). Adapting quality of life instruments. *Value in Health, 7*(1, Suppl.), S27–S30. https://doi.org/10.1007/s11336-009-9135-y

Tsai, T. I., Luck, L., Jefferies, D., & Wilkes, L. (2018). Challenges in adapting a survey: Ensuring cross-cultural equivalence. *Nurse Researcher, 26*(1), 28–32. https://doi.org/10.7748/nr.2018.e1581

Weeks, A., Swerissen, H., & Belfrage, J. (2007). Issues, challenges, and solutions in translating study instruments. *Evaluation Review, 31*(2), 153–165. https://doi.org/10.1177/0193841x06294184

Wild, D., Grove, A., Martin, M., Eremenco, S., McElroy, S., Verjee-Lorenz, A., Erikson, P., & ISPOR Task Force for Translation and Cultural Adaptation. (2005). Principles of good practice for the translation and cultural adaptation process for patient-reported outcomes (PRO) measures: Report of the ISPOR task force for translation and cultural adaptation. *Value in Health, 8*(2), 94–104. https://doi.org/10.1111/j.1524-4733.2005.04054.x

Willis, G. B. (2015a). *Analysis of the cognitive interviewing in questionnaire design*. Oxford University Press.

Willis, G. B. (2015b). Research synthesis: The practice of cross-cultural cognitive interviewing. *Public Opinion Quarterly, 79*, 359–395. https://doi.org/10.1093/poq/nfu092

5

Does Jaundice in Newborn Infants Affect Exclusivity and Duration of Breastfeeding in Taiwan?

Kuei-Hui CHU[1] • Sen-Wen TENG[2] • Chen-Jei TAI[3] • Ching-Mei CHANG[4] • Li-Yin CHIEN[5*]

ABSTRACT

Background: Cases of breastfeeding- and breast-milk-related jaundice tend to increase with increased rates of breastfeeding. Diagnoses of jaundice often lead mothers to discontinue breastfeeding because of assumptions that breastfeeding may exacerbate neonatal jaundice and lengthen the duration of phototherapy treatment.

Purpose: This study was designed to explore the effect of neonatal jaundice on breastfeeding duration and exclusivity during the first 4 months postpartum.

Methods: This study applied a two-group comparative and follow-up design. The two groups comprised 135 and 160 mothers of infants, respectively, with and without neonatal jaundice. All of the participants were recruited from three certified baby-friendly hospitals in northern Taiwan. Follow-up was conducted by telephone at 1 and 4 months postpartum.

Results: Mean breastfeeding duration was longer in the group of participants whose infants had neonatal jaundice (group with neonatal jaundice) than in the group whose infants did not have this condition (group without neonatal jaundice; 102.00 vs. 89.85 days, $p = .007$). The degree of breastfeeding was higher in the group with neonatal jaundice, although the difference was significant only at 1 month postpartum and not during hospitalization or at 4 months postpartum. The results of a Cox regression model showed that the group without neonatal jaundice was more likely to discontinue breastfeeding (adjusted hazard ratio = 1.68, 95% CI [1.08, 2.62]). A generalized estimating equation model suggests that infants with neonatal jaundice had a higher likelihood of being breastfed for at least half of their feedings (adjusted $OR = 1.53$, 95% CI [1.04, 2.25]).

Conclusions: On the basis of the results of this study, neonatal jaundice is not an obstacle to breastfeeding in pro-breastfeeding hospital environments. Participants whose infants developed neonatal jaundice were found in this study to breastfeed more often, which promotes breastfeeding success.

KEY WORDS:
neonatal jaundice, breastfeeding, breastfeeding duration, baby-friendly hospital initiative.

Introduction

On the basis of guidelines published by the World Health Organization (WHO) in 1989 (WHO/UNICEF, 1989), Taiwan began to publicly encourage women to breastfeed in 1992. Hospitals in Taiwan are recognized as "baby-friendly" if they meet the lactation promotion criteria adapted from the WHO/UNICEF's 10 steps to successful breastfeeding standards (Chien & Tai, 2007; Chien et al., 2007; Chiou et al., 2014; Chu et al., 2005). The breastfeeding rate at 6 months postpartum has increased from 49.9% in 2011 to 57.7% in 2018 (Health Promotion Administration, Ministry of Health and Welfare, Taiwan, ROC, 2018; Waits et al., 2018). However, a rising prevalence of infants with jaundice has been identified alongside this rising breastfeeding rate. According to one study, while the breastfeeding rate in one hospital rose from 92.2% to 97.2% since the implementation of a baby-friendly policy, the prevalence of neonatal jaundice in that hospital also rose, from 10.9% to 23.8% (Lin et al., 2008).

Breastfeeding jaundice and breast milk jaundice are two types of breastfeeding-related jaundice in newborns (Leung & Sauve, 1989). The first is frequently found among newborns who do not receive sufficient breast milk and later appear to lose weight and be dehydrated between 4 and 7 days postpartum (Preer & Philipp, 2011). Breast milk jaundice typically occurs 1 week after birth. Although this condition

[1]PhD, RN, Assistant Professor, Department of Nursing, Ching Kuo Institute of Management and Health, Taiwan, ROC • [2]MD, Attending Physician, Department of Obstetrics and Gynecology, Cardinal Tien Hospital-Hsintien, and Assistant Professor, School of Medicine, College of Medicine, Fu Jen Catholic University, Taiwan, ROC • [3]PhD, MD, Professor, Department of Obstetrics and Gynecology, School of Medicine, College of Medicine, Taipei Medical University, and Attending Physician, Department of Traditional Chinese Medicine, Taipei Medical University Hospital, Taiwan, ROC • [4]PhD, RN, Assistant Professor, Department of Nursing, Hungkuang University, Taiwan, ROC • [5]ScD, RN, Professor, Institute of Community Health Care, School of Nursing, National Yang Ming Chiao Tung University, and National Yang Ming University, Taiwan, ROC.

may last up to 12 weeks, it rarely causes complications in healthy, breast-fed infants (Prameela, 2019). More than 65% of newborns who are fed breast milk develop neonatal jaundice. Hyperbilirubinemia may be diagnosed and became severe in infants at 10–14 days postpartum, with symptoms potentially continuing for 2–3 months (Preer & Philipp, 2011). Watson (2009) posited that having neonatal jaundice is a natural process that poses no real harm to newborns, although it requires evaluation and attention to prevent large amounts of bilirubin from circulating to tissues in the brain, which may cause seizures or brain damage. Mothers and families are generally instructed to monitor for jaundice by observing the skin color of their infants and the whites of their eyes (Chuang et al., 2015).

Previous studies have shown that breastfeeding and higher levels of bilirubin at hospital discharge are two predictors of hospital readmission (Jones et al., 2018). Other similar studies have confirmed that breastfeeding may cause severe weight loss because of dehydration (Fonseca et al., 2014). Exclusively breastfed infants have been found to exhibit more-severe clinical symptoms of neonatal jaundice (Chen et al., 2012).

Phototherapy is recommended to resolve high levels of bilirubin (> 15 mg/dl) in infants (Alizadeh Taheri et al., 2014). Women in Taiwan tend to perform a customary practice, "doing-the-month," at home after giving birth (Chien et al., 2006). According to doing-the-month practices, women should be confined at home, rest as much as possible, and follow specific behavioral rules for at least 1 month after childbirth (Chien et al., 2006; Ding et al., 2020). This restrictive situation typically requires discontinuing breastfeeding and may lead to inadequate milk supply and lactation, especially when infants are required to receive phototherapy in hospital settings (Muchowski, 2014). Any postpartum separation between mother and child has been found to harm breastfeeding rates (Chang et al., 2019) because of the interruption of baby–mother attachment and breastfeeding activities during separation (Sivanandan et al., 2009).

In addition to phototherapy, a common treatment for neonatal jaundice is to prevent fluid or water deprivation by increasing liquid uptake (Becker et al., 2011; Goyal et al., 2018). Mothers are advised to increase breastfeeding times and amounts (Saeidi et al., 2009). If the condition still does not improve, health professionals may suggest using formula or liquid supplementation or even stopping breastfeeding temporarily to improve liquid uptake (Zhang et al., 2015). In these cases, mothers may consider discontinuing breastfeeding altogether because of worries that breastfeeding may exacerbate neonatal jaundice and lengthen the duration of phototherapy (Muchowski, 2014).

Attempts have been made in previous studies to further elucidate the impact of hospital breastfeeding policies on the breastfeeding rate. Breastfeeding while treating neonatal jaundice may worsen this condition. Few studies have focused on the impact of neonatal jaundice on exclusive breastfeeding and breastfeeding discontinuation. This study was designed to explore the effect of neonatal jaundice on breastfeeding duration and exclusivity in the first 4 months after giving birth.

Methods

Design

A two-group comparative and follow-up design was used in this study. The setting was three certified baby-friendly hospitals in Taipei City, Taiwan. The data were collected from September 2013 through September 2014. The study protocol was approved by the Taiwan Taipei Tzu Chi Hospital Institutional Review Board (No. 02-M03-018) on June 27, 2013.

Sample

The inclusion criteria were no severe health problems (mothers and neonates) and mothers having initiated breastfeeding during hospitalization. The mothers of infants with blood total bilirubin levels ≥ 5 mg/dl at 2–3 days postpartum were assigned to the group with neonatal jaundice, whereas all other mothers were assigned to the comparison group.

We estimated the required sample size at 177 participants (Schoenfeld, 1983) based on $\alpha = .05$, power = 0.80, hazard ratio (HR) = 1.5, a rate of breastfeeding of 22.8%, and an event rate of 85%. Presuming a 10% rate of attrition, a sample size of at least 195 participants was recruited.

We approached 141 and 210 mothers of infants with and without neonatal jaundice, respectively, to participate in this study. Ultimately, the group with neonatal jaundice included 135 participants, and the group without neonatal jaundice included 160 participants. All participating mothers of infants with neonatal jaundice were experiencing physiological neonatal jaundice.

Measurements

Structured questionnaires were used to collect the data. Information, including sociodemographic variables (maternal age, educational level, work status, and marital status), obstetrics variables (parity, delivery mode, and infant birth weight), health problems among mothers and infants, and prior breastfeeding experience, were gathered during the first few days postpartum in the hospital. Furthermore, information on breastfeeding degree, breastfeeding duration, and management of neonatal jaundice (phototherapy, formula supplementation, liquid supplementation, interruption of breastfeeding, and increase in breastfeeding amount and times, if applicable) was gathered at all three time points (during hospitalization, 1 month, and 4 months postpartum).

Degree of breastfeeding was categorized into seven levels, as follows: 100% human milk, ≥ 80% human milk and < 20% formula (2 of 10 times not fed with human milk), 51%–79% human milk (2–4 of 10 times not fed with human milk), 50% human milk (5 of 10 times not fed with human milk), 20%–49% human milk (6–7 of 10 times not fed with human milk), ≤ 19% human milk (8–9 of 10 times not fed with human milk), and 100% formula (no breastfeeding). Women were asked regarding their current infant feeding practices. Duration of breastfeeding was defined as from the time of birth to the complete cessation of breastfeeding.

Data Collection

Participants in the study provided their written consent and contact information. The participants were interviewed face-to-face during hospitalization and later by telephone at 1 and 4 months after giving birth. One hundred thirty (96.3%) participants whose infants developed neonatal jaundice and 146 (91.3%) participants whose infants did not develop neonatal jaundice completed the 1-month postpartum interview; 126 (93.3%) and 144 (90.0%) participants, respectively, completed the 4-month postpartum interview.

Data Analysis

This study used IBM SPSS Statistics Version 22.0 (IBM Inc., Armonk, NY, USA) for data analysis. Frequencies, percentages, means, and standard deviations were included. Crude comparisons between the two groups were examined using the Chi-squared test, Pearson's correlation coefficients, t tests, or one-way analysis of variance. To examine the bivariable association between degree of breastfeeding and neonatal jaundice, the degree of breastfeeding was consolidated from seven to three categories (100%, > 50%, ≤ 50%), as some cell sizes were too small to yield valid statistical results. Multivariate analyses were conducted using a Cox regression model and generalized estimating equations (GEEs) for duration of breastfeeding and degree of breastfeeding, respectively. In the GEE model, the degree of breastfeeding (dependent variable) was recategorized as a binomial variable (> 50% breastfeeding and ≤ 50% breastfeeding). In the Cox regression model, time from birth to discontinuance of breastfeeding was used as the dependent variable. Only variables with two-sided p values ≤ .05 were retained in the final multivariate model.

Results

As shown in Table 1, no significant difference was found between the two groups in terms of demographics, obstetrics variables, and maternal and child health. In the group with neonatal jaundice, the bilirubin level ranged from 9.93 to 13.60 mg/dl at 2–7 days postpartum and 45 (33.3%) were prescribed phototherapy. In terms of jaundice management, in the group with neonatal jaundice, 43 infants (37.7%) received formula supplementation, two (1.8%) received liquid supplementation, 10 (8.8%) received interruption of breastfeeding, and 83 (72.8%) received an increase in breastfeeding amounts and times.

Breastfeeding duration and degree of breastfeeding by group are presented in Table 2. The mean duration of breastfeeding was 102 (SD = 32.8) and 89.9 (SD = 40.9) days for the groups with and without neonatal jaundice, respectively (p = .007). At hospitalization and at 1 and 4 months postpartum, the group with neonatal jaundice had higher rates of exclusive breastfeeding and lower rates of exclusive formula feeding than the group without neonatal jaundice. However, these differences were only statistically significant at 1 month postpartum.

The GEE model showed neonatal jaundice, delivery mode, and time as significant predictors of degree of breastfeeding (Table 3). Participants who gave birth via cesarean section were significantly less likely to breastfeed for more than half of their feedings (OR = 0.33, 95% CI [0.22, 0.50]), whereas participants in the group with neonatal jaundice were significantly more likely to breastfeed for more than half of their feedings (adjusted OR = 1.53, 95% CI [1.04, 2.25]). The participants were more likely to breastfeed for more than half of their feedings during hospitalization and 1 month postpartum than at 4 months postpartum (adjusted OR = 2.20, 95% CI [1.62, 2.99], and 1.64, 95% CI [1.33, 2.02] for hospitalization and at 1 month postpartum, respectively).

The results of the Cox regression model showed that maternal age, maternal educational level, prior breastfeeding experience, and neonatal jaundice were significant predictors of breastfeeding duration (Table 4). Participants whose infants did not develop neonatal jaundice tended to stop breastfeeding (HR = 1.68, 95% CI [1.08, 2.62]). Younger participants (≤ 29 years old) were more likely than older participants (≥ 35 years old) to discontinue breastfeeding (HR = 2.39, 95% CI [1.37, 4.18]), whereas no significant difference in discontinuance was found between participants in the 30–34 years of age range and those 35 years old or older. An educational level of high school or lower was associated with a greater risk of discontinuing breastfeeding (HR = 2.14, 95% CI [1.01, 4.53]), whereas no significant difference was found among participants with higher levels of education. Likelihood of discontinuance was higher among multipara participants with no prior breastfeeding experience than among participants who gave birth for the first time (HR = 4.18, 95% CI [1.82, 9.65]), whereas no significant difference was found between primipara and multipara participants with prior breastfeeding experience. The survival curve, which illustrates the duration of breastfeeding by neonatal jaundice status, is presented in Figure 1. As shown, the survival curve for participants whose infants developed neonatal jaundice is less steep.

Discussion

This study found that participants whose infants developed breastfeeding or breast milk jaundice had a significantly longer mean duration of breastfeeding and a higher degree of breastfeeding than participants whose infants did not develop jaundice. This finding differs from a previous study that found that infants exposed to phototherapy were less likely to continue to be breastfed and be exclusively breastfed

Table 1

Characteristics of Study Participants (N = 295)

Variable	With Neonatal Jaundice (*n* = 135)		Without Neonatal Jaundice (*n* = 160)		*p*
	n	%	*n*	%	
Maternal age (years; *M* and *SD*)	32.9	3.9	33.4	4.1	.28
Maternal educational level					.70
Senior high school or lower	24	17.8	33	20.6	
University	94	69.6	104	65.0	
Postgraduate	17	12.6	23	14.4	
Maternal occupational status					.30
Full-time	88	65.2	109	68.1	
Part-time	3	2.2	8	5.0	
None	44	32.6	43	26.9	
Currently married					.15
Yes	134	99.3	155	96.9	
No	1	0.7	5	3.1	
Parity					.08
1	82	60.7	81	50.6	
≥ 2	53	39.3	79	49.4	
Delivery mode					.31
Vaginal	96	71.1	105	65.6	
Cesarean	39	28.9	55	34.4	
Maternal health problems[a]					.32
Yes	29	21.5	30	18.8	
No	106	78.5	130	81.2	
Infant birth weight (g; *M* and *SD*)	3116.2	384.1	3098.0	352.9	.67
Infant health problems besides jaundice					.16
Yes[b]	5	3.7	12	7.5	
No	130	96.3	148	92.5	
Prior experience with breastfeeding (*n* = 132)					.50
Yes	50	94.3	72	91.1	
No	3	5.7	7	8.9	

[a]Maternal health problems include vaginal bleeding (*n* = 9), preeclampsia (*n* = 8), pregnancy-induced hypertension (*n* = 5), gestational diabetes (*n* = 30), hydramnios (*n* = 1), virus infection (*n* = 2), and other (Group B streptococci or placenta previa, etc.; *n* = 8).
[b]Infant health problems include infection (*n* = 3), heart problem (*n* = 10), ear problem (*n* = 1), perineum problem (*n* = 2), and dermatitis (*n* = 1).

than infants who were not exposed to phototherapy during the first 4 months of life (Waite & Taylor, 2016). This finding also disagrees with another study showing that postdischarge breastfeeding rates for infants diagnosed with jaundice were not significantly different than the general infant population (Pound & Gaboury, 2009). The findings of this study should be viewed in the context of the ongoing Baby-Friendly Hospital Initiative in Taiwan (Health Promotion Administration, Ministry of Health and Welfare, Taiwan, ROC, 2019). In certified baby-friendly hospitals, women whose infants are diagnosed with neonatal jaundice may be encouraged to increase the amount and frequency of breastfeeding as a way to promote bilirubin metabolism. The results of past studies indicate that breastfeeding more than 8 times a day reduces the risk of high bilirubin (Chen et al., 2015). In addition, staff at baby-friendly hospitals may provide more assistance when breastfeeding-related problems such as latching or sucking occur. Ineffective sucking behaviors may suppress lactation (Mizuno et al., 2004) and have been identified as important predictors of breastfeeding jaundice and early discontinuance of breastfeeding (Almqvist-Tangen et al., 2012). The findings of this study suggest that, with the assistance of health professionals, mothers should be able to breastfeed successfully even if their infants have breastfeeding-related jaundice. Healthcare workers should encourage mothers of infants with neonatal jaundice to breastfeed and provide appropriate care and guidance.

The findings of previous studies indicate that mothers know little about neonatal jaundice and do not expect breastfeeding problems until their infant requires bilirubin-level monitoring and treatment (Chu et al., 2019; Zhang et al., 2015). In this study, the participants adopted strategies such as increased

Table 2

Breastfeeding During the First 4 Months of Birth by Mothers of Infants With Neonatal Jaundice and Mothers of Infants Without Neonatal Jaundice (N = 295)

Variable	With Neonatal Jaundice		Without Neonatal Jaundice		*p*
	n	%	*n*	%	
Breastfeeding during hospitalization	135	45.8	160	54.2	.30
100%	56	41.5	58	36.3	
> 50%	40	29.6	42	26.3	
≤ 50%	39	28.9	60	37.4	
Breastfeeding at 1 month (*n* = 276)	130	47.1	146	52.9	.03
100%	59	45.4	54	37.0	
> 50%	32	24.6	24	16.4	
≤ 50%	27	20.8	40	27.4	
None	12	9.2	28	19.2	
Breastfeeding at 4 months (*n* = 270)	126	46.7	144	53.3	.10
100%	57	45.2	49	34.0	
> 50%	12	9.5	16	11.1	
≤ 50%	22	17.5	20	13.9	
None	35	27.8	59	41.0	
Breastfeeding duration (*n* = 270)	126	46.7	144	53.3	.03
≤ 30 days	11	8.7	31	21.5	
31–60 days	15	11.9	17	11.8	
61–90 days	6	4.8	8	5.6	
≥ 91 days	94	74.6	88	61.1	
Duration of breastfeeding (*M* and *SD*)	102.0	32.8	9.9	40.9	.01

Note. Different value for *n* is because of loss of follow-up.

breastfeeding duration and frequencies (72.8%), formula feeding (37.7%), and temporary stoppage of breastfeeding (8.8%) in response to a diagnosis of neonatal jaundice. Previous studies have reported that temporary cessation of breastfeeding to treat neonatal jaundice increased the risk of breastfeeding discontinuation (Alizadeh Taheri et al., 2014; Muchowski, 2014). However, the results of this study

Table 3

Generalized Estimating Equation Model on Factors Associated With More Than Half of the Feeding Being Breastfeeding During the First 4 Months Postpartum (N = 295)

Variable	Odds Ratio	95% CI	*p*
Delivery mode			
Caesarean	0.33	[0.22, 0.50]	< .01
Vaginal	1.00		
Neonatal jaundice			
No	1.00		
Yes	1.53	[1.04, 2.25]	.03
Time			
During hospitalization	2.20	[1.62, 2.99]	< .01
1 month postpartum	1.64	[1.33, 2.02]	< .01
4 months postpartum	1.00		

Note. Working correlation matrix is unstructured.

Table 4

Cox Proportional Hazards Model for Factors Associated With Duration of Breastfeeding During the First 4 Months Postpartum (N = 295)

Variable	Hazard Ratio	95% CI	*p*
Neonatal jaundice			
No	1.68	[1.08, 2.62]	.020
Yes	1.00		
Maternal age (years)			
≤ 29	2.39	[1.37, 4.18]	.002
30–34	0.94	[0.58, 1.54]	.810
≥ 35	1.00		
Maternal educational level			
High school or lower	2.14	[1.01, 4.53]	.047
Vocational school	1.07	[0.38, 2.98]	.910
University	0.98	[0.51, 1.89]	.950
Postgraduate	1.00		
Breastfeeding experience			
Multipara without breastfeeding experience	4.18	[1.82, 9.65]	.001
Multipara with breastfeeding experience	1.05	[0.67, 1.66]	.830
Primipara	1.00		

Figure 1
Duration of Breastfeeding Based on Whether Infants have Neonatal Jaundice

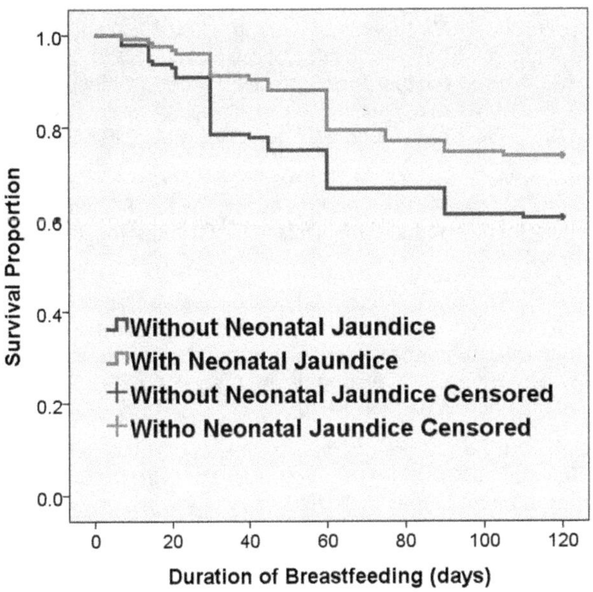

suggest that these practices did not result in negative breastfeeding outcomes during the first 4 months postpartum. In addition, intention to increase breastfeeding duration and frequencies may be an underlying reason why the mothers in the group with neonatal jaundice obtained better breastfeeding outcomes. Therefore, healthcare workers should encourage mothers to increase breastfeeding times, recommend appropriate precautions, and suggest appropriate responses to potential problems, for example, recommending formula milk supplementation when infant weight loss exceeds 7%, when human milk expression is insufficient, and when newborn infants experience decreased stool frequencies. These actions may help ensure that infants are discharged as scheduled and avoid separation, which may cause maternal anxiety and failure in breastfeeding (O'Brien et al., 2008).

To avoid the negative impact of neonatal jaundice on breastfeeding, healthcare workers must allay the doubts of new mothers regarding breastfeeding and neonatal jaundice and assure them that jaundice is a temporary condition. For example, healthcare workers may provide information about neonatal jaundice, teach women how to express human milk when breastfeeding stops temporarily during phototherapy or when supplementary formula is given, and help extend the duration of breastfeeding sessions. In addition, healthcare workers may provide dietary suggestions to help women improve lactation. Furthermore, they may teach new mothers to express milk and save their milk while their infants receive phototherapy.

In addition to neonatal jaundice, the study found associations between cesarean delivery and reduced levels of breastfeeding during the first 4 months postpartum. In addition, young maternal age, low educational level, and no prior experience of breastfeeding were associated with a shorter breastfeeding duration. These findings are similar to those of previous studies (Colombo et al., 2018; Holowko et al., 2016; Kitano et al., 2015). Breastfeeding promotion programs should especially target younger mothers (< 30 years old), plan breastfeeding with pregnant women who are going to have a cesarean delivery, provide more assistance to mothers who undergo cesarean delivery, and improve breastfeeding-friendly environments to help prepare working mothers to continue breastfeeding after returning to work.

Limitations

Newborn babies with high levels of bilirubin during the first 2 or 3 days of life based on skin probing results were assigned to the group with jaundice. Infants who experienced jaundice after discharge were not included in the study. All of the infants in the group with neonatal jaundice were diagnosed with physiological jaundice, as pathological jaundice fell beyond the scope of this study. Information on breastfeeding outcomes and jaundice management were obtained using self-administered questionnaires. Thus, data may be misleading or erroneous if participants did not answer questions honestly or did not accurately recall information. More than 80% of the participants in this study held a college degree or higher, which suggests that the average breastfeeding duration may be longer among study participants than in the general population.

Conclusions

In this study, conducted in certified baby-friendly hospitals, participants whose infants developed neonatal jaundice reported a longer duration and a higher degree (> 50%) of breastfeeding. Neonatal jaundice was not found to be an obstacle to breastfeeding in the pro-breastfeeding environment that prevailed in the study settings. The infants with neonatal jaundice were breastfed more often, which resulted in a greater rate of breastfeeding success for this group. Future research may explore whether different approaches to managing neonatal jaundice such as hospitalization, length of phototherapy, and liquid/formula supplementation influence breastfeeding outcomes differently. In addition, studies that track changes in bilirubin level longitudinally over a longer follow-up period are warranted.

Acknowledgment

This study was funded by the Taiwan Nurses Association (Grant No. 1022022).

Author Contributions

Study conception and design: KHC, LYC
Data collection: SWT, KHC, CMC,
Data analysis and interpretation: KHC, LYC, CJT
Drafting of the article: KHC SWT, LYC
Critical revision of the article: KHC, LYC

References

Alizadeh Taheri, P., Sadeghi, M., & Sajjadian, N. (2014). Severe neonatal hyperbilirubinemia leading to exchange transfusion. *Medical Journal of the Islamic Republic of Iran, 28,* Article 64.

Almqvist-Tangen, G., Bergman, S., Dahlgren, J., Roswall, J., & Alm, B. (2012). Factors associated with discontinuation of breastfeeding before 1 month of age. *Acta Paediatrica, 101*(1), 55–60. https://doi.org/10.1111/j.1651-2227.2011.02405.x

Becker, G. E., Remmington, S., & Remmington, T. (2011). Early additional food and fluids for healthy breastfed full-term infants. *Cochrane Database of Systematic Reviews, 2011*(12), CD006462. https://doi.org/10.1002/14651858.CD006462.pub2

Chang, P.-C., Li, S.-F., Yang, H.-Y., Wang, L.-C., Weng, C.-Y., Chen, K.-F., Chen, W., & Fan, S.-Y. (2019). Factors associated with cessation of exclusive breastfeeding at 1 and 2 months postpartum in Taiwan. *International Breastfeeding Journal, 7*(14), Article 18. https://doi.org/10.1186/s13006-019-0213-1

Chen, Y.-J., Chen, W.-C., & Chen, C.-M. (2012). Risk factors for hyperbilirubinemia in breastfed term neonates. *European Journal of Pediatrics, 171*(1), 167–171. https://doi.org/10.1007/s00431-011-1512-8

Chen, Y.-J., Yeh, T.-F., & Chen, C.-M. (2015). Effect of breastfeeding frequency on hyperbilirubinemia in breast-fed term neonate. *Pediatrics International, 57*(6), 1121–1125. https://doi.org/10.1111/ped.12667

Chien, L.-Y., & Tai, C.-J. (2007). Effect of delivery method and timing of breastfeeding initiation on breastfeeding outcomes in Taiwan. *Birth, 34*(2), 123–130. https://doi.org/10.1111/j.1523-536X.2007.00158.x

Chien, L.-Y., Tai, C.-J., Chu, K.-H., Ko, Y.-L., & Chiu, Y.-C. (2007). The number of baby friendly hospital practices experienced by mothers is positively associated with breastfeeding: A questionnaire survey. *International Journal of Nursing Studies, 44*(7), 1138–1146. https://doi.org/10.1016/j.ijnurstu.2006.05.015

Chien, L.-Y., Tai, C.-J., Ko, Y. -L., Huang, C.-H., & Sheu, S.-J. (2006). Adherence to "doing-the-month" practices is associated with fewer physical and depressive symptoms among postpartum women in Taiwan. *Research in Nursing & Health, 29*(5), 374–383. https://doi.org/10.1002/nur.20154

Chiou, S.-T., Chen, L.-C., Yeh, H., Wu, S.-R., & Chien, L.-Y. (2014). Early skin-to-skin contact, rooming-in, and breastfeeding: A comparison of the 2004 and 2011 National Surveys in Taiwan. *Birth, 41*(1), 33–38. https://doi.org/10.1111/birt.12090

Chu, K.-H., Sheu, S.-J., Hsu, M.-H., Liao, J., & Chien, L.-Y. (2019). Breastfeeding experiences of Taiwanese mothers of infants with breastfeeding or breast milk jaundice in certified baby-friendly hospitals. *Asian Nursing Research, 13*(2), 154–160. https://doi.org/10.1016/j.anr.2019.04.003

Chu, K.-H., Tai, C.-J., & Chien, L.-Y. (2005). The relationship between in-hospital breastfeeding rates and hospital type. *Hu Li Za Zhi, 52*(6), 40–48. https://doi.org/10.6224/JN.52.6.40 (Original work published in Chinese)

Chuang, S.-W., Luo, P.-J., Huang, C.-L., Li, Y.-H., Peng, H.-F., & Sheng, C.-C. (2015). Knowledge promotion and identification of skin color change in neonatal jaundice for primary caregiver by using skin color chart. *VGH Nursing, 32*(4), 343–350. https://doi.org/10.6142/VGHN.32.4.343 (Original work published in Chinese)

Colombo, L., Crippa, B. L., Consonni, D., Bettinelli, M. E., Agosti, V., Mangino, G., Bezze, E. N., Mauri, P. A., Zanotta, L., Roggero, P., Plevani, L., Bertoli, D., Giannì, M. L., & Mosca, F. (2018). Breastfeeding determinants in healthy term newborns. *Nutrients, 10*(1), Article 48. https://doi.org/10.3390/nu10010048

Ding, G., Niu, L., Vinturache, A., Zhang, J., Lu, M., Gao, Y., Pan, S., & Tian, Y., Shanghai Birth Cohort Study. (2020). "Doing the month" and postpartum depression among Chinese women: A Shanghai prospective cohort study. *Women Birth, 33*(2), e151–e158. https://doi.org/10.1016/j.wombi.2019.04.004

Fonseca, M.-J., Severo, M., Barros, H., & Santos, A.-C. (2014). Determinants of weight changes during the first 96 hours of life in full-term newborns. *Birth, 41*(2), 160–168. https://doi.org/10.1111/birt.12087

Goyal, P., Mehta, A., Kaur, J., Jain, S., Guglani, V., & Chawla, D. (2018). Fluid supplementation in management of neonatal hyperbilirubinemia: A randomized controlled trial. *Journal of Maternal-Fetal & Neonatal Medicine, 31*(20), 2678–2684. https://doi.org/10.1080/14767058.2017.1351535

Health Promotion Administration, Ministry of Health and Welfare, Taiwan, ROC. (2018). *Survey plan for breastfeeding rate in counties and cities in 2018.* https://www.grb.gov.tw/search/planDetail?id=12691859

Health Promotion Administration, Ministry of Health and Welfare, Taiwan, ROC. (2019). *Current status of breastfeeding in Taiwan.* https://www.hpa.gov.tw/Pages/Detail.aspx?nodeid=506&pid=463

Holowko, N., Jones, M., Koupil, I., Tooth, L., & Mishra, G. (2016). High education and increased parity are associated with breast-feeding initiation and duration among Australian women. *Public Health Nutrition, 19*(14), 2551–2561. https://doi.org/10.1017/S1368980016000367

Jones, E., Taylor, B., Rudge, G., MacArthu, R. C., Jyothish, D., Simkiss, D., & Cummins, C. (2018). Hospitalisation after birth of infants: cross sectional analysis of potentially avoidable admissions across England using hospital episode statistics. *BMC Pediatrics, 18*(1), Article 390. https://doi.org/10.1186/s12887-018-1360-z

Kitano, N., Nomura, K., Kido, M., Murakami, K., Ohkubo, T., Ueno, M., & Sugimoto, M. (2015). Combined effects of maternal age and parity on successful initiation of exclusive breastfeeding. *Preventive Medicine Reports, 3,* 121–126. https://doi.org/10.1016/j.pmedr.2015.12.010

Leung, A. K. C., & Sauve, R. S. (1989). Breastfeeding and breast milk jaundice. *Journal of the Royal Society of Health, 109*(6), 213–217. https://doi.org/10.1177/146642408910900615

Lin, Y.-Y., Tsao, P.-N., Hsieh, W.-S., Chen, C.-Y., & Chou, H.-C. (2008). The impact of breast-feeding on early neonatal jaundice. *Clinical Neonatology, 15*(1), 31–35. https://doi.org/10.7098/CN.200806.0031

Mizuno, K., Fujimaki, K., & Sawada, M. (2004). Sucking behavior at breast during the early newborn period affects later breast-feeding rate and duration of breast-feeding. *Pediatrics International, 46*(1), 15–20. https://doi.org/10.1111/j.1442-200X.2004.01834.x

Muchowski, K. E. (2014). Evaluation and treatment of neonatal hyperbilirubinemia. *American Family Physician, 89*(11), 873–878.

O'Brien, M., Buikstra, E., & Hegney, D. (2008). The influence of psychological factors on breastfeeding duration. *Journal of Advanced Nursing, 63*(4), 397–408. https://doi.org/10.1111/j.1365-2648.2008.04722.x

Pound, C. M., & Gaboury, I. (2009). The impact of jaundice in newborn infants on the length of breastfeeding. *Paediatrics & Child Health, 14*(7), 445–449.

Prameela, K. K. (2019). Breastfeeding during breast milk jaundice—A pathophysiological perspective. *Medical Journal of Malaysia, 74*(6), 527–533. http://www.e-mjm.org/2019/v74n6/breast-milk-jaundice.pdf

Preer, G. L., & Philipp, B. L. (2011). Understanding and managing breast milk jaundice. *Archives of Disease in Childhood. Fetal and Neonatal Edition, 96*(6), F461–F466. https://doi.org/10.1136/adc.2010.184416

Saeidi, R., Heydarian, F., & Fakehi, V. (2009). Role of intravenous extra fluid therapy in icteric neonates receiving phototherapy. *Saudi Medical Journal, 30*(9), 1176–1179. https://doi.org/10.1088/2058-7058/21/06/20

Schoenfeld, D. A. (1983). Sample-size formula for the proportional-hazards regression model. *Biometrics, 39*, 499–563. https://doi.org/10.2307/2531021

Sivanandan, S., Chawla, D., Misra, S., Agarwal, R., & Deorari, A. K. (2009). Effect of sling application on efficacy of phototherapy in healthy term neonates with nonhemolytic jaundice: A randomized controlled trial. *Indian Pediatrics, 46*(1), 23–28. https://www.indianpediatrics.net/jan2009/23.pdf

Waite, W. M., & Taylor, J. A. (2016). Phototherapy for the treatment of neonatal jaundice and breastfeeding duration and exclusivity. *Breastfeeding Medicine, 11*(4), 180–185. https://doi.org/10.1089/bfm.2015.0170

Waits, A., Guo, C. Y., & Chien, L. Y. (2018). Evaluation of factors contributing to the decline in exclusive breastfeeding at 6 months postpartum: The 2011–2016 National Surveys in Taiwan. *Birth, 45*(2), 184–192. https://doi.org/10.1111/birt.12340

Watson, R. L. (2009). Hyperbilirubinemia. *Critical Care Nursing Clinics of North America, 21*(1), 97–120. https://doi.org/10.1016/j.ccell.2008.11.001

World Health Organization/UNICEF. (1989). *Archived: Protecting, promoting and supporting breast-feeding.* https://www.who.int/nutrition/publications/infantfeeding/9241561300/en/

Zhang, L., Hu, P., Wang, J., Zhang, M., Zhang, Q. L., & Hu, B. (2015). Prenatal training improves new mothers' understanding of jaundice. *Medical Science Monitor, 21*, 1668–1673. https://doi.org/10.12659/MSM.893520

6

Depression in Nonhospitalized Jordanian Patients with Coronary Artery Disease

Ibtisam M. AL-ZARU[1]* • Fadwa ALHALAIQA[2] • Heyam Fawaz DALKY[3] • Kholoud Ali ARRAMADAN[4] • Abdul-Monim BATIHA[2]

ABSTRACT

Background: Patients with coronary artery disease (CAD) are likely to experience depression, which contributes to the burden of disease and is a risk factor for mortality. Patients in outpatient clinics in Jordan are not routinely screened for depression. Significant relationships among patient characteristics must be determined to ascertain the predictors of depression.

Purpose: The aims of this research were to assess the level of depression symptoms in nonhospitalized patients with CAD; to examine the relationships between depression and relevant sociodemographic, self-reported health history, and patient health perception variables; and to identify possible predictors of depression in Jordan.

Methods: This cross-sectional study recruited a convenience sample (N = 174) of nonhospitalized outpatients who had been diagnosed with CAD. Self-reported demographic, health history, and health perception information (independent variables) were provided by the participants. The depression scores (dependent variable) for the participants were assessed using the Cardiac Depression Scale. Data were analyzed using descriptive statistics, the chi-square test, Pearson's correlations, and multiple linear regressions.

Results: Half of the participants reported mild to moderate depression, with 37% reporting severe depression. Predictors of depression included gender (being female), having a concomitant chronic disease, prior surgery, irregular exercise, impaired sexual activity, and self-perceived poor psychological health.

Conclusions/Implications for Practice: To improve patient outcomes, clinical personnel should screen patients with CAD for depression and offer a combined pharmaceutical and therapeutic treatment intervention. An easy-to-administer instrument to detect depression may be included in the standard patient checkup routine used in clinics. Several patient characteristics were found to significantly affect depression and health outcomes.

KEY WORDS:
Jordan, coronary artery disease, depression, health assessment, demographic predictors of depression.

Introduction

Coronary artery disease (CAD) is a worldwide health problem and the leading cause of mortality (World Health Organization [WHO], 2014). On the basis of WHO statistics, CAD affects 110 million people and is the cause of 8.9 million deaths annually. CAD causes 15.9% of deaths each year and is the most common cause of death globally (GBD 2015 Mortality and Causes of Death Collaborators, 2016). The prevalence of CAD is predicted to reach 23.6 million people worldwide in 2030 (WHO, 2017). CAD is the main cause of death in Jordan, where it is responsible for 19.8% of all deaths in the country (WHO, 2014). Seventy-five percent of CAD deaths occur in low- to middle-income countries because of increases in the prevalence of cardiovascular disease risk factors (Mehta, Wei, & Wenger, 2015; WHO, 2014).

Depression is a widely recognized problem in patients with CAD (O'Neil, 2013), with at least 14% of patients with CAD believed to experience depression, of which 20% experience minor depression (Blumenthal, 2008; Huffman, Celano, Beach, Motiwala, & Januzzi, 2013). A German study on depression in patients with coronary heart disease found that 22% of the participants had been diagnosed with depression (Konrad, Jacob, Rapp, & Kostev, 2016). Similarly, a Jordanian study found that 25% of patients who complained of physical illness had symptoms of depression (Hamdan-Mansour et al., 2014). Depression has been associated with increased morbidity, mortality, and healthcare costs and a lower quality of life (Celano & Huffman, 2011; May et al., 2017; Sher, Lolak, & Maldonado, 2010). One study in Taiwan found a 21% prevalence of depression and suggested that depression functions as an independent factor that worsens the quality of life of patients (Huang, Chi, Sousa, Wang, & Pan, 2011). According to WHO, depression is a global phenomenon that affects some 350 million people worldwide, is a major cause of disability, and contributes greatly to the economic burden of disease (WHO, 2016).

[1]*PhD, RN, Associated Professor, Faculty of Nursing, Department of Adult Health, Jordan University of Science and Technology, Jordan* • [2]*PhD, RN, Associate Professor, Faculty of Nursing, Philadelphia University, Jordan* • [3]*PhD, RN, Associate Professor, Faculty of Nursing, Department of Community/Mental Health, Jordan University of Science and Technology, Jordan* • [4]*MSN, RN, Ministry of Health, Jordan.*

Depression is a risk factor for ischemic heart disease (May et al., 2017). However, the burden of depression has been widely underestimated (Charlson et al., 2013). A study conducted in Canada found depression among patients with CAD to be higher than in the normal population and identified depression as a potential predictor of otherwise healthy individuals developing CAD (Frasure-Smith & Lespérance, 2010). Konrad et al. (2016) studied CAD as a predictor of depression, and Bayat et al. (2011) identified CAD as a predictor of depression in a large scale, cross-sectional study in Iran.

A literature review that investigated the relationship between CAD and depression suggests a bidirectional relationship, with CAD a risk factor for depression and depression a risk factor for CAD (Khawaja, Westermeyer, Gajwani, & Feinstein, 2009). The findings in the literature suggest that depression is a serious problem in patients with CAD and that the relationship between CAD and depression should be examined further (O'Neil, 2013).

In one Jordan study, 25% of patients (n = 850) who complained of physical illnesses also showed symptoms of depression (Hamdan-Mansour et al., 2014). The authors noted that, among patients with CAD, 30% had mild depression and 29.3% had moderate-to-severe depression. Moreover, CAD was highly correlated with gender and employment status. However, patients with cancer reported the highest mean level of depression, followed by patients with more than one disease (e.g., diabetes mellitus and CAD). The authors also noted that having one or more chronic illness was stressful and that stress may affect how patients manage their diseases. In addition, psychosocial status may be a factor in compliance behavior, which in turn may affect patient health outcomes (Hamdan-Mansour et al., 2014).

The findings of the several studies worldwide that have investigated the risk factors for depression in patients with CAD suggest that being female, having a history of cardiac catheterization, and having other concomitant chronic diseases increase the risk of depression in this population (Huffman et al., 2013; Khawaja et al., 2009; Konrad et al., 2016; May et al., 2017). Other studies have claimed that erectile dysfunction increases risk of depression in patients with CAD (Clouse et al., 2003; Vlachopoulos, Jackson, Stefanadis, & Montorsi, 2013). The conclusions of an Irish study stated that the perception of psychological well-being among patients with heart failure has not been sufficiently examined (Morgan, Villiers-Tuthill, Barker, & McGee, 2014), noting that a regression analysis (n = 91) showed that patients' perception of illness versus well-being accounted for a larger proportion of variance in depression than either sociodemographic characteristics or functional status. Furthermore, the authors suggested that the negative perceptions of patients affected health outcomes and increased the risk of health complications (Morgan et al., 2014). Physical activities play an important role in reducing the risk of depression in the general population and among patients with CAD (Peterson, Charlson, Wells, & Altemus, 2014). Finally, another study suggested that older patients with CAD face a higher risk of developing depression than younger patients with CAD (Konrad et al., 2016). The relationship between the sociodemographic and clinical characteristics of patients with CAD, respectively, and depression remains unclear in the literature and therefore requires further study and clarification.

Depression Screening for Patients With Coronary Artery Disease

A number of widely used screening tools for depression are available. The Beck Depression Inventory-II (Beck, Steer, & Brown, 1996) was previously used in a study in Jordan to detect depression among patients diagnosed with physical illnesses (Hamdan-Mansour et al., 2014). The American Heart Association recommends the use of a two- and nine-item Patient Health Questionnaire, although its validity as a screening tool remains unclear and no evidence currently supports the use of this tool to improve cardiac patients' outcomes (Huffman et al., 2013). Neither of the aforementioned two instruments has been used directly on cardiac patients. The Cardiac Depression Scale (CDS; Hare & Davis, 1996) has been used to assess depression in cardiac patients in Iran, with results showing the CDS to be a reliable and sensitive tool in this population (Gholizadeh et al., 2010; Kiropoulos et al., 2012). On the basis of this experience, the CDS was used in this study to screen for depression.

Limited medical resources necessitate the prioritization of medical expenditures on the leading causes of death and disabilities. Jordan has an advanced healthcare system and is a major international destination for medical tourism. However, the focus of the healthcare system on the physical aspects of disease to the detriment of the psychological aspects is evident from the small budget devoted to mental health. The general lack of awareness among nurses in Jordan of the importance of assessing depression in patients with CAD likely prolongs hospitalization and increases treatment costs. Thus, predictors of depression in patients with CAD should be considered in future intervention programs.

Depression has been studied in patients with CAD in many Western countries, but few studies have been conducted in Arab countries such as Jordan. Only one Jordanian study in this category, a study on depression in patients with physical illnesses, including coronary vascular disease, was identified in the literature (Hamdan-Mansour et al., 2014).

This study aimed to assess level of depression symptoms in outpatients with CAD and to examine the relationships between depression and various sociodemographic, self-reported health history, and patient health perception variables to identify possible predictors of depression in this patient population in Jordan.

Methods

Design and Sample

A cross-sectional design was used to conduct a one-time assessment of depression and of self-reported health history in a convenience sample of nonhospitalized patients with coronary heart disease attending an outpatient clinic in a Jordanian hospital. Medical records were examined to identify patients who met the inclusion criteria, which included (a) ≥ 18 years old and (b) a diagnosis of CAD for at least 6 months before data collection. The exclusion criteria included (a) previous diagnosis of depression or psychatric disease, (b) showing symptoms of cognitive impairment, and (c) and currently taking antidepressent medications. Patients typically presented at the clinic with chest pain, electrocardiogram changes, and elevated troponin and other cardiac enzymes.

Using G* Power software, a minimum sample of 169 was estimated as necessary to identify statistically significant relationships of moderate magnitude ($p < .05$). The number of participants for this study was set at 250 to allow for potential withdrawals and for incomplete questionnaires.

Measures

The instruments used for data collection were self-administered in the clinic. Three of the data collection forms were developed by the author, and one was the Arabic version of a widely used scale. The data collection forms are listed hereinafter.

Sociodemographic data form

This form was used to collect information on the gender, marital status, professional status, education status, family monthly income, and health insurance status of the participant.

Health history form

This form was used to collect information on the clinical characteristics and medical/surgical history (e.g., comorbidities, cardiac catheterization history, duration of cardiac disease, medication compliance, smoking status, and physical exercise habits) of the participant.

Health perception form

This form was used to collect self-rated information on physical, psychological, and sexual health since developing a coronary problem. Items are scored using a 5-point scale, with 1 = *excellent* and 5 = *weak*.

The Cardiac Depression Scale

The questionnaire, developed by Hare and Davis (1996) in Australia to measure depression of individuals with cardiac diseases, is a 26-item or six-subscale tool with a developer-reported Cronbach's α of .9. An instrument validation study by Kiropoulos et al. (2012) reported internal consistency α coefficients for the six subscales (from .62 to .82) and found the instrument to be reliable for assessing depression in cardiac patients. Permission to use and translate the CDS into Arabic was obtained from the authors.

Using the CDS, participants rated their feelings toward each of the 26 items using a 7-point scale ranging from 1 = *strongly disagree* to 7 = *strongly agree*. The total score range for the CDS is 26–182, with scores < 90 indicating no depression, between 90 and 99 indicating mild/moderate depression, and > 100 indicating severe depression (Gholizade et al., 2010). A panel of bilingual and bicultural experts developed the Arabic version of the CDS using a back-translation technique. The initial Arabic version of CDS was pilot tested on 20 cardiac patients and found to be clear and understandable, with a Cronbach's α coefficient of .89.

Data Collection

Data collection was conducted from August to September 2015. After obtaining university and hospital approval, the hospital director gave permission to collect data. The purpose of the study was explained to the head nurse and the physician of the cardiac outpatient clinic, and permission was received to review the relevant medical records in the outpatient clinic. Patients who met the inclusion criteria were then identified, and potential participants were sent a cover letter with information sheets and a reply envelope. Those who returned the completed information form were met by the principal investigator and her assistants, who answered their potential participant concern questions and explained policies regarding protecting participant rights. Participants completed the questionnaires after providing verbal and written consent. Participants completed the instruments while in the waiting room of the hospital clinic and returned them to a research team member. The principal investigator and her assistants were available to answer any questions.

Ethical Consideration

The Jordan University of Science and Technology Institutional Review Board approved this study (216-2013). Data collection began after a patient provided written informed consent to participate. Before obtaining the consent form, the researcher explained the purpose, method, and process of this study to patients. Patients were assured that participation status would not affect the services they received at the clinic, that they had the right to withdraw at any time, and that individual responses would be kept confidential.

Statistical Analysis

SPSS for Windows Version 19.0 (IBM, Armonk, NY, USA) was used to obtain descriptive and correlational values. Relationships between sociodemographic characteristics and depression scores were determined using chi-square analysis and determining Pearson's r correlation coefficients. In addition, multiple linear regressions were used to identify the significant predictors of depression in the sample. In this study, "depression predictors" refer to all demographic, health history, and self-perceived health (physical, psychological, and sexual) variables that potentially predict depression, whereas "clinical characteristics" refer to both health history and health perception variables. Statistical advice was reached to make all multiple linear regressions' test requirements achieved before data analysis.

Results

Participant Characteristics

Of the 250 patients who met the inclusion criteria, 40 declined to participate and 36 patients returned incomplete questionnaires, leaving 174 patients who were enrolled as participants. The mean age of participants was 58.6 years (*SD* = 10.2), and 134 (77%) were married. Half of the participants were male (*n* = 90, 51.7%) and unemployed (*n* = 87, 50%). Most were literate (*n* = 146, 84%), and almost two thirds reported having a moderate family monthly income (*n* = 108, 62.1%). Sociodemographic data are shown in Table 1.

Health History

Most of the participants reported having a concomitant chronic disease (typically diabetes or hypertension; *n* = 157, 90.2%) and having undergone a cardiac catheterization procedure (94.2%). A small number (*n* = 19, 10.9%) reported receiving five or more cardiac catheterization procedures. Half had a history of prior surgery (*n* = 97, 55.7%; mostly appendectomies and gall bladder stone removals), and 25.9% (*n* = 45) reported smoking cigarettes, with 62% of this number (*n* = 28) smoking at least one pack per day.

Nearly all of the participants (*n* = 170, 97.7%) complied with their medical prescriptions, and almost two thirds (*n* = 112, 64.4%) reported experiencing a shocking or stressful event during the last year such as the death of a family member or an acute health problem. Frequency and percentage data are shown in Table 2. Although some of the patients self-reported that they had depression and anxiety and had taken related medications (see Table 2), their files did not corroborate this information. However, because their family members confirmed the depression or anxiety to be a short episode of sadness because of bereavement, these data were included in the analysis.

TABLE 1.

Frequency Distribution of the Sociodemographic Variables (N = 174)

Variable	*n*	%
Age (*M* and *SD*)	58.6	10.2
Gender		
Male	90	51.7
Female	84	48.3
Marital status		
Single	10	5.2
Married	134	77.0
Divorced	3	1.7
Widowed	27	15.5
Educational level		
Illiterate	28	16.1
Can read and write	28	16.1
Secondary degree or less	60	34.5
More than secondary degree	58	33.3
Employment status		
Working	49	28.1
Retired	38	21.8
Unemployed	87	50.0
Monthly income		
Low	58	33.3
Moderate	108	62.1
High	8	4.6
Health insurance		
Yes	133	76.4
No	41	23.6

Note. Age range: 38–81 years.

Health Perceptions

About half of the participants rated their physical health as less than good (*n* = 97, 55.74%), and 14.4% (*n* = 25) rated their health as excellent or very good. Less than half (*n* = 77, 44.3%) perceived their psychiatric or mental health to be less than good (fair or weak). Although 29 participants did not respond to the query on sexual behavior, almost two thirds of the patients reported that having a coronary disease affected their sexual activity (*n* = 121, 69.5%). The most prevalent problem noted was erectile dysfunction (*n* = 33, 19.0%).

Depression Symptoms

The CDS was found to be valid and reliable in this study (Cronbach's α = .75). The total CDS mean score was 91.9 (*SD* = 26.5), indicating a mild/moderate level of depression. Using the frequency distribution of depression symptoms as measured by CDS, approximately half of the participants reported depressive symptoms (*n* = 93, 53.4%), with a relatively small number reporting mild/moderate depression (*n* = 31, 17.8%) and a larger number (*n* = 62, 35.6%) reporting severe depressive symptoms (see Table 3).

Relationship Between Depression and Sociodemographic and Clinical Characteristic Variables

The results of chi-square analyses are shown in Table 4. A significant difference was found for gender (χ^2 = 4.66, *p* = .03), with more female patients (51.7%) showing depressive symptoms than male patients. CDS total scores were categorized as "no depression" (< 90), "mild/moderate depression" (90–99), and "severe depression" (> 100). A relationship was found between having concomitant chronic diseases and having a CAD diagnosis (90.2%; χ^2 = 8.40, *p* = .004) and between previously having surgery and having a CAD diagnosis (55.7%; χ^2 = 6.20, *p* = .01). Moreover, a significant difference was found for exercise (χ^2 = 9.90, *p* < .001), with nonregular exercisers reporting higher depression scores (proportion: 60.5%). In addition, a relationship was found

TABLE 2.
Frequency Distribution of the Self-Reported Health History of the Patients (N = 174)

Variable	*n*	%
Chronic disease		
No chronic diseases	17	9.8
Hypertension (HTN)	24	13.8
Diabetes mellitus (DM)	9	5.2
DM and HTN	34	19.5
DM and HTN and hyperlipidemia	20	11.5
DM and HTN and heart failure	16	9.2
Other (e.g., cancer, thyroid disease)	54	31.0
Coronary catheterization history		
Yes	164	94.2
No	10	5.8
Frequencies of coronary catheterization		
No previous catheterization	10	5.8
1–2 times	105	60.3
3–4 times	40	23.0
5–6 times	11	6.3
> 6 times	8	4.6
Surgical history		
Yes	97	55.7
No	77	44.3
Smoking history		
Yes	45	25.9
No	129	74.1
Coronary heart disease (duration; years)		
6 months to < 1	34	19.5
1–5	96	55.2
6–10	23	13.2
> 10	21	12.1
Previous diagnosis of depression[a]		
Yes	8	4.6
No	166	95.4
Previous diagnosis of anxiety[a]		
Yes	11	6.3
No	163	93.7
Previous use of antidepressant medication[a]		
Yes	9	5.2
No	165	94.8
Previous use of antianxiety medication[a]		
Yes	8	4.6
No	166	95.4
Current medication compliance		
Yes	170	97.7
No	4	2.3
Regular exercise		
Yes	69	39.5
No	105	60.5
Sexual activity since diagnosis		
Affected	121	69.8
Not affected	53	30.2
Shocking/stressful event within last year		
Health problem	44	25.3
Family member death	26	14.9
Family member travelling	18	10.3
Problem with relatives	7	4.0
Other	17	9.9
Nothing	62	35.6

[a]Self-reported.

for influence of impaired sexual activity (proportion: 69.8%; $\chi^2 = 8.40$, $p < .001$). The participants who reported that heart disease affected their sexual activity had higher depression scores. No significant relationships were found between CAD diagnosis and other sociodemographic, health history, or physical and psychological health perception variables.

In terms of self-rated health, Pearson *r* correlation results showed a statistically negative relationship between depression and perceived physical health ($r = -.28$, $p < .001$; small relationship) and perceived psychological health ($r = -.48$, $p < .001$; medium relationship; Pallant, 2003). A negative relationship was noted because the health perception scores were reversed, with 1 corresponding to excellent and 5 corresponding to weak. Thus, participants who perceived their physical or psychiatric health as fair or weak registered higher depression scores than those who perceived their health as very good or excellent.

Predictors of Depression

The statistically significant predictors of depression identified in this study include weak/fair self-rated psychological health, impaired sexual activity, one or more prior surgeries, being female, and lack of regular exercise ($F = 20.2$, $p < .001$, adjusted $R^2 = .36$, $p < .05$; Table 5). The regression model explained 36% of the variance in depression severity.

Discussion

This study aimed to assess depression symptoms in Jordanian outpatients with CAD and to describe the relationships

TABLE 3.
Frequency Distribution of Depression Symptoms as Measured by the Cardiac Depression Scale (N = 174)

Cardiac Depression Scale Score	*n*	%
Not depressed	81	46.6
Depressed		
Mild/moderate depression	31	17.8
Severe depression	62	35.6

TABLE 4.

Chi-Square Analysis of Relationship Between Depression Scores and Selected Sociodemographic and Clinical Characteristics (N = 174)

Variable	n	%	χ^2	df	p
Gender			4.66	1	.030
Female	90	51.7			
Male	84	48.3			
Marital status			0.89	1	.340
Married	164	94.3			
Not married	10	5.7			
Educational status			4.20	1	.500
Low	116	66.7			
High	58	33.3			
Working status			1.16	1	.280
Work	87	50.0			
Not working	87	50.0			
Presence of health insurance			0.06	1	.870
Yes	133	76.4			
No	41	23.6			
Chronic diseases			8.40	1	.004
Yes	157	90.2			
No	17	9.8			
Previous coronary catheterization			0.00	1	.940
Yes	164	94.2			
No	10	5.8			
Surgical history			6.20	1	.010
Yes	97	55.7			
No	77	44.3			
Smoking			0.13	1	.700
Yes	45	25.9			
No	129	74.1			
Last month's cardiac hospitalization			0.99	1	.300
Yes	79	45.4			
No	95	54.6			
Coronary heart disease duration			1.48	1	.200
6 months to ≤ 5 years	130	74.7			
> 5 years	44	25.3			
Regular exercise			9.90	1	< .001
Yes	69	39.7			
No	105	60.3			
Sexual activity since diagnosis			8.40	1	< .001
Affected	121	69.8			
Not affected	53	30.2			

Note. Clinical characteristics refer to health history and patient physical and psychological health perception variables.
*$p < .05$.

between depression and various sociodemographic, self-reported health history, and patient health perception variables. Furthermore, this study identified those variables that predicted depression in the sample. Half of the participants reported mild-to-moderate depression, and nearly one third reported severe depression. Being female and having one or more concomitant chronic diseases were two of the clinical predictors of depression identified in this study. The following section presents detailed information about the levels of depression, associated factors, and possible predictors identified in this study.

Level and Severity of Depression Symptoms

About 30% of the patients with CAD in Hamdan-Mansour et al. (2014) were affected by mild to moderate levels of depression. In this study, only 17.8% of participants were reported to be in the mild-to-moderate range. However, the percentage of participants reporting in the high range in this study exceeded that found by Hamdan-Mansour and colleagues (35.6% vs. 30%, respectively). This may be because the earlier study included patients with any physical illness (e.g., respiratory diseases, CAD, cancer), whereas this study focused exclusively on patients with CAD. Echoing this study, a study of patients with stable/unstable angina and myocardial infarction found a similarly high incidence (31%–45%) of "significant" depression (Huffman et al., 2013), and a study in Iran found that 65.9% of participants reported depressive symptoms 24 months after experiencing a myocardial infarction (Hosseini et al., 2011). In a meta-analysis of patient data, depression was identified as a risk factor for mortality, although the authors noted that the severity of depression lessened over time because of patient adjustment (Meijer et al., 2013).

In terms of total CDS scores (summed across 26 items using a 7-point agreement scale), the overall mean was in the mild-to-moderate range (91.9 ± 26.5, range: 26–182), which is higher than the mean score of the original CDS study in Australia (80.3 ± 27.8; Hare & Davis, 1996) and less than the mean reported in an Iranian study (101.37 ± 25.72; Gholizadeh et al., 2010). The higher scores for those studies conducted in Middle Eastern countries than in Australia may be attributable to political, socioeconomic, and cultural differences.

TABLE 5.

Multiple Linear Regression to Test the Significant Predictors of Depression According to Selected Sociodemographic and Clinical Characteristics (N = 174)

Variable	β	p	R^2	F
Psychological health self-evaluation	−.36	< .001	.36	20.20
Regular exercises	.20	.001	.36	20.20
Sexual activity affected	.32	< .001	.36	20.20
Gender	.16	.010	.36	20.20
Surgical history	.14	.020	.36	20.20

Note. Clinical characteristics refer to health history and patient physical and psychological health perception variables.

Relationships Between Sociodemographic Variables and Depression

This study revealed significant relationships between depression and the sociodemographic variables of gender (being female), concomitant chronic diseases (having one or more), surgical history (previous surgeries), exercise (lacking regular exercise), and sexual activity (impaired). The relatively higher depression scores for women in this study may be because of the traditional role of Jordanian women as responsible for their family, which is often a source of stress. Moreover, in Jordanian culture, the actions of women are more likely to be criticized than those of men. In addition, having one or more chronic diseases in addition to CAD and one or more prior surgeries may affect patients negatively and inhibit the effective management of their diseases.

In this study, patients who self-reported as not exercising regularly had higher depression scores than those who did. Physical inactivity and lack of regular exercise have been shown to affect depression, with a long-term, large-scale study on outpatients with cardiac diseases in the United States concluding that lack of exercise is a mediator between depression and negative coronary heart disease outcomes (Whooley et al., 2008). Furthermore, physical activity is recognized as a positive influence on both mental and physical health as well as a means of relieving stress, which promotes good health and positive behavioral outcomes (WHO, 2011).

Associations have been found among depression, CAD, and sexual health. One review noted that, although depression contributes to impaired sexual activity in patients with heart disease and often results in erectile dysfunction or fear of heart attack during performance, further research is needed, especially in women and older adults (Nascimento et al., 2013).

Many studies have reported that being unmarried and unemployed increase the risk of depression in patients with CAD (Al-Abbudi, Lami, & Wady, 2018; Bjørnnes et al., 2018; Eng et al., 2011). A study conducted by Al-Abbudi et al. (2018) at an outpatient clinic and sharing the same purpose as this study found a significant relationship between depression and marital status (being unmarried), employment (not having a job), and education (being illiterate; Al-Abbudi et al., 2018). However, this study found no significant relationship between depression and these three variables. One possible explanation for this discrepancy is that the entire sample in this study was educated, with around half reporting a low level of education. Another possible explanation is the faith in God in this study professed by participants of all educational levels, which may help them acquiesce to their current condition as "God's will."

This study found no significant relationship between age and depression, which contrasts with the finding in Konrad et al. (2016) that older patients with CAD faced a higher risk for depression than their younger peers. The more regular participation of older people than younger people in religious activities in Muslims countries such as Jordan may help older people in these countries accept their current condition.

Predictors of Depression in Outpatients With Coronary Artery Disease

The predictors of depression identified in this study include gender, prior surgery, exercise, sexual activity, and perceived psychological health. These variables, with the addition of perceived psychological health and the absence of concomitant chronic diseases, are the same as those that were found to be significantly related to depression. Although, because disease management was not investigated, compliance with medications was not identified as a significant issue in this study, nonadherence to CAD self-management routines likely contributes to depression as well (Khawaja et al., 2009).

A statistically significant relationship was identified between depression and self-perceived psychological health. This finding is consistent with prior studies in which patients with CAD with poor self-perceived mental health statuses reported more depressive symptoms than those who perceived their mental health as good (Kent & Shapiro, 2009; Morgan et al., 2014). Patients who hold negative images of themselves may be more likely to rate their mental state as lower than their stabler or better-adjusted peers. Negative self-image may increase stress in patients and lead to more depressive symptoms. In addition, coronary disease and the commonly prescribed medications for this disease are known to cause psychophysiological changes that the patient may perceive as unhealthy or mentally debilitating, which may exacerbate stress and increase depression.

Limitations

This study was conceived as an initial attempt to study depression among patients with CAD in Jordan. There are several limitations to this study. First, the cross-sectional design approach that was used addresses only one point in time. Second, the convenience sampling technique may introduce a bias because the participants may not be representative of the general Jordanian population. Third, the lack of a theoretical framework may affect the clarity of the results. Fourth, the use of self-ratings is inherently subjective, and participant responses are likely to be affected by bias. All of the participants were attending the outpatient clinic and presumably had some degree of pain or anxiety that may have negatively affected their perceptions. Conducting follow-up studies would further enhance scholarly understanding of the variables that affect perception. All of these limitations may affect the generalizability of the results (Brennan, 2001), which should be considered and applied with caution. Research into this topic must be further advanced by developing interventions that combine psychobehavioral techniques with pharmacological interventions to treat heart disease and depression concurrently.

Conclusions/Implications for Practice

The nonhospitalized patient population with CAD in Jordan is affected by a relatively high prevalence of depression. However, depression is not routinely diagnosed or treated. Screening for depression using an easy-to-use, reliable instrument such as the CDS and then treating both heart disease and depression simultaneously may be expected to improve medical outcomes and reduce the overall cost of treating these diseases.

Certain sociodemographic and health-related factors were shown in this study to be statistically significant predictors of depression in patients with CAD and should be considered by healthcare providers. Patients with CAD who are female, who do not exercise regularly, and who rate their psychological health as poor are more likely to be severely depressed than their peer patients with CAD. Furthermore, having a history of surgeries and having one or more concomitant chronic diseases (e.g., diabetes, hypertension) are likely to be significant contributors to depression.

Future studies should identify additional variables that predict depression and use all of the identified variables to build CAD patient treatment guidelines. The results of this study support the need for specialized intervention programs to enhance the quality of life for patients with CAD.

On the basis of the findings of this study, healthcare organizations and health policymakers should consider using CDS as a screening tool for depression to detect and treat depression earlier, which may reduce overall costs of treatment, reduce mortality, and reduce comorbidities.

Authors Contributions

Study conception and design: IMA
Data collection: KAA
Data analysis and interpretation: IMA, FA
Drafting of the article: All authors
Critical revision of the article: HFD

References

Al-Abbudi, S. J., Lami, F. H., & Wady, Z. A. (2018). Prevalence and assessment of severity of depression among ischemic heart disease patients attending outpatient cardiology department baghdad teaching hospital, Baghdad, Iraq. *Journal of Psychiatry, 21*(2), 438. https://doi.org/10.4172/2378-5756.1000438

Bayat, N., Alishiri, G. H., Salimzadeh, A., Izadi, M., Saleh, D. K., Lankarani, M. M., & Assari, S. (2011). Symptoms of anxiety and depression: A comparison among patients with different chronic conditions. *Journal of Research in Medical Sciences, 16*(11), 1441–1447.

Beck, A. T., Steer, R. A., & Brown, G. K. (1996). *Manual for the Beck Depression Inventory-II.* San Antonio, TX: Psychological Corporation.

Bjørnnes, A. K., Parry, M., Lie, I., Falk, R., Leegaard, M., & Rustøen, T. (2018). The association between hope, marital status, depression and persistent pain in men and women following cardiac surgery. *BMC Women's Health, 18*(1), 2. https://doi.org/10.1186/s12905-017-0501-0

Blumenthal, J. A. (2008). Depression and coronary heart disease: Association and implications for treatment. *Cleveland Clinic Journal of Medicine, 75*(Suppl. 2), S48–5S3.

Brennan, R. L. (2001). *Generalizability theory.* New York, NY: Springer-Verlag.

Celano, C. M., & Huffman, J. C. (2011). Depression and cardiac disease: A review. *Cardiology in Review, 19*(3), 130–142. https://doi.org/10.1097/CRD.0b013e31820e8106

Charlson, F. J., Moran, A. E., Freedman, G., Norman, R. E., Stapelberg, N. J., Baxter, A. J., ... Whiteford, H. A. (2013). The contribution of major depression to the global burden of ischemic heart disease: A comparative risk assessment. *BMC Medicine, 11*, 250. https://doi.org/10.1186/1741-7015-11-250

Clouse, R. E., Lustman, P. J., Freedland, K. E., Griffith, L. S., McGill, J. B., & Carney, R. M. (2003). Depression and coronary heart disease in women with diabetes. *Psychosomatic Medicine, 65*(3), 376–383. https://doi.org/10.1097/01.PSY.0000041624.96580

Eng, H. S., Yean, L. C., Das, S., Letchmi, S., Yee, K. S., Bakar, R. A., ... Choy, C. Y. (2011). Anxiety and depression in patients with coronary heart disease: A study in a tertiary hospital. *Iranian Journal of Medical Sciences, 36*(3), 201–206.

Frasure-Smith, N., & Lespérance, F. (2010). Depression and cardiac risk: Present staus and future directions. *Heart, 96*(3), 173–176. https://doi.org/10.1136/hrt.2009.186957

GBD 2015 Mortality and Causes of Death Collaborators. (2016). Global, regional, and national life expectancy, all-cause mortality, and cause-specific mortality for 249 causes of death, 1990–2015: A systematic analysis for the Global Burden of Disease Study 2015. *The Lancet, 388*(10053), 1459–1544. https://doi.org/10.1016/S0140-6736(16)31012-168

Gholizadeh, L., Salamonson, Y., Davidson, P. M., Parvan, K., Frost, S. A., Chang, S., & Hare, D. L. (2010). Cross-cultural validation of the cardiac depression scale in Iran. *British Journal of Clinical Psychology, 49*(4), 517–528. https://doi.org/10.1348/014466509X478709

Hamdan-Mansour, A. M., Ghannam, B. M., Abeiat, D. D., Badawi, T. H., Thultheen, I. N., & Shamali, I. M. (2014). Predicting depression among Jordanian patients diagnosed with physical illnesses. *Psychology, 5*(19), 2120–2130. https://doi.org/10.4236/psych.2014.519214

Hare, D. L., & Davis, C. R. (1996). Cardiac depression scale: Validation of a new depression scale for cardiac patients. *Journal of Psychosomatic Research, 40*(4), 379–386. https://doi.org/10.1016/0022-3999(95)00612-5

Hosseini, S. H., Yousefnejad, K., Tabiban, S., Nesarhoseyni, V., Bagheri, B., Kiasari, A. M., ... Mokhberi, V. (2011). Effects of depression and anxiety symptoms on cardiac mortality following myocardial infarction: A 2-year follow-up. *International Journal of Psychiatry in Clinical Practice, 15*(2), 91–96. https://doi.org/10.3109/13651501.2010.538065

Huang, C. Y., Chi, S. C., Sousa, V. D., Wang, C. P., & Pan, K. C. (2011). Depression, coronary artery disease, type 2 diabetes, metabolic syndrome and quality of life in Taiwanese adults from a cardiovascular department of a major hospital in Southern Taiwan. *Journal of Clinical Nursing, 20*(9-10), 1293–1302. https://doi.org/10.1111/j.1365-2702.2010.03451.x

Huffman, J. C., Celano, C. M., Beach, S. R., Motiwala, S. R., & Januzzi, J. L. (2013). Depression and cardiac disease: Epidemiology, mechanisms, and diagnosis. *Cardiovascular Psychiatry and Neurology, 2013*, 695925. https://doi.org/10.1155/2013/695925

Kent, L. K., & Shapiro, P. A. (2009). Depression and related psychological factors in heart disease. *Harvard Review of Psychiatry, 17*(6), 377–388. https://doi.org/10.3109/10673220903463333

Khawaja, I. S., Westermeyer, J. J., Gajwani, P., & Feinstein, R. E. (2009). Depression and coronary artery disease: The association, mechanisms, and therapeutic implications. *Psychiatry (Edgmont), 6*(1), 38–51.

Kiropoulos, L. A., Meredith, I., Tonkin, A., Clarke, D., Antonis, P., & Plunkett, J. (2012). Psychometric properties of the cardiac depression scale in patients with coronary heart disease. *BMC Psychiatry, 12*, 216. https://doi.org/10.1186/1471-244X-12-216

Konrad, M., Jacob, L., Rapp, M. A., & Kostev, K. (2016). Depression risk in patients with coronary heart disease in Germany. *World Journal of Cardiology, 8*(9), 547–552. https://doi.org/10.4330/wjc.v8.i9.547

May, H. T., Horne, B. D., Knight, S., Knowlton, K. U., Bair, T. L., Lappé, D. L., ... Muhlestein, J. B. (2017). The association of depression at any time to the risk of death following coronary artery disease diagnosis. *European Heart Journal. Quality of Care & Clinical Outcomes, 3*(4), 296–302. https://doi.org/10.1093/ehjqcco/qcx017

Mehta, P. K., Wei, J., & Wenger, N. K. (2015). Ischemic heart disease in women: A focus on risk factors. *Trends in Cardiovascular Medicine, 25*(2), 140–151. https://doi.org/10.1016/j.tcm.2014.10.005

Meijer, A., Conradi, H. J., Bos, E. H., Anselmino, M., Carney, R. M., Denollet, J., & de Jonge, P. (2013). Adjusted prognostic association of depression following myocardial infarction with mortality and cardiovas and cardiovascular events: Individual patient data meta-analysis. *The British Journal of Psychiatry, 203*(2), 90–102. https://doi.org/10.1192/bjp.bp.112.111195

Morgan, K., Villiers-Tuthill, A., Barker, M., & McGee, H. (2014). The contribution of illness perception to psychological distress in heart failure patients. *BMC Psychology, 2*(1), 50. https://doi.org/10.1186/PREACCEPT-1583576822131822

Nascimento, E. R., Maia, A. C., Pereira, V., Soares-Filho, G., Nardi, A. E., & Silva, A. C. (2013). Sexual dysfunction and cardiovascular diseases: A systematic review of prevalence. *Clinics (São Paulo, Brazil), 68*(11), 1462–1468. https://doi.org/10.6061/clinics/2013(11)13

O'Neil, A. (2013). The relationship between coronary heart disease (CHD) and major depressive disorder (MDD): Key mechanisms and the role of quality of life. *Europe's Journal of Psychology, 9*(1), 163–184. https://doi.org/10.5964/ejop.v9i1.466

Pallant, J. (2003). *SPSS survival manual: A step by step guide to data analysis using SPSS for windows* (2nd ed.). Philadelphia, PA: Open University Press.

Peterson, J. C., Charlson, M. E., Wells, M. T., & Altemus, M. (2014). Depression, coronary artery disease, and physical activity: How much exercise is enough? *Clinical Therapeutics, 36*(11), 1518–1530. https://doi.org/10.1016/j.clinthera.2014.10.003

Sher, Y., Lolak, S., & Maldonado, J. R. (2010). The impact of depression in heart disease. *Current Psychiatry Reports, 12*(3), 255–264. https://doi.org/10.1007/s11920-010-0116-8

Vlachopoulos, C., Jackson, G., Stefanadis, C., & Montorsi, P. (2013). Erectile dysfunction in the cardiovascular patient. *European Heart Journal, 34*(27), 2034–2046. https://doi.org/10.1093/eurheartj/eht112

Whooley, M. A., de Jonge, P., Vittinghoff, E., Otte, C., Moos, R., Carney, R. M., ... Browner, W. S. (2008). Depressive symptoms, health behaviors, and risk of cardiovascular events in patients with coronary heart disease. *JAMA, 300*(20), 2379–2388. https://doi.org/10.1001/jama.2008.711

World Health Organization. (2011). *Global atlas on cardiovascular disease prevention and control*. Geneva, Switzerland: Author.

World Health Organization. (2014). *Noncommunicable disease (NCD) country profiles 2014*. Retrived from https://apps.who.int/iris/bitstream/handle/10665/128038/9789241507509_eng.pdf

World Health Organization. (2016). *Mental health—Depression: Let's talk*. Retrived from https://www.who.int/mental_health/management/depression/en/

World Health Organization. (2017). *Cardiovascular diseases: Key facts*. Retrieved from https://www.who.int/cardiovascular_diseases/about_cvd/en/

Effect of Life Review on Quality of Life in Terminal Patients

Mei-Hua HUANG[1] • Ruey-Hsia WANG[2] • Hsiu-Hung WANG[3]*

ABSTRACT

Background: Enhancing quality of life takes precedence in the terminal stage of a disease, when a cure is considered impossible and all alternative methods to prevent disease progression have been exhausted. Life review, involving appreciating accomplishments and resolving conflicts, is widely considered to be an effective approach to bringing peace to terminal patients.

Purpose: This study was conducted to assess the effects of life review on quality of life in terminal patients.

Methods: The Cochrane Library, PubMed, MEDLINE, CINAHL, CEPS, and ProQuest databases were searched for original studies published between 2007 and July 2018. Studies that used experimental designs to assess the effects of life review on quality of life in terminal patients, involved patients aged >18 years, and were published in English or Chinese were considered eligible for inclusion. Studies that measured quality of life in individuals other than patients as well as unpublished papers or data were excluded. The search terms used included "life review," "end of life," "terminal or terminally ill," "advanced cancer," "palliative," "hospice," and "quality of life." The quality of each included study was assessed using the Downs and Black checklist.

Results: Six studies with 296 patients were included in the review. The participants in the included studies were from multiple countries. Life review was found to affect quality of life significantly (95% CI [0.147, 0.668], $Z = 3.062$, $p < .05$). The selected studies exhibited moderate heterogeneity ($I^2 = 42.407$, $p > .1$).

Conclusions: Life review was found to affect quality of life significantly in the participants in the included studies. The feasibility and safety of applying life review interventions should be considered for terminal patients, and implementers of these interventions should be trained and qualified. Only a few studies in the literature have evaluated the effects of life review therapy in terminal patients. Further studies that use stricter selection criteria are necessary to evaluate the efficacy of the life review intervention before its adoption in clinical practice.

Key Words:
life review, terminal-stage patients, end-of-life care, quality of life, meta-analysis.

Introduction

The terminal stage of a disease is defined as the stage at which a patient's disease is not amenable to cure, health progressively deteriorates, and survival is not expected by the health professionals providing care. The main goal of end-of-life care is to provide the highest quality of life (QOL) to patients and their relatives (World Health Organization, 1990). End-of-life care strives to add "life to years" instead of years to life (Tang & McCorkle, 2002). The relationship between spiritual well-being and QOL in patients with cancer has been increasingly studied in recent years. Most healthcare researchers and clinicians suggest that QOL should consider symptoms, functioning, psychological and social well-being, and, to a lesser extent, meaning and fulfillment (Kaasa & Loge, 2003).

An approach that improves the QOL of patients who are facing problems related to life-threatening diseases and their families by controlling pain and other symptoms and satisfying their psychological, social, and spiritual needs is desirable (Bennett & Closs, 2008; Choi & Kim, 2017). Cohen and Mount (1992) strongly advocated that, in end-of-life care, QOL is not only a primary concern but also the main objective of every intervention. Kissane and Kelly (2000) described "demoralization syndrome" in patients with terminal illness as a triad of hopelessness, loss of meaning, and desire for death. Psychotherapeutic interventions designed for patients who desire death must reinforce meaning and purpose, thereby reducing the desire for death and overall suffering for these patients who experience hopelessness (Chochinov et al., 2004).

Life review is considered an effective psychospiritual intervention for people facing death (Leung et al., 2015). Therapeutic life review may assist people to cope with loss, guilt, conflict, and defeat and may enable them to discover meaning in their accomplishments (Haber, 2006). Therapeutic life

[1]*MS, RN, Director, Department of Nursing, Jhong Jheng Spine & Orthopedic Hospital, and Doctoral Student, College of Nursing, Kaohsiung Medical University* • [2]*PhD, RN, Professor, College of Nursing, Kaohsiung Medical University* • [3]*PhD, RN, FAAN, Professor, College of Nursing, Kaohsiung Medical University.*

review is a procedure of recalling, evaluating, and integrating life experiences that aims to achieve ego integrity in the final stage of life (Trueman & Parker, 2006). The differences between life review and reminiscence must be emphasized because many researchers have conflated these concepts (Haight & Burnside, 1993). Reminiscence is a descriptive activity that involves thoughts about a patient's life and recalls prominent events from the past. During reminiscence, memory is more an affective function than a cognitive function. It may be structured or unstructured and undertaken either individually or in a group setting (Haight & Burnside, 1993; Keall, Clayton, & Butow, 2015). By contrast, life review is typically structured around one or more life themes, with lifetime family experiences and work experiences being the most common (Haber, 2006). In contrast to reminiscence, life review is an appraisal activity that involves investigating and, if possible, resolving a specific conflict. Life review functions at a deeper level than reminiscence with a goal of helping patients seek meaning from life events. This may help patients face death through achieving a sense of peace through resolving conflicts and providing a feeling of achievement in life tasks (Haber, 2006). Aspects of the process of life review such as individuality, structure, and evaluation distinguish this process from reminiscence and give it therapeutic value, with evaluation being the most crucial aspect (Haight & Burnside, 1993).

Several studies have investigated life review in older adults. Life review has been reported to pacify individuals through the process of life evaluation, which involves both appreciating accomplishments and resolving conflicts (Bohlmeijer, Smit, & Cuijpers, 2003). Moreover, the positive effects of life review interviews on depression (Haight, Michel, & Hendrix, 1998; Hanaoka & Okamura, 2004; Korte, Bohlmeijer, Cappeliez, Smit, & Westerhof, 2012; Pot et al., 2010) and self-esteem (Chiang, Lu, Chu, Chang, & Chou, 2008; Haight, Michel, & Hendrix, 2000) have been reported. However, few investigations or empirical studies on psychotherapeutic interventions for end-of-life patients have been published. Results from these previous studies provide critical underpinnings for psychotherapeutic approaches. The clinical effects of life review have been investigated in many practical studies. For example, one systematic review of the effects of therapeutic life review found that it is difficult to use therapeutic life review effectively with patients with life-threatening diseases (Keall et al., 2015). As the effects of using life review on terminal patients are inconsistent in the literature, this systematic review and meta-analysis of quantitative evaluations of life review interventions was conducted to improve the QOL domains in terminal patients.

Methods

Search Strategies and Screening Process

A systematic review and meta-analysis was conducted to examine the effects of life review on QOL in terminally ill patients.

This study adopted the Preferred Reporting Items for Systematic Reviews and Meta-Analyses, and systematic database searches were conducted in August 2018. Five electronic databases covering the realms of biomedicine science, social science, and general references were screened, including Cochrane Library, PubMed, MEDLINE, CINAHL, CEPS, and ProQuest. The search terms used included "life review," "end of life," "terminal or terminally ill," "advanced cancer," "palliative," "hospice," and "quality of life." The results were saved to a citation manager in Endnote X6. Figure 1 presents the flowchart of this systematic review according to the Preferred Reporting Items for Systematic Reviews and Meta-Analyses (Moher, Liberati, Tetzlaff, & Altman, 2009).

The inclusion criteria were studies that (a) employed experimental designs that are suitable for assessing the effects of life review in terminally ill patients who lived for less than 6 months or received palliative care, (b) included terminally ill patients aged >18 years, (c) were original studies published in English or Chinese, (d) used life review as an intervention, and (e) used QOL as an outcome measure. Studies that assessed QOL in populations other than patients (e.g., patient caretakers or relatives) and unpublished papers or data were excluded from this study.

Assessment of Study Quality

The quality of the included studies was assessed using the Downs and Black checklist, a quality index with high internal consistency, high retest reliability, and good interrater reliability (Downs & Black, 1998). This checklist consists of 27 items that are distributed over the five subscales of reporting, external validity, internal validity: bias, internal validity: confounding, and power. The Downs and Black checklist may be used to assess the methodological quality of both randomized controlled trials (RCTs) and nonrandomized studies, with scores greater than or equal to 20 considered good, between 15 and 19 considered fair, and 14 or below considered poor (Kennelly, 2011). Two investigators selected original studies on the basis of the inclusion criteria and reviewed the quality of each. Any disagreement between the two investigators regarding the extracted data was resolved through discussion. As study quality was the issue of concern, the score for each of the included studies should exceed 14.

Meta-Analysis

After the eligible studies were identified, each study was analyzed using the Comprehensive Meta-Analysis software program. Heterogeneity was assessed using forest plots that used both Q (a significant result that indicates statistic heterogeneity; Hwu & Lin, 2014) and I^2 (a significant result that indicates methodological heterogeneity) statistics. Values of 25%, 50%, and 75% indicate low, moderate, and high heterogeneity, respectively (Higgins, Thompson, Deeks, & Altman,

2003). A fixed-effects model was adopted for analysis when $p > .1$ and $I^2 < 50\%$ (because of trial homogeneity), whereas a random-effects model was adopted when $p < .1$ and $I^2 \geq 50\%$. The magnitude and significance of the effects of life review on QOL were calculated and are presented as odds ratios with 95% confidence intervals.

Results

After searching and screening the literature, six original studies that had been published in international journals in English were included in this review. The characteristics of participants, research design, settings, outcome measurements, and quality were analyzed (Table 1). The six studies in this review included 296 participants in total and were conducted in Japan (n = 1), the United States (n = 1), Canada (n = 1), Hong Kong (n = 1), Australia (n = 1), and China (n = 1). An analysis of research design found that four of the studies used an RCT design (Studies 2–4 and 6) and that two used a one-group pretest–posttest design (Studies 1 and 5). An analysis of research settings revealed that the intervention periods were 1–3 weeks (Studies 2 and 4–6) and 24 weeks (Study 1), with the intervention period for Study 3 varied according to the physical and psychological capacities of each patient. Moreover, differences were observed in terms of numbers of sessions, with one study (Study 4), three studies (Studies 2 and 5–6), and two studies (Studies 1 and 3) involving two, three, and four sessions, respectively. The investigators in these studies included psychologists (Studies 1 and 3), nurses (Studies 5–6), and research assistants (Study 2). The specialist background of the investigators in Study 4 was not specified.

Furthermore, the outcome measurement instruments differed among the six studies. The questionnaires used

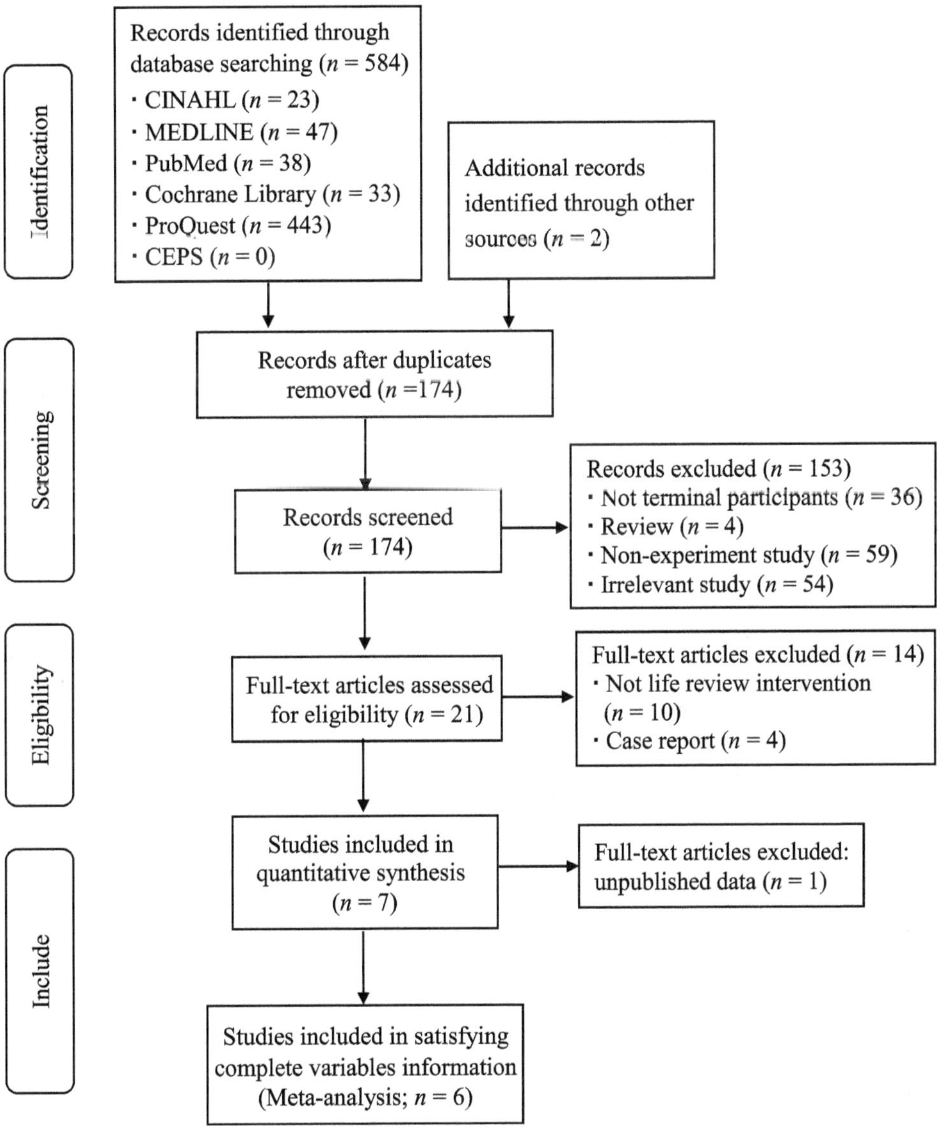

Figure 1. Preferred Reporting Items for Systematic Reviews and Meta-Analyses flow diagram. CINAHL = Cumulative Index to Nursing and Allied Health Literature; CEPS = Chinese Electronic Periodicals Service.

TABLE 1.
Literature Matrix

Author (Year)/ Country	Participant	Study Design	Delivery Personnel/ Setting	Intervention Duration/ Frequency/Complexity
1. Ando, Tsuda, & Morita (2007)/ Japan	1. *n* = 12; participants who receive palliative care 2. Age: 63 years (avg) 3. Gender: female (10), male (2) 4. Diseases: no data	One-group pretest–posttest design (no control group)	Psychologist/ palliative care unit patients	1. No explanation how to perform four sessions and the duration 2. Four sessions 3. Span: 24 weeks
2. Steinhauser et al. (2008)/ United States	1. *n* = 82 (includes lost to follow-up) palliative care or hospice setting patients 2. Age: range of 28–96; E = 26, relaxation = 26, C = 26 3. Gender: female (38), male (44) 4. Disease: cancer (48), heart disease (5), lung disease (10), other (19)	1. Randomly assigned 2. Blinded to subjects' intervention group assignment	Research assist/ inpatient and outpatient	1. 45 minutes to 1 hour 2. One session for 1 week/two sessions 3. Span: 3 weeks
3. Henry et al. (2010)/ Canada	1. *n* = 24 (includes lost to follow-up) participants were diagnosed with advance ovarian cancer (Stage 3 or 4) within the last 2 months. 2. Age: no explanation (eligibility criteria: >18 years); E = 12, C = 12 3. Gender: no explanation	1. Randomly assigned 2. Blind to data analysis	Psychologists	1. 30–90 minutes 2. Individualized to respect the patient 3. Four sessions
4. Mok, Lau, Lai, & Ching (2012)/ Hong Kong	1. *n* = 84 (includes lost to follow-up 2. Age: no explanation (eligibility criteria: >18 years) 3. Gender: female (5), male (5) 4. Disease: cancer type: breast (5), prostate (4), lung (1)	Randomly assigned	No explanation	1. First session span 2. 30–60 minutes, 15–30 minutes for the second session/2–3 days between sessions 3. Two sessions
5. Keall, Butow, Steinhauser, & Clayton (2013)/ Australia	1. *n* = 14 (includes lost to follow-up) 2. Age: no explanation (eligibility criteria: >18 years) 3. Gender: female (5), male (5) 4. Disease: cancer type: breast (5), prostate (4), lung (1)	Quasi study one-group pretest–posttest design (no control group)	Experienced palliative care nurse	1. 40–150 minutes 2. 1 week 3. Three sessions
6. Xiao, Kwong, Pang, & Mok (2013)/ China	1. *n* = 80; Chinese patients with advanced cancer 2. Age: E = 40; 59.78 years (avg) C = 40; 58.53 years (avg) 3. Gender: female (38), male (42) 4. Participants' diseases: 50% gastrointestinal cancer	Randomized clinical trial/single blind (data collector)	Nurse/home-based hospital participants	1. No explanation of duration for once life review 2. Three weekly life review program/three sessions 3. Span: 3 weeks

Note. n = number; avg = average; Sig = significant; NS = nonsignificant improvements; E = experimental group; C = control group; QOL = quality of life; SELT-M = Skalen zur Erfassung von Lebens qualitat beiTumorkranken–Modified version; QOLC-E = Quality-of-Life Concerns in the End-of-Life; QUAL-E = Quality of Life at the End of Life; MQOL = McGill Quality of Life Questionnaire.

TABLE 1.
Literature Matrix, Continued

Outcome Measure and Follow-Up Frequency	Result	Quality Assessment Score	Reason for Dropout	Drop Rate
1. Pretest/posttest (immediately) 2. Overall QOL (one item) is a part of SELT-M	Overall QOL: pretest–posttest, $p = .013$	20	Nine participants withdrew Reason: unexpectedly deteriorated ($n = 7$), inappropriate candidates for life review interviews due to the obsessive and compressive reminiscence type ($n = 1$), and serious depression ($n = 1$).	42.86% (9/21)
Pretest/posttest 1 week later/ posttest 2 weeks later/ QUAL-E	QUAL-E: NS in all measurements	16	40 participants withdrew Reason: no explanation.	48.78% (40/82)
Pretest/posttest 1 month/ posttest 3 months/MQOL	MQOL total: NS in all measurements	22	Four participants withdrew Reasons: Participants did not receive full MMI because of longer-than-expected surgery recovery or did not want to face emotions related to diagnosis ($n = 2$); patients who lost to follow-up at 3 months ($n = 2$).	14.29% (4/28)
Pretest/posttest 1 day later/ posttest 2 weeks later	QOLC-E total $p = .025$	21	26 participants withdrew Reasons: Discharged and could not be found by phone ($n = 10$), died ($n = 12$), became cognitively impaired ($n = 2$), refused to participate ($n = 1$), became too weak to communicate ($n = 1$).	30.95% (26/84)
Pretest/posttest 1 week later	QUAL-E: end-of-life preparation subscale (NS in all measurements) QUAL-E: life completion (NS in all measurements)	21	Four participants withdrew Reasons: deteriorated before the intervention ($n = 2$); participant deteriorated cognitively during the intervention ($n = 1$); no explanation ($n = 1$).	28.57% (4/14)
Pretest/posttest (baseline and immediately after the program and at a 3-week follow-up)/ overall QOL	Overall QOL: C and E at posttest ($p < .001$) and follow-up ($p < .001$)	25	30 participants withdrew Reason: physical discomfort ($n = 10$), death ($n = 15$), cognitive impairment ($n = 5$)	37.50% (30/80)

included the overall Quality of Life scale (Studies 1 and 6), Quality of Life at the End of Life scale (Studies 2 and 5), McGill Quality of Life Questionnaire total scale (Study 3), and Quality-of-Life Concerns in the End-of-Life scale (Study 4). Three of the six studies (Studies 1, 4, and 6) found that life review improved QOL ($p < .05$). Furthermore, the attrition rate in these studies ranged from 14% to 49%, and scores on the quality index checklist ranged between 16 and 25 (Table 1).

These six studies exhibited moderate heterogeneity ($I^2 = 42.407$, $p > .1$). No harmful effects of the life review intervention were identified on the reported outcome measures. The six studies all found a significantly improved QOL in the intervention group over the control group (95% CI [0.147, 0.668], $Z = 3.062$, $p < .05$; Table 2). Because of the wide variation in posttest duration, only data from the first posttest were considered in this review to distinguish between immediate and prolonged effects and to avoid the high participant dropout rates over time.

Discussion

The studies included in this review found that life review enhanced QOL in terminal patients. QOL is affected by the overall self-assessment of her or his life, whereas life review is a procedure of recalling, evaluating, and integrating life experiences with the goal of achieving ego integrity (Trueman & Parker, 2006). Life review intervention assists participants to identify and examine past experiences and achievements to find meaning, resolve conflicts, make amends with friends and family, and finish incomplete work. Life review is consistent with Erickson's developmental theory, which culminates in resolving the conflict between integrity and despair in the last stage of life. Life review provides an evaluative opportunity to achieve life integrity (Haight & Burnside, 1993) and facilitates acceptance of a single life cycle with few or no regrets. Furthermore, life review enables individuals to integrate memories into a meaningful whole and achieve satisfaction.

The meta-analysis conducted in this review of six studies showed crucial and direct results of life review for terminal patients. Four of these studies were compared with another meta-analysis, which found the posttest effect on QOL to be significant (Wang, Chow, & Chan, 2017). In addition, two other meta-analyses found that life review interventions are often flexible and incorporate individualized performance settings. According to Keall et al. (2015), assessing the effectiveness of life reviews in patients with advanced life-threatening diseases is difficult. Differences among studies in terms of implementers, procedures, and the format of meetings employed in the life reviews may influence the effectiveness of the review. However, this meta-analysis overcame these potential problems. Life review is primarily an assessment activity that investigates issues and, when possible, resolves conflicts. It requires profound reflection, and participants seek meaning in their life events. Because of the risks of negative effects, life review should not be considered a harmless approach because it may affect the resilience of participants and foster feelings of victimization during the review process (Korte, Bohlmeijer, & Smit, 2009). In other words, the implementing researcher should be an expert who is able to guide participants to reflect while being aware of potential harm. Wang et al. (2017) completed a rigorously designed systematic review of RCTs that set strict criteria for the testing method, including a large scale, distinct definitions, multicenter samples, and sensitive measurements.

Limitations

This review was affected by several limitations. First, studies published only in English or Chinese were included. Second, only the short-term effects of life review were considered. Third, although the included studies applied a variety of operative processes for life review, the study

TABLE 2.
Effect Size and 95% CIs of the Included Studies (N = 6)

	Statistic for Each Study							
Study (Year)	Std Diff in Means	*SE*	Variance	Lower Limit	Upper Limit	*Z*	*p*	Std Diff in Means and 95% CI
Xiao et al. (2013)	0.240	0.240	0.058	−0.231	0.710	0.997	.319	
Steinhauser et al. (2008)	−0.177	0.350	0.122	−0.862	0.508	−0.506	.613	
Ando et al. (2007)	1.219	0.445	0.198	0.348	2.091	2.743	.006	
Henry et al. (2010)	0.167	0.388	0.151	−0.594	0.927	0.430	.667	
Mok et al. (2012)	0.755	0.271	0.073	0.224	1.286	2.788	.005	
Keall et al. (2013)	0.484	0.420	0.176	−0.339	1.307	1.152	.249	
Total (95% CI)	0.407	0.133	0.018	0.147	0.668	3.062	.002	

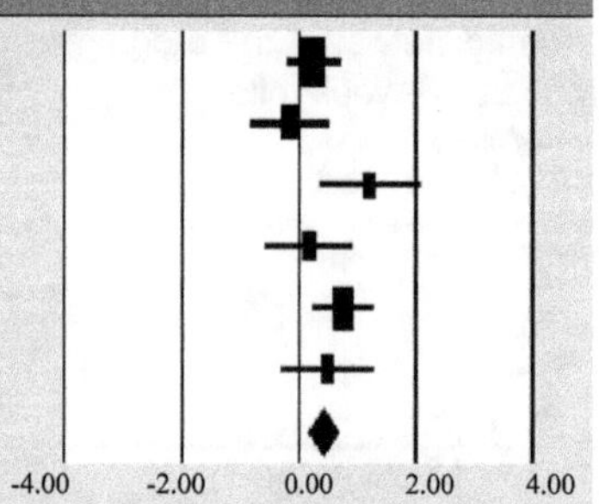

Note. CI = confidence interval; Std Diff = standard difference.

design did not assess which process was the most effective and suitable for terminal patients. Fourth, although the search term "life review" was used, other related terms such as "storytelling" and "forgiveness" were not used because of considerations of method consistency. Thus, some otherwise eligible studies may not have been identified and included in this review.

Conclusions

Few studies have evaluated the effect of life review therapy in terminal patients. Because of the low probability of survival, life review therapy may best be used as a short-term procedure in this patient population. However, more studies are required to confirm its efficacy. Furthermore, as many practical studies have employed different session regimes, periods, and therapy durations, future studies should conduct comparisons of different operative methods. Nurses are in an ideal position to offer life review because of their qualities of leadership, creativity, and empathy, which are essential to providing psychosocial care to terminal patients. However, greater consideration should be given to the psychological and emotional needs of terminal patients.

Author Contributions

Study conception and design: MHH, HHW
Data collection: MHH, HHW
Data analysis and interpretation: All authors
Drafting of the article: MHH, HHW
Critical revision of the article: All authors

References

*Reference marked with an asterisk indicate studies included in the meta analysis.

*Ando, M., Tsuda, A., & Morita, T. (2007). Life review interviews on the spiritual well-being of terminally ill cancer patients. *Support Care Cancer, 15*(2), 225–231. https://doi.org/10.1007/s00520-006-0121-y

Bennett, M. I., & Closs, S. J. (2008). Clinical assessment and measurement. In S. Payne, J. Seymore, & C. Ingleton (Eds.), *Palliative nursing: Principles and evidence for practice* (2nd ed., pp. 145–158). London, England: McGraw-Hill.

Bohlmeijer, E., Smit, F., & Cuijpers, P. (2003). Effects of reminiscence and life review on late-life depression: A meta-analysis. *International Journal of Geriatric Psychiatry, 18*(12), 1088–1094. https://doi.org/10.1002/gps.1018

Chiang, K. J., Lu, R. B., Chu, H., Chang, Y. C., & Chou, K. R. (2008). Evaluation of the effect of a life review group program on self-esteem and life satisfaction in the elderly. *International Journal of Geriatric Psychiatry, 23*(1), 7–10. https://doi.org/10.1002/gps.1824

Chochinov, H. M., Hack, T., Hassard, T., Kristjanson, L. J., McClement, S., & Harlos, M. (2004). Dignity and psychotherapeutic considerations in end-of-life care. *Journal of Palliative Care, 20*(3), 134–142. https://doi.org/10.1017/S1478951511000526

Choi, S., & Kim, M. Y. (2017). End-of -life care for elderly with terminal stage chronic illnesses: A literature review. *International Information Institute, 20*(1), 339–346.

Cohen, S. R., & Mount, B. M. (1992). Quality of life in terminal illness: Defining and measuring subjective well-being in the dying. *Journal of Palliative Care, 8*(3), 40–45.

Downs, S. H., & Black, N. (1998). The feasibility of creating a checklist for the assessment of the methodological quality both of randomised and non-randomised studies of health care interventions. *Journal of Epidemiology of Community Health, 52*(6), 377–384. https://doi.org/10.1136/jech.52.6.377

Haber, D. (2006). Life review: Implementation, theory, research, and therapy. *The International Journal of Aging and Human Development, 63*(2), 153–171. https://doi.org/10.2190/DA9G-RHK5-N9JP-T6CC

Haight, B. K., & Burnside, I. (1993). Reminiscence and life review: Explaining the differences. *Archives of Psychiatric Nursing, 7*, 91–98. https://doi.org/10.1016/S0883-9417(09)90007-3

Haight, B. K., Michel, Y., & Hendrix, S. (1998). Life review: Preventing despair in newly relocated nursing home residents short- and long-term effects. *The International Journal of Aging and Human Development, 47*(2), 119–142. https://doi.org/10.2190/A011-BRXD-HAFV-5NJ6

Haight, B. K., Michel, Y., & Hendrix, S. (2000). The extended effects of the life review in nursing home residents. *The International Journal of Aging and Human Development, 50*(2), 151–168. https://doi.org/10.2190/QU66-E8UV-NYMR-Y99E

Hanaoka, H., & Okamura, H. (2004). Study on effects of life review activities on the quality of life of the elderly: A randomized controlled trial. *Psychotherapy and Psychosomatics, 73*(5), 302–311. https://doi.org/10.1159/000078847

*Henry, M., Cohen, S. R., Lee, V., Sauthier, P., Provencher, D., Drouin, P., ... Mayo, N. (2010). The meaning-making intervention (MMi) appears to increase meaning in life in advanced ovarian cancer: A randomized controlled pilot study. *Psycho-Oncology, 19*(12), 1340–1347. https://doi.org/10.1002/pon.1764

Higgins, J. P., Thompson, S. G., Deeks, J. J., & Altman, D. G. (2003). Measuring inconsistency in meta-analyses. *British Medical Journal, 327*(7414), 557–560. https://doi.org/10.1136/bmj.327.7414.557

Hwu, Y. J., & Lin, F. Y. (2014). Effectiveness of propolis on oral health: A meta-analysis. *The Journal of Nursing Research, 22*(4), 221–230. https://doi.org/10.1097/jnr.0000000000000054

Kaasa, S., & Loge, J. H. (2003). Quality of life in palliative care: Principles and practice. *Palliative Medicine, 17*(1), 11–20. https://doi.org/10.1191/0269216303pm662ra

*Keall, R. M., Butow, P. N., Steinhauser, K. E., & Clayton, J. M. (2013). Nurse-facilitated preparation and life completion interventions are acceptable and feasible in the Australian palliative care setting: Results from a phase 2 trial. *Cancer Nursing, 36*(3), E39–E46. https://doi.org/10.1097/NCC.0b013e3182664c7a

Keall, R. M., Clayton, J. M., & Butow, P. N. (2015). Therapeutic life review in palliative care: A systematic review of quantitative evaluations. *Journal of Pain and Symptom Management, 49*(4), 747–761. https://doi.org/10.1016/j.jpainsymman.2014.08.015

Kennelly, J. (2011). Methodological approach to assessing the evidence. In A. Handler, J. Kennelly, & N. Peacock (Eds.), *Reducing racial/ethnic disparities in reproductive and perinatal outcomes* (1st ed., pp. 7–19). Boston, MA: Springer. https://doi.org/10.1007/978-1-4419-1499-6_2

Kissane, D. W., & Kelly, B. J. (2000). Demoralisation, depression and desire for death: Problems with the Dutch guidelines for euthanasia of the mentally ill. *Australian and New Zealand Journal of Psychiatry, 34*(2), 325–333. https://doi.org/10.1046/j.1440-1614.2000.00692x

Korte, J., Bohlmeijer, E. T., Cappeliez, P., Smit, F., & Westerhof, G. J. (2012). Life review therapy for older adults with moderate depressive symptomatology: A pragmatic randomized controlled trial. *Psychological Medicine, 42*(6), 1163–1173. https://doi.org/10.1017/S0033291711002042

Korte, J., Bohlmeijer, E. T., & Smit, F. (2009). Prevention of depression and anxiety in later life: Design of a randomized controlled trial for the clinical and economic evaluation of a life-review intervention. *BMC Public Health, 9*, 250. https://doi.org/10.1186/1471-2458-9-250

Leung, P. P. Y., Wan, A. H. Y., Lui, J. Y. M., Ho, A. H. Y., Liu, K. H., So, A., ... Chan, C. L. W. (2015). The effects of a positive death education group on psycho-spiritual outcomes for Chinese with chronic illness: A quasi-experimental study. *Illness Crisis & Loss, 23*(1), 5–19. https://doi.org/10.2190/IL.23.1.b

Moher, D., Liberati, A., Tetzlaff, J., & Altman, D. G. (2009). Preferred reporting items for systematic reviews and meta-analyses: The PRISMA statement. *Annals of Internal Medicine, 151*(4), 264–269. https://doi.org/10.7326/0003-4819-151-4-200908180-00135

*Mok, E., Lau, K. P., Lai, T., & Ching, S. (2012). The meaning of life intervention for patients with advanced-stage cancer: Development and pilot study. *Oncology Nursing Forum, 39*(6), E480–E488. https://doi.org/10.1188/12.ONF.E480-E488

Pot, A. M., Bohlmeijer, E. T., Onrust, S., Melenhorst, A. S., Veerbeek, M., & De Vries, W. (2010). The impact of life review on depression in older adults: A randomized controlled trial. *International Psychogeriatrics, 22*(4), 572–581. https://doi.org/10.1017/S104161020999175X

*Steinhauser, K. E., Alexander, S. C., Byock, I. R., George, L. K., Olsen, M. K., & Tulsky, J. A. (2008). Do preparation and life completion discussions improve functioning and quality of life in seriously ill patients? Pilot randomized control trial. *Journal of Palliative Medicine, 11*(9), 1234–1240. https://doi.org/10.1089/jpm.2008.0078

Tang, S. T., & McCorkle, R. (2002). Appropriate time frames for data collection in quality of life research among cancer patients at the end of life. *Quality of Life Research, 11*(2), 145–155. https://doi.org/10.1023/A:1015021531112

Trueman, I., & Parker, J. (2006). Exploring community nurses' perceptions of life review in palliative care. *Journal of Clinical Nursing, 15*(2), 197–207. https://doi.org/10.1111/j.1365-2702.2006.01244x

Wang, C. W., Chow, A. Y., & Chan, C. L. (2017). The effects of life review interventions on spiritual well-being, psychological distress, and quality of life in patients with terminal or advanced cancer: A systematic review and meta-analysis of randomized controlled trials. *Palliative Medicine, 31*(10), 883–894. https://doi.org/10.1177/0269216317705101

World Health Organization. (1990). *Cancer pain relief and palliative care—Report of a WHO Expert Committee.* Technical Report Series, 804 (p. 11). Geneva, Switzerland: Author.

*Xiao, H., Kwong, E., Pang, S., & Mok, E. (2013). Effect of a life review program for Chinese patients with advanced cancer. *Cancer Nursing, 36*(4), 274–283. https://doi.org/10.1097/NCC.0b013e318268f7ba

8

Effects of Massage and Acupressure on Relieving Labor Pain, Reducing Labor Time and Increasing Delivery Satisfaction

Ilknur Munevver GÖNENÇ[1]* • Füsun TERZIOĞLU[2]

ABSTRACT

Background: Several recent studies have documented the effects of massage and acupressure in reducing labor pain and labor time and in satisfaction with the delivery. However, few studies have investigated the comparative effects of these two therapies.

Purpose: The aim of this study was to compare the effects of massage and acupressure on labor-related pain management, duration, and satisfaction with delivery.

Methods: This randomized controlled trial (n = 120) included three intervention groups (massage only, acupressure only, and massage + acupressure) and one control group, in which patients received no massage or acupressure treatment. A personal information form, Pregnant Watch Form, and Visual Analog Scale (VAS) were used to collect data. Frequency and percentage calculations, chi-square test, Student's t test, Tukey's honestly significant difference test, and one-way variance analysis were used for data analysis.

Results: In the latent phase of labor, the mean VAS scores of the massage-only group and massage + acupressure group were lower (4.56 ± 1.36 and 4.63 ± 1.52, respectively) than that of the control group (6.16 ± 1.46; $p < .01$). In the active and transition phases, the mean VAS scores of the massage-only group, acupressure-only group, and massage + acupressure group were significantly lower than that of the control group ($p < .01$ and $p < .001$, respectively). During postpartum, the mean VAS score of the massage + acupressure group was lower (2.30 ± 0.70) than that of the control group (2.96 ± 0.72; $p = .003$). Cervical dilatation completion time and 1- and 5-minute Apgar scores were similar among all of the groups ($p > .05$). The three intervention groups reported relatively more positive feelings than the control group, and all three of the interventions were found to be effective in improving satisfaction.

Conclusions/Implications for Practice: The results of this study indicate that the dual application of massage and acupressure is relatively more effective than either therapy applied alone and that massage is more effective than acupressure.

KEY WORDS:
labor pain, massage, acupressure, labor time, mother's satisfaction.

Introduction

Labor is a special experience for a mother and her family. However, not only is labor pain one of the most painful conditions that women typically experience in life, the stress related to uncontrolled labor pain also has a negative impact on the mother, the fetus, and the newborn (Perry, Hockenberry, Lowdermilk, & Wilson, 2014). Therefore, pain relief during labor is an essential aspect of obstetrical care. Labor pain relief methods are categorized into pharmacological (inhalation anesthesia, regional anesthesia, opioids such as pethidine) and nonpharmacological (hypnosis, laboring in water, acupuncture, massage) methods (Jones et al., 2012). Nonpharmacological applications may be performed by a midwife and a nurse independently in cooperation with the pregnant woman. Using nonpharmacologic pain-relief measures such as touch, massage, aromatherapy, and acupressure are important because assessing labor pain and applying appropriate nonpharmacologic interventions make midwives and nurses responsible for managing the labor process.

Massage, one of the oldest nonpharmacological methods of controlling labor pain, creates physiological and psychological effects on organisms through systematic manipulations that stimulate soft tissues mechanically (Brosseau et al., 2012). Massage induces relaxation during labor, reduces the severity of pain, relaxes muscle spasms, increases physical activity, channels the attention of the mother, and contributes to overall relaxation (Mortazavi, Khaki, Moradi, Heidari, & Vasegh Rahimparvar, 2012). By contrast, acupressure, the application of pressure to acupuncture points, is grounded in the meridian theory, which holds that acupressure incites the meridians that compose the network of energy routes throughout the body, augmenting the flow of qi (bioenergy) and thus changing the symptom experience. Fingers, towels, acupressure bands, and tennis balls are commonly used to apply acupressure (Simkin & O'hara, 2002). Acupressure has four basic effects on the body: analgesic, homeostatic, immunity enhancement, and sedative/psychological. The pain relief effect of acupressure has been explained using gate control, nociceptive afferent, and

[1]*PhD, RN, Assistant Professor, Faculty of Nursing, Department of Midwifery, Ankara University, Ankara, Turkey* • [2]*PhD, RN, Professor, Faculty of Health Sciences, Department of Nursing, Atılım University, Ankara, Turkey.*

endorphin theories. Gate control theory holds that applying pressure to acupuncture points stimulates thick C fibers without myelin, which are touch and pressure receptors, thus preventing pain stimuli from reaching the cortex. Nociceptive afferent theory holds that acupressure inhibits the transmission of pain to the brain by stimulating mechanoreceptors. Endorphin theory holds that acupressure stimulates endorphin secretions, a natural analgesic (Dung, Clogston, & Dunn, 2004; Ma, Ma, & Cho, 2005; Sandifer, 1997).

The most commonly used acupressure points during the birth process are Sanyinjiao (SP6), He Gu (LI4), Zhi Yin (BL67), and Ci Liao (BL32). In this study, Acupoint SP6 was selected as it is the acupoint typically preferred in gynecology (Chen & Chen, 2004). Yu et al. (2015) indicated that Sanyinjiao (SP6) is one of the most commonly used acupressure points and may have better therapeutic effects than lesser used or unused acupuncture points. A meta-analysis found that labor pain severity after an SP6 intervention was lower in the acupressure-only group than in the touch group (Najafi, Jaafarpour, Sayehmiri, & Khajavikhan, 2018). Sanyinjiao is strongly related to the uterus. Pressing or needling SP6 promotes the flow of qi and blood to the uterus, improving nourishment and relieving pain in this organ (Yu et al., 2015). Sanyinjiao is easy for women to locate and for practitioners to apply pressure to without medical assistance. The application of acupressure to SP6 increases the pain threshold and blood flow and stimulates the release of endorphins. Studies have shown that pressure applied to the SP6 point decreases perceived pain and shortens delivery duration in pregnant women (Lee, Chang, & Kang, 2004; Makvandi, Mirzaiinajmabadi, Sadeghi, Mahdavian, & Karimi, 2016).

When administered to pregnant women, massage and acupressure have both been shown to reduce perceived pain (Jones et al., 2012; Smith, Levett, Collins, & Jones, 2012), anxiety, drug administration during labor (Chaillet et al., 2014; Levett, Smith, Bensoussan, & Dahlen, 2016), and the rate of cesarean section (Chaillet et al., 2014; Kashanian & Shahali, 2009) as well as shorten delivery duration and length of time spent in the hospital (Lee et al., 2004). These benefits help reduce hospital costs and the healthcare burden on the economy.

Systematic reviews support massage as a potentially effective approach to pain relief as well as a practical approach to pain management, providing increased satisfaction and reducing medication use. Nevertheless, the literature on this subject recommends further research (Smith, Collins, Crowther, & Levett, 2011; Smith et al., 2012).

Massage and acupressure are effective, nonpharmacological methods that may be applied during the labor process (Deepak & Chopra, 2013; Lee et al., 2004; Pilevarzadeh, Salari, & Shafiei, 2002; Simkin & O'hara, 2002). The beneficial effects of these methods may increase when used concurrently. Pressure may be administered to acupressure points during massage sessions. Although some studies have investigated these methods separately, no studies investigating the concurrent application of these two methods during pregnancy and birth were found in the literature. Furthermore, only a few published studies examined the comparative efficacy of massage and acupressure (Hajiamini, Masaoud, Ebadi, Mahboubh, & Matin, 2012).

Objective and Hypothesis

This study was designed to assess the effects of massage and acupressure on labor pain management during the first stage of delivery, duration of labor, and satisfaction with delivery in a sample of pregnant women.

This study formulated the following hypotheses:

H_1: Perceived labor pain will differ among the four groups.

H_2: Duration of labor will differ among the four groups.

H_3: Satisfaction with delivery will differ among the four groups.

Methods

Participants

This randomized controlled trial was carried out in a women's health, education, and research hospital between August 8, 2012, and March 8, 2013.

The participant groups were formed using 2^2 factorial trial levels, and four groups were used in the study. The sample size was estimated using G*Power 3.1.3 software (Heinrich Heine Universitat, Dusseldorf, Germany). The 120 (4 × 30) participants were sufficient to identify differences among the groups with a 5% margin of error and 100% power.

The inclusion criteria were as follows: having an indication for vaginal birth, being primiparous, between 20 and 30 years old, having less than 4-cm cervical dilatation, being at 38–42 weeks of gestation, having a single and healthy fetus in the vertex position, lack of complications that may cause dystocia during labor, and no analgesia or anesthesia used during the first phase of labor.

Procedures

This research was designed as a clinical trial. The participants were assigned randomly to the three intervention groups and one control group. Those in the control group continued to receive routine care from the hospital. The simple full randomization method was used for group assignments. To determine the order of application, the names of the study groups were written on a piece of paper 30 times by the researcher and the groups were selected randomly by drawing lots. The massage and acupuncture interventions were conducted by a single researcher to ensure uniformity.

Massage-only group

A 30-minute massage session was administered to participants in the massage-only group during the latent (cervical dilatation of 3–4 cm), active (cervical dilatation of 6–7 cm), and transition (cervical dilatation of 8–9 cm) phases. The head, neck, shoulder, back, arms, hands, legs, and feet were massaged during each session in the same manner and duration.

Acupressure group

A 30-minute acupressure session using acupressure bands on the Sanyinjiao (SP6) acupressure points was administered to participants in the acupressure-only group during the latent, active, and transition phases. The SP6 points are located 3 kun (approximately 4 cm) above the inner malleolus. Researchers located the SP6 points using an acupoint device and marked them with a pencil. The acupoint device emits a green light when the correct site is touched. The acupressure bands used in this study (MedicMate Alternative Medicine Products, Colorado, USA) are a commercially available model featuring an elastic band with a small plastic button used for applying pressure. The band is adjustable to the size of the body area targeted for pressure application. This protruding plastic button is located on the SP6 point. One band was used for each individual.

Massage + acupressure group

Massage and acupressure were simultaneously administered to the participants in the massage + acupressure group during the latent, active, and transition phases. As noted above, an acupoint device was used to locate the SP6 points, a pencil was used to mark them, and an acupressure band was attached. The massage session began as soon as the acupressure band was attached.

All of the participants gave informed consent before participation. Contraction and fetal heart rate were monitored using electronic fetal monitoring before the intervention. The duration, severity, and frequency of uterine contractions were monitored continuously during the interventions using a tocodynamometer. Furthermore, the participants were monitored continuously for labor progress, vital signs, and general well-being until their transfer to a postpartum care room. A one-on-one interview with each participant was conducted within 8 hours of delivery to elicit participants' feelings, opinions, and perceptions about the intervention and the birth experience. Thirteen of the participants were delivered by cesarean section, seven received meperidine, and two received epidural anesthesia. Thus, 22 of the 142 participants were excluded from data collection, leaving data on 120 participants available for analysis.

Measures

Data for this study were collected using a personal information form, Pregnant Watch Form, Questionnaire Related to Applied Methods, and Visual Analog Scale (VAS). The personal information form, Pregnant Watch Form, and Questionnaire Related to Applied Methods were all developed by the researchers in line with the literature (Chaillet et al., 2014; Chang, Wang, & Chen, 2002; Hajiamini et al., 2012; Janssen, Shroff, & Jaspar, 2012; Kashanian & Shahali, 2009; Lee et al., 2004; Simkin & O'hara, 2002; Smith et al., 2012) and adjusted to reflect the recommendations of three experts. The personal information form collected sociodemographic information (12 questions), pregnancy status information (13 questions), and labor-related experience and coping methods information (five questions). The Pregnant Watch Form collected data on the intervention application. The Questionnaire Related to Applied Methods gathered data on massage and acupressure (e.g., satisfaction level, reuse status) as used to reduce labor pain. The VAS, first developed by Price, McGrath, Rafii, and Buckingham (1983), is used to self-evaluate perceived pain on a 10-cm ruler scale, with the analgesia indicator at one end and the most severe pain indicator at the other end (Tulunay & Tulunay, 2000). The VAS was administered immediately before and immediately after the interventions at 3–4, 6–7, and 8–9 cm of cervical dilation and during the postpartum period. Each participant was asked to mark her current level of perceived pain along the scale, with the number corresponding to the marked point recorded as the pain score.

A preliminary study was conducted with 10 of the participants, whose data were excluded from the study; their comments and results were used to revise the final version of the forms. On the basis of input from the preliminary study, the question "How many times did you go to control?" was replaced by the question "Did you take a regular antenatal follow-up?" Because the participants were unable to provide a response upon the onset of pain, the question was removed from the questionnaire.

Ethical Consideration

Written permission was obtained from the ethics board of Ankara University and from the institution where the research was conducted (date: July 23, 2012; Resolution No. 12-390-12). Written informed consent was also obtained from the participants.

Statistical Analyses

Analyses were performed using IBM SPSS Statistics Version 22.0 (IBM Inc., Armonk, NY, USA). All analyses of the research were made based on a 95% confidence level and 5% Type I error. Frequency and percentage calculations, chi-square test, Tukey's honestly significant difference (HSD) test, and one-way variance analysis were used to analyze the data.

Results

The participants had a mean age of 23.4 years and a mean marriage duration of 20.8 months. More than three quarters (79.2%) had not reached the 40th gestational week of pregnancy, and 96.7% of the pregnancies were planned. Almost all reported not attending any antenatal preparatory training (98.3%) or receiving education about how to deal with labor (95%). Three quarters (76.7%) reported being afraid of labor, 74.5% reported being afraid of severe pain, 54.3% reported being afraid that their baby's health would deteriorate, and 24.5% reported being afraid of the delivery room. Although most participants stated a fear of labor pain, 91.7% did not have a coping plan. Oxytocin was used in 32.5% of the participants in this study.

TABLE 1.
Distribution of Sociodemographic and Obstetric Characteristics

	Massage (M) Group		Acupressure (A) Group		M + A Group		Control Group		Total		
Characteristic	*M*	*SD*	*M*	*SD*	*M*	*SD*	*M*	*SD*	*M*	*SD*	*p*
Age	23.4	3.2	24.1	3.4	23.7	2.9	22.4	3.0	23.4	3.2	.169
Duration of marriage (months)	20.6	9.9	23.1	13.3	19.2	9.1	20.3	8.5	20.8	10.2	.487
Gestational week	39.3	0.9	39.3	1.0	39.4	1.0	39.3	1.1	39.3	1.0	.925
	n	%	*n*	%	*n*	%	*n*	%	*n*	%	*p*
Pregnancy											—
Planned	29	96.7	28	93.3	29	96.7	30	100.0	116	96.7	
Unplanned	1	3.3	2	6.7	1	3.3	0	0.0	4	3.3	
Follow-up examinations											—
Yes	28	93.3	30	100.0	29	96.7	29	96.7	116	96.7	
No	2	6.7	0	0.0	1	3.3	1	3.3	4	3.3	
Experiencing fear of birth											.619
Yes	23	76.7	25	83.3	21	70.0	23	76.7	92	76.7	
No	7	23.3	5	16.7	9	30.0	7	23.3	28	23.3	
No plan to proactively cope with labor pain											—
Yes	3	10.0	3	10.0	2	6.7	2	6.7	10	8.3	
No	27	90.0	27	90.0	28	93.3	28	93.3	110	91.7	
Oxytocin											.134
Used	6	20.0	11	36.7	8	26.7	14	46.7	39	32.5	
Did not use	24	80.0	19	63.3	22	73.3	16	53.3	81	67.5	

The groups were similar in terms of age, duration of marriage, gestational week, state of pregnancy planning, pregnancy follow-up examinations, fear of birth experience, and use of oxytocin (Table 1).

No statistical difference in VAS score was identified among the groups at pretest ($p > .05$; Table 2). In the latent phase, the massage-only and massage + acupressure groups reported lower postintervention mean VAS scores than the control group ($p < .01$; Table 3). In the active and transition phases, all of the intervention groups reported significantly lower preintervention and postintervention mean labor pain scores than the control group ($p < .01$ and $p < .001$, respectively; Table 3). In the postpartum period, the lowest VAS score (2.30) was recorded for the massage + acupressure group, whereas the highest VAS score (2.96) was recorded for the control group. The difference among the groups in terms of mean VAS scores was statistically significant ($p < .01$; Table 3).

TABLE 2.
Distribution of VAS Scores by Study Group

		VAS Score in Latent Phase						VAS Score in Active Phase			
		Preintervention		Postintervention				Preintervention		Postintervention	
Group	*n*	*M*	*SD*	*M*	*SD*	*t*	*p*	*M*	*SD*	*M*	*SD*
Massage-only group	30	6.36	1.10	4.56	1.36	8.523	< .010	8.10	0.96	7.23	1.33
Acupressure-only group	30	5.87	1.63	5.43	1.85	1.531	.141	7.97	1.40	7.53	1.50
Massage + acupressure group	30	5.83	1.49	4.63	1.52	5.410	< .001	8.10	1.03	6.93	1.23
Control group	30	5.80	1.40	6.16	1.46	−3.612	< .001	9.20	0.89	9.40	0.77
F		1.100		7.042				8.408		24.131	
p		.352		.001				.001		.001	

Note. VAS = Visual Analog Scale.

The massage-only group had the shortest cervical dilatation completion time (245 minutes), and the control group had the longest (350 minutes), although the differences among the groups were not significant ($p > .05$; Figure 1). The massage-only group had the highest 1- and 5-minute APGAR scores (7.03 and 9.03, respectively), and the control group had the lowest (6.97 and 8.97, respectively), although the differences among the groups were not significant ($p > .05$, data not shown).

The percentage of participants receiving oxygen treatment in the control group was higher than that in the other groups (Table 1).

In terms of satisfaction with their intervention, 96.8% in the massage-only group, 93.3% in the acupressure-only group, and 100% of the massage + acupressure group expressed satisfaction with their intervention and intent to use in their next delivery. Furthermore, nearly all intervention group participants stated that they would recommend these applications to the other pregnant women. In the massage-only group, 89.3% reported decreased pain, 53.6% reported experiencing relaxation with positive feelings, and 14.3% reported that the intervention shortened delivery duration. In the acupressure-only group, 82.5% reported decreased pain, 25% reported accelerated delivery with frequent birth pangs, and 17.9% reported experiencing relaxation with positive feelings. In the massage + acupressure group, 96.7% reported decreased pain, 46.7% reported experiencing relaxation with positive feelings, and 13.3% reported a facilitated birth experience accompanied by a sense of confidence.

All of the massage-only group, 90% of the acupressure-only group, and 93.3% of the massage + acupressure group reported no experience of difficulties during the interventions. Mild pain because of the intervention was reported by two participants from the acupressure-only group and one participant from the massage + acupressure group, whereas one participant each from the acupressure-only and massage + acupressure groups reported itching because of the acupressure band.

Discussion

Level of pain perceived varied during the latent, active, and transition phases of the first stage of delivery (Perry et al., 2014). Thus, this study applied different interventions and evaluated the levels of perceived pain across these phases. The massage-only group earned the lowest postintervention mean VAS score in the latent phase, whereas the score for the massage + acupressure group was only slightly higher. To the authors' knowledge, no study in the literature assesses the comparative effectiveness of massage and SP6-point acupressure in reducing labor pain. A study on the comparative effects on labor pain of ice massage and acupressure interventions applied to the same point at 3–4 cm of cervical dilation found a lower VAS score in the massage group after 30 minutes of application (Hajiamini et al., 2012). Similar to this study, a previous investigation of the effectiveness of massage treatments on labor pain that implemented a 30-minute massage intervention on pregnant women during each of the three phases of delivery found a lower VAS score in the intervention group than in the control (no intervention) group in the latent phase (Chang et al., 2002). Moreover, the findings of other studies in the literature are similar to the results of this study, indicating that massage treatments given in the latent phase are effective in controlling labor pain (Chang et al., 2002; Janssen et al., 2012; Khodakarami, Safarzadeh, & Fathizadeh, 2005). However, one study that used a similar approach to examine the effects of acupressure on labor pain found an insignificant difference in VAS score between the acupressure group and no-acupressure group (Heydari, Mojdeh, Mazloum, Tanbakuei, & Judaki, 2008). Other studies using a different approach identified positive effects of acupressure on perceived labor pain during the latent phase (Lee et al., 2004; Park et al., 2003). The results of this study reveal that massage therapy applied during the latent phase of delivery effectively reduces labor pain and that acupressure therapy applied during this phase has no significant labor-pain-reduction effect.

		VAS Score in Transition Phase						VAS Score in Postpartum	
		Preintervention		Postintervention					
t	*p*	*M*	*SD*	*M*	*SD*	*t*	*p*	*M*	*SD*
4.419	< .010	9.13	0.63	8.18	1.02	6.238	< .010	2.53	0.57
2.359	.025	9.33	0.71	9.10	0.85	1.882	.070	2.60	0.62
6.484	< .001	9.33	0.18	8.73	0.69	5.288	< .001	2.30	0.70
−2.693	.012	9.96	0.25	9.93	0.25	1.000	.326	2.96	0.72
		10.947		28.159				4.923	
		.001		< .001				.003	

TABLE 3.

Between-Group Comparison of VAS Scores (Tukey's HSD Test)

Item/Group	*n*	Massage-Only Group (M) *p*	Acupressure Group (A) *p*	M + A Group *p*	Control Group *p*
VAS score in latent phase					
Preintervention					
Massage-only group	30	–	.512	.456	.401
Acupressure-only group	30	.512	–	1.000	.998
Massage + acupressure group	30	.456	1.000	–	1.000
Control group	30	.401	.998	1.000	–
Postintervention					
Massage-only group	30	–	.143	.998	.001
Acupressure-only group	30	.143	–	.199	.268
Massage + acupressure group	30	.998	.199	–	.001
Control group	30	.001	.268	.001	–
VAS score in active phase					
Preintervention					
Massage-only group	30	–	.964	1.000	.001
Acupressure-only group	30	.964	–	.964	< .001
Massage + acupressure group	30	1.000	.964	–	.001
Control group	30	.001	< .001	.001	–
Postintervention					
Massage-only group	30	–	.784	.784	< .001
Acupressure-only group	30	.784	–	.244	< .001
Massage + acupressure group	30	.784	.244	–	< .001
Control group	30	< .001	< .001	< .001	–
VAS score in transition phase					
Preintervention					
Massage-only group	30	–	.571	.571	< .001
Acupressure-only group	30	.571	–	1.000	< .001
Massage + acupressure group	30	.571	1.000	–	< .001
Control group	30	< .001	< .001	< .001	–
Postintervention					
Massage-only group	30	–	< .001	.029	< .001
Acupressure-only group	30	< .001	–	.245	< .001
Massage + acupressure group	30	.029	.245	–	< .001
Control group	30	< .001	< .001	< .001	–
VAS score in postpartum					
Massage-only group	30	–	.981	.549	.072
Acupressure group	30	.981	–	.326	.165
Massage + acupressure group	30	.549	.326	–	.001
Control group	30	.072	.165	.001	–

Note. HSD = honestly significant difference; VAS = Visual Analog Scale.

In comparing the mean active-phase VAS scores of the intervention groups, the lowest scores were reported by the massage + acupressure group, followed by the massage-only group and the acupressure-only group, with the control group reporting the highest mean VAS score ($p < .05$). The findings of this study support a positive effect for both massage and acupressure on pain management during the active phase of delivery. Hajiamini et al. (2012) compared the effectiveness of hand ice massage and acupressure interventions in controlling labor pain, finding ice massage to be more effective than acupressure. Some studies found massage treatments to be effective in managing labor pain (Chang, Chen, & Huang, 2006; Janssen et al., 2012; Lee et al., 2004) and in delaying the use of epidural analgesia (Janssen et al., 2012). A study conducted by Chang et al. (2006) on 60 pregnant women found both physical and mental calming effects for a massage intervention.

Mafetoni and Shimo (2016) and Hjelmstedt et al. (2010) found that an acupressure intervention targeting the SP6 point in the active phase of delivery reduced labor pain

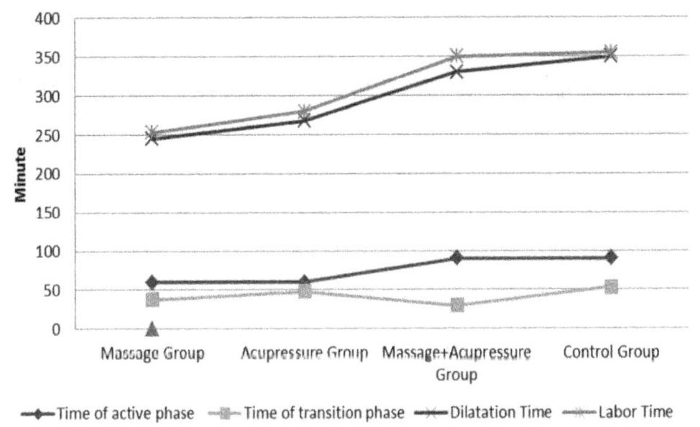

Figure 1. Distribution of durations during the stages of labor.

($p < .05$) and that the acupressure-treated groups earned lower pain scores than the nontreated group. Sehhatie-Shafaie, Kazemzadeh, Amani, and Heshmat (2013) and Deepak and Chopra (2013) indicated that acupressure reduced the labor pain perceived in the active phase of delivery and recommended the use of acupressure during labor. Moreover, massage and acupressure were found to be effective in managing labor pain in the active phase of delivery whether administered together or separately. The authors of this study believe that both massage and acupressure stimulate the door control mechanism, induce relaxation, and help pregnant women to "unwind" through the increased release of endorphins and the distraction effect.

The mean transition-phase VAS scores for the massage + acupressure group and the massage-only group were lower than that for the acupressure-only group, suggesting that massage is more effective than acupressure during the transition phase. The effects of massage and acupressure applied on the SP6 point during the transition phase of delivery have not been reported in the literature. Prior studies confirm that massage treatments administered during the transition phase reduce labor pain (Khodakarami et al., 2005; Mortazavi et al., 2012), decrease the cesarean section rate (Khodakarami et al., 2005), and improve the birth experience of the mother (Janssen et al., 2012). In Chang et al. (2006), no changes in VAS scores were found in either the massage or no-massage groups during the transition phase of delivery. In Chung, Hung, Kou, and Huang (2003), an investigation of 127 primipara pregnant women found no difference in VAS scores between the acupressure and no-acupressure groups. This study found all of the three investigated methods to be effective in controlling labor pain when applied during the transition phase, with the massage-only and massage + acupressure interventions having more significant effects than the acupressure-only intervention.

In this study, the massage and acupressure interventions did not affect time of dilatation, similar to results from Janssen et al. (2012), who found no difference in dilatation time between the massage and no-massage groups during the first and second phases of delivery. In addition, one study found no relationship between a massage intervention and duration of delivery (Chang et al., 2002), whereas another found that SP6-point acupressure did not affect the duration of either the first or second stage of labor (Park et al., 2003). Conversely, several studies showed that acupressure affects the duration of the active phase of labor (Kashanian & Shahali, 2009), dilatation time (Lee et al., 2004), and duration of labor (Kim, Chang, Lee, & Maeng, 2002). The results of this study do not support the effectiveness of massage or acupressure during some phases of delivery.

The massage and acupressure interventions in this study did not affect the APGAR scores of the newborns. Similarly, other studies in the literature highlight statistically insignificant differences in newborn APGAR scores between acupressure and no-acupressure groups (Hjelmstedt et al., 2010; Kashanian & Shahali, 2009; Mortazavi et al., 2012). Moreover, there were no adverse effects from the interventions on the health of newborns.

In this study, participants in the massage + acupressure group experienced increased positive feelings about their delivery, and both interventions positively affected satisfaction. These results may be associated with the effects of massage and acupressure applications in terms of reducing tension, relieving anxiety, and reducing pain as well as the personal support given by midwives during labor. In terms of the respective effects of the interventions on satisfaction, the participants were very satisfied with all three interventions and both confirmed interest in using them during their next delivery and expressed intent to recommend them to others. The participants in all of the intervention groups identified reduced labor pain as the most important reason for their satisfaction. No research in the literature has investigated the satisfaction level of pregnant women with these interventions. A study on couples regarding the effects of massage during delivery by Chang et al. (2002) reported strong satisfaction with the intervention. Some studies have found that massage reduces labor pain, provides psychological support, and improves the labor experience (Pilevarzadeh et al., 2002). In a study by Moradi et al. (2012), which applied acupressure to the GB-21 and SP6 points during the active phase of delivery, higher satisfaction rates and better birth experiences were reported in the acupressure group. In contrast with this study, one study found an acupressure intervention on the SP6 point to have a statistically insignificant effect on the labor experience. The findings of this study confirm that massage and acupressure interventions increased maternal satisfaction and improved the overall labor experience for participants.

Limitations

The following limitations of this study should be considered. This study was carried out in a single obstetrics clinic on a homogeneous population. The seven participants (two women in the massage-only group, one woman in the acupressure-only group, one woman in the massage + acupressure group, and three women in the control group) who received meperidine and the two participants in the control group who received epidural anesthesia were excluded from the study because of the potential effects of these medications on labor pain, labor time, and satisfaction. Therefore, the effects of acupressure and massage on those concurrently using analgesia or anesthesia in labor were not evaluated. A future study should investigate this issue.

Conclusions

In this study, the massage intervention significantly reduced the perceived labor pain of participants during all phases of delivery, whereas the acupressure intervention significantly reduced the perceived labor pain during the active and transition phases of labor only. Both interventions effectively increased maternal satisfaction. Therefore, the following conclusions may be drawn based on these findings: (a) Massage and acupressure interventions are a safe approach for women to use to manage labor pain; (b) primary care personnel should be properly trained in massage and acupressure methods to provide good care to women in labor; and (c) families should receive training on massage during the antenatal period, and a suitable environment should be provided for the application of these methods.

Acknowledgments

We are grateful to all of the women who participated in this study. This study is based on a Hacettepe Institute of Health Sciences doctoral dissertation (year: 2013; No. 339 431).

Author Contributions

Study design: IMG, FT
Data collection: IMG
Data analysis: IMG, FT
Article writing: IMG, FT

References

Brosseau, L., Wells, G. A., Poitras, S., Tugwell, P., Casimiro, L., Novikov, M., ... Cohoon, C. (2012). Ottawa Panel evidence-based clinical practice guidelines on therapeutic massage for low back pain. *Journal of Bodywork and Movement Therapies, 16*(4), 424–455. https://doi.org/10.1016/j.jbmt.2012.04.002

Chaillet, N., Belaid, L., Crochetière, C., Roy, L., Gagnè, G. P., Moutquin, J. M., ... Bonapace, J. (2014). Nonpharmacologic approaches for pain management during labor compared with usual care: A meta-analysis. *Birth, 41*(2), 122–137. https://doi.org/10.1111/birt.12103

Chang, M. Y., Chen, C. H., & Huang, K. F. (2006). A comparison of massage effects on labor pain using the McGill Pain Questionnaire. *The Journal of Nursing Research, 14*(3), 190–197. https://doi.org/10.1097/01.JNR.0000387577.51350.5f

Chang, M. Y., Wang, S. Y., & Chen, C. H. (2002). Effects of massage on pain and anxiety during labour: A randomized controlled trial in Taiwan. *Journal of Advanced Nursing, 38*(1), 68–73. https://doi.org/10.1046/j.1365-2648.2002.02147.x

Chen, H. M., & Chen, C. H. (2004). Effects of acupressure at the Sanyinjiao point on primary dysmenorrhoea. *Journal of Advanced Nursing, 48*(4), 380–387. https://doi.org/10.1111/j.1365-2648.2004.03236.x

Chung, U. L., Hung, L. C., Kuo, S. C., & Huang, C. L. (2003). Effects of LI4 and BL 67 acupressure on labor pain and uterine contractions in the first stage of labor. *The Journal of Nursing Research, 11*(4), 251–260. https://doi.org/10.1097/01.JNR.0000347644.35251.c1

Deepak, A. K. R., & Chopra, S. (2013). Effect of acupressure on intensity of labour pains and duration of first stage of labour among primigravida mothers. *Nursing and Midwifery Research Journal, 9*(4), 178–186.

Dung, H., Clogston, C. P., & Dunn, W. J. (2004). *Acupuncture: An anatomical approach.* London, England: CRP Press.

Hajiamini, Z., Masoud, S. N., Ebadi, A., Mahboubh, A., & Matin, A. A. (2012). Comparing the effects of ice massage and acupressure on labor pain reduction. *Complementary Therapies in Clinical Practice, 18*(3), 169–172. https://doi.org/10.1016/j.ctcp.2012.05.003

Heydari, P., Mojdeh, F., Mazloum, S. R., Tanbakuei, K., & Judaki, K. (2008). The effect of SP6 acupressure on length of labor. *The Iranian Journal of Obstetrics, Gynecology and Infertility, 11*(2), 15–22.

Hjelmstedt, A., Shenoy, S. T., Stener-Victorin, E., Lekander, M., Bhat, M., Balakumaran, L., & Waldenström, U. (2010). Acupressure to reduce labor pain: A randomized controlled trial. *Acta Obstetricia et Gynecologica Scandinavica, 89*(11), 1453–1459. https://doi.org/10.3109/00016349.2010.514323

Janssen, P., Shroff, F., & Jaspar, P. (2012). Massage therapy and labor outcomes: A randomized controlled trial. *The International Journal of Therapeutic Massage & Bodywork, 5*(4), 15–20.

Jones, L., Othman, M., Dowswell, T., Alfirevic, Z., Gates, S., Newburn, M., ... Neilson, J. P. (2012). Pain management for women in labour: An overview of systematic reviews. *Cochrane Database of Systematic Reviews*, 3, CD009234. https://doi.org/10.1002/14651858.CD009234.pub2

Kashanian, M., & Shahali, S. (2009). Effects of acupressure at the sanyinjiao point (SP6) on the process of active phase of labor in nulliparas women. *The Journal of Maternal-Fetal & Neonatal Medicine, 15*, 1–4. https://doi.org/10.3109/14767050903277662

Khodakarami, N., Safarzadeh, A., & Fathizadeh, N. (2005). Effect of massage therapy on pain severity and labor of primipara women. *Iranian Journal of Nursing and Midwifery Research, 10*(3), 6–9.

Kim, Y. R., Chang, S. B., Lee, M. K., & Maeng, W. J. (2002). Effects on labor pain and length of delivery time for primipara women treated by san-yin-jian (SP-6) acupressure and hob-gog (LI-4) acupressure. *Korean Journal of Women Health Nursing, 8*(2), 244–256.

Lee, M. K., Chang, S. B., & Kang, D. H. (2004). Effects of SP6 acupressure on labor pain and length of delivery time in women during labor. *Journal of Alternative and Complementary*

Medicine, 10(6), 959–965. https://doi.org/10.1089/acm.2004.10.959

Levett, K. M., Smith, C. A., Bensoussan, A., & Dahlen, H. G. (2016). Complementary therapies for labour and birth study: A randomised controlled trial of antenatal integrative medicine for pain management in labour. *BMJ Open, 6*(7), e010691. https://doi.org/10.1136/bmjopen-2015-010691

Ma, Y. T., Ma, M., & Cho, Z. H. (2005). *Biomedical acupuncture for pain management: An integrative approach.* St. Louis, MO: Elsevier Churchill Livingstone.

Mafetoni, R. R., & Shimo, A. K. (2016). The effects of acupressure on labor pains during child birth: Randomized clinical trial. *Revista Latino-Americana de Enfermagem, 24*, e2738. https://doi.org/10.1590/1518-8345.0739.2738

Makvandi, S., Mirzaiinajmabadi, K., Sadeghi, R., Mahdavian, M., & Karimi, L. (2016). Meta-analysis of the effect of acupressure on duration of labor and mode of delivery. *International Journal of Gynecology & Obstetrics, 135*(1), 5–10. https://doi.org/10.1016/j.ijgo.2016.04.017

Moradi, Z., Akbarzadeh, M., Zare, N., Hadian, F., Mohamad, J., & Jowkar, A. (2012). Comparative study of effect of two-staged acupressure at GB-21 and SP-6 points on the labor pain of active phase in nulliparous women. *Iranian Journal of Obstetrics, Gynecology & Infertility, 15*(26), 21–29.

Mortazavi, S. H., Khaki, S., Moradi, R., Heidari, K., & Vasegh Rahimparvar, S. F. (2012). Effects of massage therapy and presence of attendant on pain, anxiety and satisfaction during labor. *Archives of Gynecology and Obstetrics, 286*(1), 19–23. https://doi.org/10.1007/s00404-012-2227-4

Najafi, F., Jaafarpour, M., Sayehmiri, K., & Khajavikhan, J. (2018). An evaluation of acupressure on the Sanyinjiao (SP6) and Hugo (LI4) points on the pain severity and length of labor: A systematic review and meta-analysis study. *Iranian Journal of Nursing and Midwifery Research, 23*(1), 1–7. https://doi.org/10.4103/ijnmr.IJNMR_184_15

Park, Y., Cho, J., Kwon, J., Ahn, E., Lim, J., & Chang, S. (2003). The effect of san-yin-Jiao (SP6) acupressure on labor progression. *American Journal of Obstetrics and Gynecology, 189*(6, Suppl.), 209. https://doi.org/10.1016/j.ajog.2003.10.556

Perry, S. E., Hockenberry, M. J., Lowdermilk, D. L., & Wilson, D. (2014). *Maternal child nursing care* (5th ed., pp. 356–380). Toronto, Ontario, Canada: Elsevier Limited.

Pilevarzadeh, M., Salari, S., & Shafiei, N. (2002). Effect of massage on reducing pain and anxiety during labour. *Journal of Reproduction & Infertility, 3*(4), 42–46.

Price, D. D., McGrath, P. A., Rafii, A., & Buckingham, B. (1983). The validation of visual analogue scales as ratio scale measures for chronic and experimental pain. *Pain, 17*(1), 45–56. https://doi.org/10.1016/0304-3959(83)90126-4

Sandifor, J. (1997). *Acupressure: For health, vitality and first aid.* Boston, MA: Element Book.

Sehhatie-Shafaie, F., Kazemzadeh, R., Amani, F., & Heshmat, R. (2013). The effect of acupressure on sanyinjiao and hugo points on labor pain in nulliparous women: A randomized clinical trial. *Journal of Caring Sciences, 2*(2), 123–129. https://doi.org/10.5681/jcs.2013.015

Simkin, P. P., & O'hara, M. (2002). Nonpharmacologic relief of pain during labor: Systematic reviews of five methods. *American Journal of Obstetrics and Gynecology, 186*(5, Suppl. Nature), S131–S159.

Smith, C. A., Collins, C. T., Crowther, C. A., & Levett, K. M. (2011). Acupuncture or acupressure for pain management in labour. *Cochrane Database of Systematic Reviews*, 7, CD009232. https://doi.org/10.1002/14651858.CD009232

Smith, C. A., Levett, K. M., Collins, C. T., & Jones, L. (2012). Massage, reflexology and other manual methods for pain management in labour. *Cochrane Database of Systematic Reviews*, 2, CD009290. https://doi.org/10.1002/14651858.CD009290.pub2

Tulunay, M., & Tulunay, F. C. (2000). Pain assessment and pain measurements. In S. Erdine (Ed.), *Pain* (1st ed., pp. 91–107). İstanbul, Turkey: Alemdar Ofset. (Original work published in Turkish)

Yu, S., Yang, J., Yang, M., Gao, Y., Chen, J., Ren, Y., ... Hu, Y. (2015). Application of acupoints and meridians for the treatment of primary dysmenorrhea: A data mining-based literature study. *Evidence-based Complementary and Alternative Medicine, 2015*, 752194. https://doi.org/10.1155/2015/752194

9

Effects of Aerobic Exercise on Cognitive Function in Women with Methamphetamine Dependence in a Detoxification Program in Tianjin, China

Jingjing LIU[1] • Chen CHEN[1] • Maojie LIU[1] • Shumei ZHUANG[2]*

ABSTRACT

Background: Cognitive impairment is prevalent among individuals, especially women, with methamphetamine dependence. Although aerobic exercise has been shown to affect cognitive function in humans and animals, few related studies have focused on subjects with methamphetamine dependence.

Purpose: The aim of this study was to assess the detoxification-related effects of aerobic exercise on cognitive function in women with methamphetamine dependence.

Methods: A randomized controlled trial was used with 98 women with methamphetamine dependence undergoing a detoxification program at a mental hospital. The women were distributed using a computer-generated grouping random method into either the study or control group. The investigator conducting the baseline questionnaire, the neuropsychologist assessing the cognitive function, and the data analyst were blinded to group assignment. In addition to hospital routine care, the study group received an aerobic exercise intervention for 3 months. The control group only received hospital routine care. Attention and working memory were measured using the Trail Making Test and Digit Span Test, verbal memory was measured using Logical Memory (LM) and Memory for Persons Data (MPD), and executive function was measured using the Color-Word Stroop Test.

Results: Forty-nine participants were randomized into each group, and the valid data of 43 participants in the study group and 46 in the control group were analyzed. The study group showed significantly more improvement over time in terms of Digit Span Test, Trail Making Test, LM-delayed, MPD-5 minutes delayed, MPD-30 minutes delayed, and Color-Word Stroop Test than the control group ($p < .05$). LM-immediate and MPD-immediate scores showed that the effects of time and the interaction between time and group were significant but that the main effect of group was not.

Conclusions/Implications for Practice: Women undergoing detoxification for methamphetamine dependence may practice aerobic exercise to improve attention, working memory, executive function, and parts of verbal memory. Aerobic exercise may be incorporated into detoxification treatment programs to facilitate the recovery of cognitive functions in women.

KEY WORDS:
aerobic exercise, cognitive function, intervention studies, methamphetamine dependence, women.

Introduction

Drug use is a serious problem worldwide, and global deaths directly related to the use of drugs have been increasing (United Nations Office on Drugs and Crime, 2018). The range of drugs being used illicitly has expanded from heroin and opium to new psychoactive substances (e.g., piperazines) and amphetamine-type stimulants (e.g., methamphetamine; Luo et al., 2018). When used recreationally, methamphetamine leads to increased energy and euphoria, which gives this drug a high potential for abuse and addiction (Panenka et al., 2013). Long-term use of methamphetamine may result in neurotoxic side effects (Long et al., 2017), whereas abuse of this drug has been associated with the shrinkage of the prefrontal cortex and hippocampus damage in the brain, which are related to cognitive disorders (Golsorkhdan et al., 2020; Long et al., 2017). Most previous studies have found that the cognitive function scores of people with methamphetamine addiction are lower than those of healthy controls in the categories of attention, working memory, verbal memory, and executive function (Potvin et al., 2018). Working memory is a temporary and limited storage system for basic information related to other complex tasks (Fattore & Diana, 2016). Executive function refers to be the product of coordinated operation of various processes conducted to achieve specific objectives flexibly (Shuai et al., 2017). Verbal memory refers to the memory of orally expressed information (Kilciksiz et al., 2020).

Studies have shown that the duration required to become addicted to drugs is shorter in women than in men because of the distinct effects of different sex hormones on brain structures (Zhou et al., 2016). Compared with men, women have

[1]BSN, RN, Graduate Student, School of Nursing, Tianjin Medical University, China • [2]PhD, RN, Associate Professor, School of Nursing, Tianjin Medical University, China.

more difficulty quitting drugs and are more likely to relapse after abstinence (Zhou et al., 2016). Moreover, female methamphetamine users may be more vulnerable to related brain damage, especially in terms of hippocampus-related cognitive disorders (Du et al., 2015). Abuse of methamphetamine in women affects not only their own physical and psychological health but also that of their offspring (Dong et al., 2018). Furthermore, methamphetamine-dependence-related cognitive disorders have frequently been associated with suicidal/violent behaviors (Y. Zhang et al., 2020), which harm the individual users, their families, and the society. Despite the strong evidence supporting the more-potent effects of methamphetamine in women than men (Prakash et al., 2017) and the known negative effects of methamphetamine-induced cognitive impairment on daily functions, no standard treatment is currently available for cognitive impairment in patients with methamphetamine dependence. In addition, few studies have been published on how to effectively improve cognitive function in this population.

The American College of Sports Medicine defines aerobic exercise as to include the wide range of sports that repeatedly and rhythmically use large muscle groups (as cited in Bidonde et al., 2017). It is well documented that exercise not only enhances cardiopulmonary function but also improves brain function (Wilke et al., 2019). Previous studies of the effects of exercise on cognitive function have reported that aerobic exercise programs improve cognitive function in adults with craniocerebral injury (Chin et al., 2015), Type 2 diabetes mellitus (Podolski et al., 2017), and Parkinson's disease (da Silva et al., 2018). Although similar cognitive-function benefits of aerobic exercise have been evidenced in humans and animals (Pietrelli et al., 2018), few studies have been conducted in methamphetamine-dependent populations, with even fewer addressing the subcategory of women. As abusing methamphetamine causes significant harm in women, adopting effective interventions to improve cognitive function in women who abuse methamphetamines is important. In this randomized controlled trial focused on women with methamphetamine dependence enrolled in a detoxification program, aerobic exercise was adopted as the independent variable, and attention, working memory, verbal memory, and executive function were adopted as the dependent variables. The objective of this study was to explore the effects of an aerobic exercise program on cognitive function at two points in time: (a) immediately after completion of the exercise program and (b) at 3 months postintervention.

Methods

Trial Design

This was a randomized controlled trial. Participants were randomly allocated into two groups (1:1), with the study group receiving a 3-month aerobic exercise program in addition to routine medical care in a hospital and the control group receiving routine medical care in a hospital only.

Sample Size

The sample size was calculated using G*Power 3.1.9.7 software, with α set to .05, power set to 0.9, and the value of effect set to 0.25. Estimating a 20% lost-to-follow-up rate, at least 36 participants were required in each group.

Participants

This study was conducted between December 2016 and October 2018 at a mental hospital in Tianjin, China, where eligible women under detoxification treatment were recruited as participants. Before conducting the intervention, the researchers received professional and unified training and were instructed in the purpose of this study and the inclusion and exclusion criteria in detail. The inclusion and exclusion criteria were evaluated by the researchers using medical records, hospital urine test reports, professional physician diagnoses, and admission assessment reports. Qualified patients were recruited according to their order of hospital admission. Inclusion criteria included (a) being female, (b) age between 18 and 65 years, (c) having a positive methamphetamine urine test result, (d) having received at least 3 months of therapy at the study hospital, (e) having a low-exercise lifestyle (no regular exercise or exercising less than twice weekly), and (f) ability to speak Mandarin and write and read in Chinese. Exclusion criteria included (a) having a physical contradiction that prevents participation such as bone metastases, asthma, hypertension, heart disease, anemia, decreased white blood cell count, imbalance, severe pain, and diabetes mellitus; (b) having other brain-dysfunction-related conditions such as stroke, Alzheimer's disease, dementia, or brain injury; and (c) having serious psychiatric or neurologic sequelae.

Interventions

Aerobic exercise intervention

The aerobic exercise intervention was a supervised, moderate-intensity exercise program conducted in the hospital that was designed jointly by a team of professional rehabilitation therapists, sports coaches, doctors, and nurses. Informed consent was obtained from all of the participants before the intervention. Before the formal intervention, a preexperiment was conducted to ensure the safety of the experimental protocol. An aerobic exercise coach with over 10 years of experience in aerobic exercise practice coached each participant in the movements to ensure the effect of the intervention. In addition, each participant was provided with a guidebook and DVD specially made for the aerobic exercise intervention to help them master the aerobic exercise movements.

The supervision team, which took responsibility for ensuring participant adherence to the intervention, was composed of trained and professional rehabilitation therapists, sports coaches, doctors, and nurses. The doctors and nurses in charge of the patient assumed supervision responsibilities from Monday to Friday to urge the participants to carry out their aerobic exercises in a timely manner. The supervision team also helped ensure participant safety by making sure that participants stopped exercising and received appropriate treatments immediately if they experienced symptoms of discomfort.

The participants attended aerobic exercise sessions in the hospital 5 times every week for 3 months. The study group was divided into three subgroups of 14–16 participants each. At 10 a.m. from Monday to Friday, the participants performed the aerobic exercise intervention at the same time in three spacious rooms. The exercise intervention was not conducted on Saturdays or Sundays. The supervision team visited the three rooms during the intervention sessions to ensure that each participant completed the exercise accurately and similarly.

During each session, the participants completed the whole aerobic exercise under the guidance of the order and sound from the same video made for the aerobic exercise intervention. Each session began with a 5-minute warm-up to ensure exercise safety and lasted for 40 minutes. The participants practiced a series of aerobic exercises for the next 30 minutes, including head movements, shoulder movements, chest movements, waist movements, upper limb movements, and lower limb movements. The sessions ended with 5 minutes of relaxation movements. The participants exercised at a rate that achieved 55%–69% of the maximal heart rate, which could be estimated as the number 220 minus the age of the participant. We used a sports bracelet (model: Mi Band 2) to monitor the heart rate of the participants during each session. Each participant's heart rate reached the ideal heart rate during the intervention.

Routine care group

The participants in the control group received hospital routine care only. Hospital routine care comprised medication care, diet care (nutritional support), health checkup, manual labor (assembling plastic flowers and so on), and discipline education.

Data Collection

Baseline information was collected using face-to-face interviews as soon as the group allocation process was completed. All of the cognitive function tests were administered by a trained neuropsychologist at baseline, immediately after completion of the exercise program (Posttest 1), and 3 months after completion of the intervention (Posttest 2).

Demographic Status

Demographic factors measured in this study included age, educational level, employment status, and marital status. All of the variables except age were categorical.

Clinical Characteristics

Clinical information about methamphetamine abuse included the method of synthetic drug use, daily dose of methamphetamine use, duration of methamphetamine abuse, and duration of abstinence. Cognitive measurements included attention and working memory by Trail Making Test (TMT) and Digit Span Test (DST), verbal memory by Logical Memory (LM) and Memory for Persons Data (MPD), and executive function by Color-Word Stroop Test (CWST).

Attention and Working Memory

DST, designed to measure attention and working memory (Aumont et al., 2019), was derived from the Wechsler Memory Scale-Revised. In the first test, participants were required to recall the numbers forward after being read a series of computer-generated numbers. In the second test, participants were required to recall the same numbers backward. The test finished when participants were not able to recall the digits for two tests in a row. The mean number of the longest span of numbers was recorded as the final score. The test lasted about 5 minutes.

TMT, a subtest of the Wechsler Memory Scale-Third Edition, consists of two parts (TMT-A and TMT-B). TMT-A requires respondents to connect an array of numbers in ascending order in 150 seconds, whereas TMT-B asks respondents to sort an array of numbers and letters in numerical and alphabetical order in 300 seconds. The numbers of correct connections are respectively recorded for the two parts, with lower scores indicating severer cognitive impairment.

Verbal Memory

LM was designed to assess verbal memory from the Wechsler Memory Scale-Third Edition (McDonald et al., 2014). In the LM, respondents are asked to recall a story immediately (LM-I) and once again at 30 minutes (LM-D) after the story was presented. The rate of correctness of the two recalls is recorded.

MPD is also used to assess verbal memory. In the MPD, 15 items are presented. If the respondents are able to immediately recall all of the items correctly in the first two trials, the tests are ended. If this condition is not met, two additional trials are administered until the respondents are able to immediately recall all of the items correctly (MPD-immediate [MPD-1]). After 5 minutes, the respondents are required to recall all of the items (MPD-5 minutes delayed [MPD-2]). After 30 minutes, the delayed recall of respondents is tested (MPD-30 minutes delayed [MPD-D]).

Executive Function

CWST is used to assess executive function. In the CWST, respondents are required to name the color of an incongruent/congruent color word that is written. The number of correct responses (colors named) in 2 minutes is recorded. It is well documented that performance on the CWST correlates with the prefrontal cortex, implicating executive function (Kujach et al., 2018).

Randomization and Blinding

All of the participants in this study were anonymized using codes and randomly assigned (1:1) into the study group or the control group using a computer-generated randomization method. The distribution results were sealed in opaque envelopes by an assistant who was not otherwise involved in this study and turned a blind eye to the identity of the participants.

As the control group did not perform the aerobic exercise, participants could not be blinded to the distribution results. The study group and the control group were assigned to two wards on the second and third floors of the hospital to prevent the two groups from communicating. The researchers, doctors, nurses, rehabilitation therapists, and sports coaches who were involved in the treatment and the intervention were aware of the grouping results of the study. The nurses and doctors involved in treatment received professional training to ensure that the routine care provided to each group was equivalent. The investigator who conducted the baseline information and the neuropsychologist who assessed the cognitive function were specially trained. They did not participate in the intervention and were not aware of the grouping allocation of the participants. In addition, the data analyst was blinded to group assignment.

Ethical Approval

In accordance with the guidance of the ethics committee of the World Health Organization, this study adhered to the relevant rules of the institutional review board and received ethical approval from the Chinese Ethics Committee of Registering Clinical Trials, An-Kang Hospital, and Tianjin Medical University (registration number: ChiCTR-ROC-15006327).

Statistical Analysis

The continuous variables were described statistically in terms of the mean and standard deviation, and the categorical variables were described statistically in terms of proportions. Data were analyzed using SPSS 16.0 (SPSS Inc., Chicago, IL, USA). The demographic and clinical characteristics of the two groups were compared using an independent sample *t* test for continuous variables and a chi-square test for categorical variables. Scores on the DST, TMT, LM, MPD, and CWST were assessed in accordance with published scoring algorithms. A general linear model repeated-measures analysis of variance was applied to evaluate the effects of the exercise intervention on the cognitive-function variables over 6 months. Time was the within-subject factor, whereas group was the between-subject factor. The result measurement at different time points was taken as the within-subject dependent variables. The main effects for time and group were determined using the three time points (baseline, Posttest 1, and Posttest 2). Sphericity assumed was used to test for a correlation among repetitive measure data. Tests of within-subject comparison were used to analyze the effects of time and the reciprocal action between time and group, and tests of between-subject effects were used to assess the group factors. To prevent false positives, Bonferroni correction was applied to the repeated measurements of paired comparisons (Meng et al., 2020). All of the significance tests were two-sided with a 5% level of significance.

Results

Participants

Of the 108 patients approached, 98 met the inclusion and exclusion criteria and expressed interest to participate. The 10 who did not participate were either ineligible (n = 8) or not interested (n = 2). Reasons for ineligibility included having dyslexia (n = 2), a serious heart disease (n = 1), hypertension (n = 1), severe bone metastases (n = 1), or less than 3 months of scheduled therapy at this hospital (n = 3). Before the formal intervention, the rehabilitation coach gave guidance to each participant on aerobic exercise. Some participants (n = 3) withdrew from the study because of discomfort.

After 3 months, six participants withdrew from the program. The data of the 89 participants (43 in the study group and 46 in the control group) who completed the study were used in the analysis (Figure 1).

As shown in Table 1, most participants had a middle school education (66.3%), were single (79.8%), and were unemployed (78.7%). Regarding drug abuse history, all reported using inhalation/smoking/sniffing. The average methamphetamine abuse time was around 8 years. The statistical tests showed an even distribution of participants across the groups.

Cognitive Outcomes at Baseline

Comparisons of baseline cognitive functioning by DST, TMT, LM, MPD, and CWST scores between the two groups are shown in Table 2. No significant difference was found at baseline in any measure between the two groups (all *p*s > .05).

Effects of Aerobic Exercise

Attention and working memory

The DST scores of study group participants rose significantly from 7.37 (SD = 1.51) at baseline to 8.63 (SD = 1.20) at completion of the exercise program (Posttest 1) and continued to increase to 9.19 (SD = 1.33) at 3 months after completion of the exercise program (Posttest 2). Postintervention working memory scores as measured by DST were found to be significantly higher in the study group than the control group (F = 5.09, p = .027; Figure 2-A).

A statistically significant difference between the two groups was also found for TMT-A and TMT-B (F = 4.05, p = .047 [Figure 2-B]; F = 4.11, p = .046 [Figure 2-C]). For the study group, there was a rise from 33.23 (SD = 12.16) to 42.14 (SD = 11.90) at Posttest 1 and to 46.19 (SD = 11.38) at Posttest 2 in TMT-A. A similar change was observed for TMT-B as well.

Figure 1

Randomization Process Used in this Study

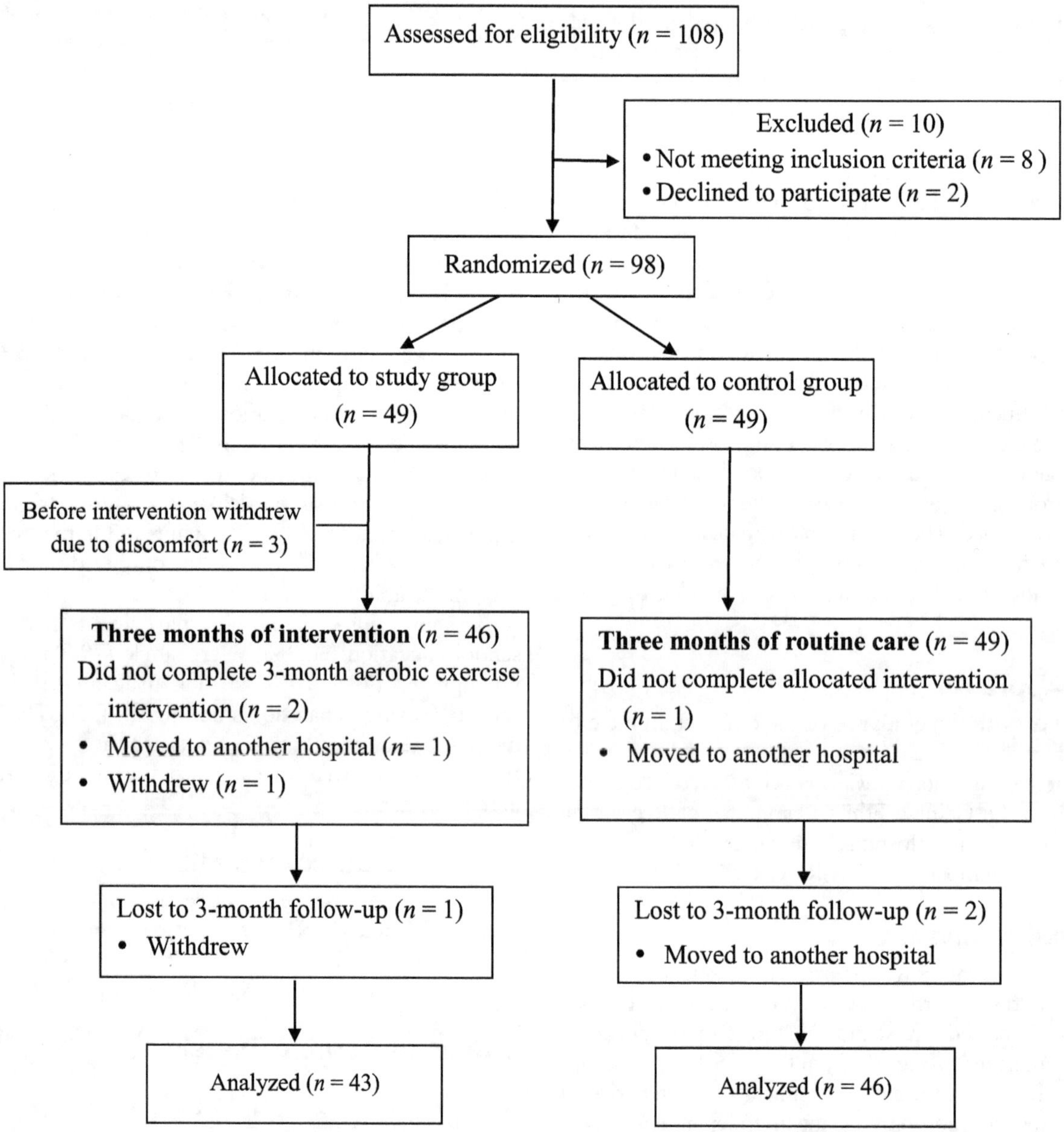

Verbal memory

LM-D performance in the study group began at 28.63 (SD = 12.59) at baseline and increased by about 12 points at Posttest 1 and by another 5 points at Posttest 2, with the magnitude of increase exceeding that of the control group (F = 4.10, p = .046; Figure 2-E).

The study group had significantly better posttest MPD-2 scores (F = 5.62, p = .020) than the control group, improving from 9.74 (SD = 1.58) at baseline to 11.40 (SD = 1.14) at Posttest 1 and to 12.00 at Posttest 2 (SD = 0.93; Figure 2-G). Similar to MPD-2, the study group had significantly improved posttest MPD-D scores, with no significant change observed in the control group (F = 4.81, p = .031). In the study group, MPD-D scores rose from 9.74 (SD = 1.58) at baseline to 11.35 (SD = 1.11) and 11.93 (SD = 1.01) at Posttests 1 and 2, respectively (Figure 2-H). Interestingly, no significant differences in scores between the two groups were found for LM-I (Figure 2-D) and MPD-1 (Figure 2-F).

Executive function

The effect of aerobic exercise on executive function was dramatically greater in the study group than in the control group (F = 4.09, p = .046), with the CWST score in the study group rising from 32.02 (SD = 12.20) at baseline to 42 at Posttest 2 (Figure 2-I).

Discussion

This was the first randomized controlled trial study to explore the effects of aerobic activity on cognitive function in

Table 1

Between-Group Comparison of Baseline Demographic Status and Clinical Characteristics

Characteristic	Control Group (*n* = 46)		Study Group (*n* = 43)		Total		t/χ^2	*p*
	n	%	*n*	%	*n*	%		
Educational level							0.10	.95
Primary school	12	26.1	10	23.3	22	24.7		
Middle school	30	65.2	29	67.4	59	66.3		
High middle school	4	8.7	4	9.3	8	9.0		
Marital status							0.14	.93
Unmarried	26	56.5	25	58.1	51	57.3		
Married	10	21.7	8	18.6	18	20.2		
Divorced	10	21.7	10	23.3	20	22.5		
Employment status							0.89	.35
Employed	8	17.4	11	25.6	19	21.3		
Unemployed	38	82.6	32	74.4	70	78.7		
	M	*SD*	*M*	*SD*	*M*	*SD*		
Age (years)	28.96	8.27	29.93	7.91	29.43	8.07	0.57	.57
Daily dose of methamphetamine use (mg)	0.98	0.33	1.04	0.37	1.01	0.35	0.81	.42
Duration of using methamphetamine (years)	7.82	3.57	8.05	3.84	7.93	3.68	0.29	.77
Duration of abstinence (years)	2.69	0.72	2.81	0.80	2.75	0.76	0.75	.46
Attention and working memory								
DST	7.26	1.76	7.37	1.51			0.32	.75
TMT								
TMT-A	33.50	14.44	33.23	12.16			−0.09	.93
TMT-B	34.09	14.77	34.60	14.18			0.17	.87
Verbal memory								
LM								
LM-I	33.39	15.09	33.02	16.25			−0.11	.91
LM-D	30.61	14.80	28.63	12.59			−0.68	.50
MPD								
MPD-1	8.24	2.71	8.05	3.15			−0.31	.76
MPD-2	10.20	1.26	9.74	1.58			−1.50	.14
MPD-D	10.20	1.26	9.74	1.58			−1.50	.14
Executive function								
CWST	32.72	14.19	32.02	12.20			−0.24	.81

Note. All of the patients in this study used inhalation/smoking/sniffing for methamphetamine. Thus, data on the major method of methamphetamine use were not analyzed. DST = Digit Span Test; TMT = Trail Making Test; LM = Logical Memory; LM-I = LM-immediate; LM-D = LM-delayed; MPD = Memory for Persons Data; MPD-1 = MPD-immediate; MPD-2 = MPD-5 minutes delayed; MPD-D = MPD-30 minutes delayed; CWST = Color-Word Stroop Test.

women with methamphetamine dependence and to evaluate changes in these effects over time. The findings of this study are discussed below.

The most significant finding in this study is that the aerobic exercise had significantly beneficial effects on attention, working memory, and executive function and that these beneficial effects were sustained over the 3 months after intervention. This finding was consistent with the outcome from prior animal studies on the effects of exercise (Ghodrati-Jaldbakhan et al., 2017). There are several explanations for the observed changes in attention, working memory, and executive function. First, exercise boosts brain neurotransmitter system efficiency. Neurotransmitters have the function of information transmission among neurons. Brain-derived neutrophil factor (BDNF), which is widely expressed in the hippocampus and cerebral cortex, self-regulates its production during exercise (Walsh & Tschakovsky, 2018). The exercise-induced increase in BDNF levels may enhance attention, working memory, and executive function (de Azevedo et al., 2019; Gökçe et al., 2019). Furthermore, insulin-like growth factor 1 (IGF-1) and vascular endothelial growth factor (VEGF) may also be increased by exercise (Lin et al., 2018). Second, aerobic exercise may significantly modulate neurogenesis (Rendeiro & Rhodes, 2018). The release of VEGF, BDNF, and IGF is associated with neurogenesis (Ma et al., 2017; Rendeiro & Rhodes, 2018). Neurogenesis

Table 2

Aerobic Exercise Effects on Cognitive Function

Domain	Control Group (*n* = 46)						Study Group (*n* = 43)						Effect of Time (*F*)	Effect of Group (*F*)	Interaction Between Time and Group (*F*)
	Baseline		3 Months		6 Months		Baseline		3 Months		6 Months				
	M	*SD*	*M*	*SD*	*M*	*SD*	*M*	*SD*	*M*	*SD*	*M*	*SD*			
Attention and working memory															
DST	7.26	1.76	7.85	1.69	8.00	1.73	7.37	1.51	8.63	1.20	9.19	1.33	86.69**	5.09*	15.37**
TMT															
TMT-A	33.50	14.44	35.17	14.05	36.17	14.27	33.23	12.16	42.14	11.90	46.19	11.38	550.34**	4.05*	238.13**
TMT-B	34.09	14.77	36.65	13.83	38.13	13.33	34.60	14.18	44.05	13.58	47.74	12.75	293.51**	4.11*	82.25**
Verbal memory															
LM															
LM-I	33.39	15.09	36.54	13.73	37.83	13.33	33.02	16.25	41.33	14.43	44.56	14.60	220.53**	1.48	43.59**
LM-D	30.61	14.80	32.41	14.89	33.33	14.82	28.63	12.59	40.09	12.27	45.14	12.31	487.66**	4.10*	250.96**
MPD															
MPD-1	8.24	2.71	8.76	2.57	8.93	2.60	8.05	3.15	9.60	2.80	10.58	2.67	117.02**	1.82	37.93**
MPD-2	10.20	1.26	10.63	0.97	10.78	1.11	9.74	1.58	11.40	1.14	12.00	0.93	117.19**	5.62*	40.39**
MPD-D	10.20	1.26	10.63	0.97	10.78	1.11	9.74	1.58	11.35	1.11	11.93	1.01	104.95**	4.81*	34.90**
Executive function															
CWST	32.72	14.19	34.70	13.93	36.20	13.69	32.02	12.20	41.95	11.76	46.26	11.56	320.03**	4.09*	118.00**

Note. Statistical tests: general linear model repeated-measures analysis of variance. Tests of within-subject effects: effects of time and the reciprocal action between time and group. Tests of between-subject effects: effects of group. DST = Digit Span Test; TMT = Trail Making Test; LM = Logical Memory; LM-I = LM-immediate; LM-D = LM-delayed; MPD = Memory for Persons Data; MPD-1 = MPD-immediate; MPD-2 = MPD-5 minutes delayed; MPD-D = MPD-30 minutes delayed; CWST = Color-Word Stroop Test.

$^*p < .05$. $^{**}p < .001$.

induced by aerobic exercise may improve attention, memory, and executive function (Ma et al., 2017). Third, exercise increases synaptic plasticity. VEGF, BDNF, and IGF may significantly mediate synaptic function (Bettio et al., 2019). High levels of neuronal activation may alter the number and composition of membrane receptors as well as the number and shape of dendritic spines, which may change the structural plasticity of the synapse (Rendeiro & Rhodes, 2018). Moreover, enhanced neurogenesis may change the structural plasticity of the synapse (Bettio et al., 2019). Fourth, exercise may irritate vascular proliferation in the hippocampus and cortex (Cooper et al., 2018). VEGF may participate in angiogenesis and change of vascular plasticity (Cooper et al., 2018). Furthermore, aerobic exercise also promotes the perfusion and transportation of oxygen, nutrients, and neurotrophins to regulate the cerebral vascular system and improve brain function (Cooper et al., 2018). Finally, neurogenesis, vascular proliferation, and change of synaptic plasticity may change the structure and function of the brain, including the hippocampus and prefrontal cortex (Nouchi et al., 2014). Memory is closely related to hippocampal function (Ólafsdóttir et al., 2018), whereas executive function and working memory are closely related to the prefrontal cortex (Kujach et al., 2018; Pietrelli et al., 2018). Therefore, attention, working memory, and executive function are also improved with the improvement of brain structure and brain function.

Another significant finding of this study is that, based on changes in LM-D, MPD-2, and MPD-D, delayed repetition of verbal memory was significantly improved at the conclusion of the aerobic intervention and was sustained for 3 months afterward. In addition, studies of healthy people have shown that people who have exercised for a long time score higher on verbal memory tests (Zhao et al., 2016). This finding may be related to the increase of BDNF level induced by exercise, which may help protect hippocampal volume (Zhao et al., 2016). However, in this study, no significant difference between the study and control groups in terms of immediate repetition of verbal memory was found, with each group showing a rising trend over time, which is attributed to the changes in LM-I and MPD-1. People with methamphetamine-induced brain dysfunction exhibit specific memory disorders, including response inhibition, excessive sensitivity to the influence of interferential stimuli, and difficulties in sustaining attention (Bernhardt et al., 2020; Mizoguchi & Yamada, 2019). The effect found on immediate repetition of verbal memory may be associated with methamphetamine-induced distraction, slow response, and inefficient focus on complex tasks. Further research is necessary to verify the effect of aerobic exercise on verbal memory.

A third significant finding of this study is that cognitive function in the participants improved with duration after withdrawal, as the scores for cognitive function in the control group increased over the 6 months after withdrawal. This finding supports the results of a recent study, which found that methamphetamine-induced cognitive dysfunction would improve somewhat over time after withdrawal (Proebstl et al.,

Figure 2

The Line Chart of Change Trend of Cognitive Function's Average Scores in the Study Group and Control Group at Three Time Points

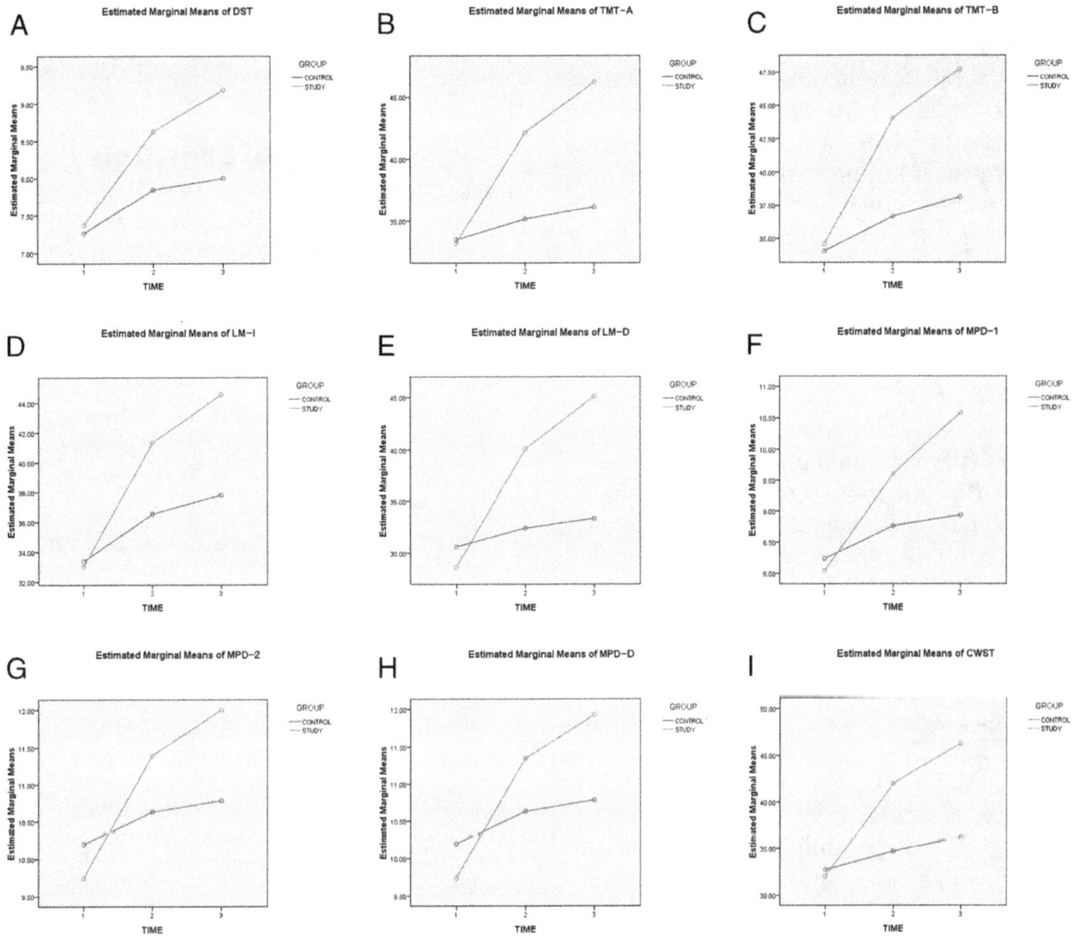

Note. DST = Digit Span Test; TMT-A = Trail Making Test, Trail A; TMT-B = Trail Making Test, Trail B; LM-I = LM-immediate; LM-D = LM-delayed; MPD-1 = MPD-immediate; MPD-2 = MPD-5 minutes delayed; MPD-D = MPD-30 minutes delayed; CWST = Color-Word Stroop Test.

2019). After abstinence, brain functions and structures related to cognitive function improve gradually (Z. Zhang et al., 2018). Therefore, methamphetamine-induced cognitive dysfunction may improve after withdrawal. In addition, the results from this study presented that the rate of improvement in cognitive function resulting from aerobic exercise decreased over the postintervention, 3-month follow-up period. BDNF protein may decrease with time because of the cessation of intervention and the decrease in exercise intensity (Mackay et al., 2017). Moreover, like BDNF, the level of other factors inspired by exercise may decline after cessation of exercise. However, it is encouraging that cognitive function in the study group continued to increase although with a smaller slope until 3 months postintervention. Given the beneficial effects of exercise, the participants may have chosen to continue exercising after the study, resulting in sustained, beneficial effects on cognitive function.

Conclusions

The findings support aerobic exercise as an effective and feasible approach to improving attention, working memory, executive function, and parts of verbal memory in women who are undergoing detoxification for methamphetamine dependence. It is recommended that aerobic exercise be considered as a part of an overall treatment program to facilitate the recovery of cognitive function in these women. Further research is required to prove the long-term efficacy of this treatment and its efficacy on men who abuse methamphetamines.

Study Limitations

Although the abovementioned findings are noteworthy, several limitations should be acknowledged. First, all of the participants were recruited from one hospital in Tianjin City. Thus, the results may not be generalizable to the entire population of women in methamphetamine rehabilitation programs in China or to similar populations in other countries. Second, the cognitive function results in this study may have been affected by subjective factors of the participants, as the control group did not participate in any intervention. However, measures were taken to control contamination between the study group and the control group as much as possible. Third, time was a confounding factor of the effect of aerobic exercise, as the cognitive function of subjects is expected improve with duration of abstinence. Fourth, this study only followed the participants for 6 months in total because of limited resources. Although the positive effect of aerobic exercise on cognitive function in patients was shown over the 6-month study period, the long-term benefits remain unknown. Further research should be conducted to explore the long-term impact of aerobic exercise on cognitive function among the methamphetamine-dependent population as well as other factors that may affect cognitive function in this population.

Implications for Nursing Practice

Clinical doctors and nurses should be conscious of damage to brain structure and function by methamphetamine and of the importance of aerobic exercise for women with methamphetamine dependence. We suggest that healthcare workers be trained in aerobic exercise theory and methods before implementing exercise therapy with patients to provide proper supervision and guidance. In the future, aerobic exercise should be included in the routine care protocol of detoxification programs for women with methamphetamine dependence to improve brain function and increase rehabilitation quality.

Acknowledgments

This study was funded by the Science &Technology Development Fund of Tianjin Education Commission for Higher Education (2017KJ234). The authors are grateful to the staff of the hospital for their great support and contributions to this study. In addition, they are grateful to the study participants for choosing to join this project.

Author Contributions

Study conception and design: SZ, CC
Data collection: CC, ML
Data analysis and interpretation: CC, ML, JL
Drafting of the article: All authors
Critical revision of the article: SZ

References

Aumont, É., Arguin, M., Bohbot, V., & West, G. L. (2019). Increased flanker task and forward digit span performance in caudate-nucleus-dependent response strategies. *Brain and Cognition, 135,* Article 103576. https://doi.org/10.1016/j.bandc.2019.05.014

Bernhardt, N., Petzold, J., Groß, C., Scheck, A., Pooseh, S., Mayer-Pelinski, R., Zimmermann, U. S., Smolka, M. N., & Pilhatsch, M. (2020). Neurocognitive dysfunctions and their therapeutic modulation in patients with methamphetamine dependence: A pilot study. *Frontiers in Psychiatry, 11,* Article 581. https://doi.org/10.3389/fpsyt.2020.00581

Bettio, L., Thacker, J. S., Hutton, C., & Christie, B. R. (2019). Modulation of synaptic plasticity by exercise. *International Review of Neurobiology, 147,* 295–322. https://doi.org/10.1016/bs.irn.2019.07.002

Bidonde, J., Busch, A. J., Schachter, C. L., Overend, T. J., Kim, S. Y., Góes, S. M., Boden, C., & Foulds, H. J. (2017). Aerobic exercise training for adults with fibromyalgia. *Cochrane Database of Systematic Reviews, 6*(6), Article CD012700. https://doi.org/10.1002/14651858.CD012700

Chin, L. M., Keyser, R. E., Dsurney, J., & Chan, L. (2015). Improved cognitive performance following aerobic exercise training in people with traumatic brain injury. *Archives of Physical Medicine and Rehabilitation, 96*(4), 754–759. https://doi.org/10.1016/j.apmr.2014.11.009

Cooper, C., Moon, H. Y., & van Praag, H. (2018). On the run for hippocampal plasticity. *Cold Spring Harbor Perspectives in Medicine, 8*(4), Article a029736. https://doi.org/10.1101/cshperspect.a029736

da Silva, F. C., Iop, R. D. R., de Oliveira, L. C., Boll, A. M., de Alvarenga, J. G. S., Gutierres Filho, P. J. B., de Melo, L. M. A. B., Xavier, A. J., & da Silva, R. (2018). Effects of physical exercise programs on cognitive function in Parkinson's disease patients: A systematic review of randomized controlled trials of the last 10 years. *PLOS ONE, 13*(2), Article e0193113. https://doi.org/10.1371/journal.pone.0193113

de Azevedo, K. P. M., de Oliveira Segundo, V. H., de Medeiros, G. C. B. S., de Sousa Mata, Á. N., García, D. A., de Carvalho Leitão, J. C. G., Knackfuss, M. I., & Piuvezam, G. (2019). Effects of exercise on the levels of BDNF and executive function in adolescents: A protocol for systematic review and meta-analysis. *Medicine (Baltimore), 98*(28), Article e16445. https://doi.org/10.1097/MD.0000000000016445

Dong, N., Zhu, J., Han, W., Wang, S., Yan, Z., Ma, D., Goh, E. L. K., & Chen, T. (2018). Maternal methamphetamine exposure causes cognitive impairment and alteration of neurodevelopment-related genes in adult offspring mice. *Neuropharmacology, 140,* 25–34. https://doi.org/10.1016/j.neuropharm.2018.07.024

Du, J., Quan, M., Zhuang, W., Zhong, N., Jiang, H., Kennedy, D. N., Harrington, A., Ziedonis, D., Fan, X., & Zhao, M. (2015). Hippocampal volume reduction in female but not male recent abstinent methamphetamine users. *Behavioural Brain Research, 289*, 78–83. https://doi.org/10.1016/j.bbr.2015.04.033

Fattore, L., & Diana, M. (2016). Drug addiction: An affective–cognitive disorder in need of a cure. *Neuroscience & Biobehavioral Reviews, 65*, 341–361. https://doi.org/10.1016/j.neubiorev.2016.04.006

Ghodrati-Jaldbakhan, S., Ahmadalipour, A., Rashidy-Pour, A., Vafaei, A. A., Miladi-Gorji, H., & Alizadeh, M. (2017). Low- and high-intensity treadmill exercise attenuates chronic morphine-induced anxiogenesis and memory impairment but not reductions in hippocampal BDNF in female rats. *Brain Research, 1663*, 20–28. https://doi.org/10.1016/j.brainres.2017.02.024

Gökçe, E., Güneş, E., & Nalçaci, E. (2019). Effect of exercise on major depressive disorder and schizophrenia: A BDNF focused approach. *Noro Psikiyatri Arsivi, 56*(4), 302–310. https://doi.org/10.29399/npa.23369

Golsorkhdan, S. A., Boroujeni, M. E., Aliaghaei, A., Abdollahifar, M. A., Ramezanpour, A., Nejatbakhsh, R., Anarkooli, I. J., Barfi, E., & Fridoni, M. J. (2020). Methamphetamine administration impairs behavior, memory and underlying signaling pathways in the hippocampus. *Behavioural Brain Research, 379*, Article 112300. https://doi.org/10.1016/j.bbr.2019.112300

Kilciksiz, C. M., Keefe, R., Benoit, J., Öngür, D., & Torous, J. (2020). Verbal memory measurement towards digital perspectives in first-episode psychosis: A review. *Schizophrenia Research. Cognition, 21*, Article 100177. https://doi.org/10.1016/j.scog.2020.100177

Kujach, S., Byun, K., Hyodo, K., Suwabe, K., Fukuie, T., Laskowski, R., Dan, I., & Soya, H. (2018). A transferable high-intensity intermittent exercise improves executive performance in association with dorsolateral prefrontal activation in young adults. *NeuroImage, 169*, 117–125. https://doi.org/10.1016/j.neuroimage.2017.12.003

Lin, T. W., Tsai, S. F., & Kuo, Y. M. (2018). Physical exercise enhances neuroplasticity and delays Alzheimer's disease. *Brain Plasticity, 4*(1), 95–110. https://doi.org/10.3233/BPL-180073

Long, J. D., Liu, Y., Jiao, D. L., Wang, Y. J., Zan, G. Y., Ju, Y. Y., Zhao, M., & Liu, J. G. (2017). The neuroprotective effect of memantine on methamphetamine-induced cognitive deficits. *Behavioural Brain Research, 323*, 133–140. https://doi.org/10.1016/j.bbr.2017.01.042

Luo, W., Hong, H., Wang, X., McGoogan, J. M., Rou, K., & Wu, Z. (2018). Synthetic drug use and HIV infection among men who have sex with men in China: A sixteen-city, cross-sectional survey. *PLOS ONE, 13*(7), Article e0200816. https://doi.org/10.1371/journal.pone.0200816

Ma, C. L., Ma, X. T., Wang, J. J., Liu, H., Chen, Y. F., & Yang, Y. (2017). Physical exercise induces hippocampal neurogenesis and prevents cognitive decline. *Behavioural Brain Research, 317*, 332–339. https://doi.org/10.1016/j.bbr.2016.09.067

Mackay, C. P., Kuys, S. S., & Brauer, S. G. (2017). The effect of aerobic exercise on brain-derived neurotrophic factor in people with neurological disorders: A systematic review and meta-analysis. *Neural Plasticity, 2017*, Article 4716197. https://www.ncbi.nlm.nih.gov/pmc/articles/PMC5625797/

McDonald, C. R., Leyden, K. M., Hagler, D. J., Kucukboyaci, N. E., Kemmotsu, N., Tecoma, E. S., & Iragui, V. J. (2014). White matter microstructure complements morphometry for predicting verbal memory in epilepsy. *Cortex, 58*, 139–150. https://doi.org/10.1016/j.cortex.2014.05.014

Meng, H. J., Zhang, L. L., Luo, S. S., Cao, N., Zhang, J., & Pi, Y. L. (2020). Modulation of hand motor skill performance induced by motor practice combined with matched or mismatched hand posture motor imagery. *Physiology & Behavior, 225*, Article 113084. https://doi.org/10.1016/j.physbeh.2020.113084

Mizoguchi, H., & Yamada, K. (2019). Methamphetamine use causes cognitive impairment and altered decision-making. *Neurochemistry International, 124*, 106–113. https://doi.org/10.1016/j.neuint.2018.12.019

Nouchi, R., Taki, Y., Takeuchi, H., Sekiguchi, A., Hashizume, H., Nozawa, T., Nouchi, H., & Kawashima, R. (2014). Four weeks of combination exercise training improved executive functions, episodic memory, and processing speed in healthy elderly people: Evidence from a randomized controlled trial. *Age (Dordrecht, Netherlands), 36*(2), 787–799. https://doi.org/10.1007/s11357-013-9588-x

Ólafsdóttir, H. F., Bush, D., & Barry, C. (2018). The role of hippocampal replay in memory and planning. *Current Biology, 28*(1), R37–R50. https://doi.org/10.1016/j.cub.2017.10.073

Panenka, W. J., Procyshyn, R. M., Lecomte, T., MacEwan, G. W., Flynn, S. W., Honer, W. G., & Barr, A. M. (2013). Methamphetamine use: A comprehensive review of molecular, preclinical and clinical findings. *Drug and Alcohol Dependence, 129*(3), 167–179. https://doi.org/10.1016/j.drugalcdep.2012.11.016

Pietrelli, A., Matkovic, L., Vacotto, M., Lopez-Costa, J. J., Basso, N., & Brusco, A. (2018). Aerobic exercise upregulates the BDNF-serotonin systems and improves the cognitive function in rats. *Neurobiology of Learning and Memory, 155*, 528–542. https://doi.org/10.1016/j.nlm.2018.05.007

Podolski, N., Brixius, K., Predel, H. G., & Brinkmann, C. (2017). Effects of regular physical activity on the cognitive performance of type 2 diabetic patients: A systematic review. *Metabolic Syndrome and Related Disorders, 15*(10), 481–493. https://doi.org/10.1089/met.2017.0120

Potvin, S., Pelletier, J., Grot, S., Hebert, C., Barr, A. M., & Lecomte, T. (2018). Cognitive deficits in individuals with methamphetamine use disorder: A meta-analysis. *Addictive Behaviors, 80*, 154–160. https://doi.org/10.1016/j.addbeh.2018.01.021

Prakash, M. D., Tangalakis, K., Antonipillai, J., Stojanovska, L., Nurgali, K., & Apostolopoulos, V. (2017). Methamphetamine: Effects on the brain, gut and immune system. *Pharmacological Research, 120*, 60–67. https://doi.org/10.1016/j.phrs.2017.03.009

Proebstl, L., Krause, D., Kamp, F., Hager, L., Manz, K., Schacht-Jablonowsky, M., Straif, M., Riebschläger, M., Neumann, S., Schreiber, A., Soyka, M., & Koller, G. (2019). Methamphetamine withdrawal and the restoration of cognitive functions—A study over a course of 6 months abstinence. *Psychiatry Research, 281*, Article 112599. https://doi.org/10.1016/j.psychres.2019.112599

Rendeiro, C., & Rhodes, J. S. (2018). A new perspective of the hippocampus in the origin of exercise–brain interactions. *Brain Structure & Function, 223*(6), 2527–2545. https://link.springer.com/article/10.1007%2Fs00429-018-1665-6

Shuai, L., Daley, D., Wang, Y. F., Zhang, J. S., Kong, Y. T., Tan, X., & Ji, N. (2017). Executive function training for children with attention deficit hyperactivity disorder. *Chinese Medical Journal, 130*(5), 549–558. https://doi.org/10.4103/0366-6999.200541

United Nations Office on Drugs and Crime. (2018). *World drug report 2018*. https://www.unodc.org/wdr2018

Walsh, J. J., & Tschakovsky, M. E. (2018). Exercise and circulating BDNF: Mechanisms of release and implications for the design of exercise interventions. *Applied Physiology, Nutrition, and Metabolism, 43*(11), 1095–1104. https://doi.org/10.1139/apnm-2018-0192

Wilke, J., Giesche, F., Klier, K., Vogt, L., Herrmann, E., & Banzer, W. (2019). Acute effects of resistance exercise on cognitive function in healthy adults: A systematic review with multilevel meta-analysis. *Sports Medicine, 49*(6), 905–916. https://link.springer.com/article/10.1007%2Fs40279-019-01085-x

Zhang, Y., Sun, Y., Yu, Z., Sun, Y., Chang, X., Lu, L., Chang, S., & Shi, J. (2020). Risk factors and an early prediction model for persistent methamphetamine-related psychiatric symptoms. *Addiction Biology, 25*(1), Article e12709. https://doi.org/10.1111/adb.12709

Zhang, Z., He, L., Huang, S., Fan, L., Li, Y., Li, P., Zhang, J., Liu, J., & Yang, R. (2018). Alteration of brain structure with long-term abstinence of methamphetamine by voxel-based morphometry. *Frontiers in Psychiatry, 9*, Article 722. https://doi.org/10.3389/fpsyt.2018.00722

Zhao, E., Tranovich, M. J., DeAngelo, R., Kontos, A. P., & Wright, V. J. (2016). Chronic exercise preserves brain function in masters athletes when compared to sedentary counterparts. *The Physician and Sportsmedicine, 44*(1), 8–13. https://doi.org/10.1080/00913847.2016.1103641

Zhou, Y., Zhao, M., Zhou, C., & Li, R. (2016). Sex differences in drug addiction and response to exercise intervention: From human to animal studies. *Frontiers in Neuroendocrinology, 40*, 24–41. https://doi.org/10.1016/j.yfrne.2015.07.001

10

Mobile-Application-Based Interventions for Patients with Hypertension and Ischemic Heart Disease

Jin Yi CHOI[1] • Heejung CHOI[2] • GyeongAe SEOMUN[3] • Eun Jung KIM[4]*

ABSTRACT

Background: Hypertension and ischemic heart disease are major causes of adult mortality. Related interventions to manage these conditions are important to implement during long, symptom-free periods. The recent proliferation of smartphones has spawned numerous health interventions that rely on mobile applications.

Purpose: This systematic review was designed to summarize and analyze research on interventions using mobile applications for patients with hypertension and ischemic heart disease.

Methods: We searched for related studies published from January 2006 to August 2017 on MEDLINE, EMBASE, CINAHL, and three Korean databases. Seventeen studies were identified and evaluated against eligibility criteria that included a focus on patients with hypertension or ischemic heart disease and a discussion of the detailed effects of a mobile-app-based intervention. All of the identified studies were evaluated qualitatively using a methodology checklist.

Results: Twelve of the 17 studies were deemed as of acceptable quality according to the Scottish Intercollegiate Guideline Network quality assessment. According to the National Institutes of Health quality assessment tool, one article was of fair quality and four articles were of poor quality. Monitoring, education, and reminders were identified as application interventions. The effects of the app interventions were analyzed according to physiological factors, cognitive and behavioral factors, and psychological factors. Of the seven studies that measured blood pressure in patients with hypertension, five studies reported that the app-based interventions reduced blood pressure. Two of three studies showed a significant decrease of body mass index in patients with ischemic heart disease after the app-based interventions compared to the control group. Five of seven studies reported a significant change in medication adherence. Several studies showed different outcomes according to the disease, but the limited number of eligible studies was insufficient to demonstrate a conclusive effect.

Conclusions: To ensure the long-term effects of mobile-application-based interventions, healthcare professionals should consider the functions of mobile applications. Moreover, because the focus of these interventions may differ based on the nature of the disease, it is recommended that the composition of interventions be tailored to the specific disease.

KEY WORDS:
mobile applications, hypertension, myocardial ischemia, systematic review.

Introduction

Cardiovascular disease is the leading cause of death among adults, contributing to about 31% of all deaths annually worldwide (World Health Organization, 2017). High blood pressure (BP) is the leading cause and risk factor of cardiovascular disease (Reboussin et al., 2018). Patients with ischemic heart disease (IHD) or hypertension experience longer symptom-free periods than symptomatic periods. Older male adults show particularly decreased awareness, self-management, and treatment compliance (Joseph et al., 2016). Self-management is essential to surviving the symptom-free period (Barnason et al., 2017; Souffront et al., 2016). Most patients with IHD or hypertension use medical services until their condition becomes severe and often have long intervals between visits. Patients with hypertension generally have high BP and high low-density lipoprotein (LDL) cholesterol and remain overweight or obese because they lack awareness of early symptoms and self-management techniques (Campbell et al., 2018; Souffront et al., 2016), such as BP and symptom monitoring and various lifestyle changes. Patients must be motivated to continue self-management (Reboussin et al., 2018), indicating the need for strategies to enhance participation and motivation.

Smartphone users have proliferated since 2007. In 2019, smartphone users were estimated to exceed 3.2 billion globally or approximately one third of the global population (Statista, 2019). Concomitant with this increase has been an increase in

[1]*PhD, RN, Assistant Professor, Department of Nursing, Konkuk University, Chungju, ROK* • [2]*PhD, RN, Professor, Department of Nursing, Konkuk University, Chungju, ROK* • [3]*PhD, RN, Professor, College of Nursing, Korea University, Seoul, ROK* • [4]*PhD, RN, Assistant Professor, Department of Nursing, Dongyang University, Yeongju, ROK.*

the number of health-related applications (apps). By 2018, around 50% of the 3.4 billion smartphone and tablet users were estimated to have downloaded health-related apps (Innovatemedtec, 2018).

Health-related mobile apps may promote self-management of chronic disease (Fu et al., 2017; Machado et al., 2016; Stuckey et al., 2017; Zhao et al., 2016). To be effective, health-related apps must contain accurate information that is developed and supervised by healthcare professionals (HCPs; Zhao et al., 2016). These apps can be used for numerous purposes, including the management of data and time, health records, and consultations; the reinforcement of self-monitoring and medication taking; data collection; clinical decision-making; patient monitoring; and education (Ventola, 2014). These apps help users save time and money by reducing the number of meetings between HCPs and patients and facilitate symptom-based decision-making by allowing HCPs to check on patient status information continually using user-entered data. Moreover, these apps enable interactive digital interventions to improve the treatment participation of patients (J. Lee et al., 2016; Ventola, 2014). Although self-management support via mobile apps, particularly those that rely on social networks and short message services (SMS), do raise concerns (Johnson et al., 2016), they provide solutions through personalized access.

Aim

Systematic literature reviews have been conducted on the topics of mobile-app-based interventions for mental health (Zhao et al., 2016), lower back pain (Machado et al., 2016), physical activities (Stuckey et al., 2017), diabetes (Brzan et al., 2016; Fu et al., 2017), and cardiovascular disease (Xie et al., 2017). However, the latter literature review study focused only on Chinese research and on patients with stroke, hypertension, or coronary artery disease. Therefore, this study was developed to contribute to evidence-based nursing by analyzing the contents and effects of mobile-app-based interventions in patients with hypertension or IHD in studies conducted in Korea or in other countries.

Methods

Eligibility Criteria

The review protocol was predefined according the Population, Intervention, Comparison, and Outcome framework using the PRISMA checklist. In this review, the population was limited to adult patients (≥ 18 years old) with hypertension or IHD; the interventions were mobile-app-based self-management apps accessed via smartphone or tablet platforms; the comparison was to a control intervention or no comparison; and the outcomes were physiological factors (e.g., BP, body mass index [BMI], and LDL), cognitive and behavioral factors (e.g., medication adherence, self-monitoring, physical activities, smoking cessation), psychological factors (e.g., quality of life [QoL], self-efficacy, stress), and satisfaction and acceptance of app. The exclusion criteria were articles that were not original articles (e.g., reviews, commentaries, or notes), studies conducted on nonhumans, studies not written in Korean or English, and qualitative studies.

Data Sources and Search Methods

MEDLINE, EMBASE, and CINAHL, three databases that met the Scottish Intercollegiate Guideline Network (SIGN) guidelines for literature searches, were searched for English language articles (SIGN, 2018). The search period was set for January 1, 2006, to August 31, 2017, and the keywords including "mobile app," "smartphone," "cell phone," "mobile phone," 'cellular phone," "portable app," "mobile technology," and "app" with "hypertension" and "myocardial ischemia" were applied in cross-searches of each of the databases to obtain optimal results. KoreaMed, Korea Education and Research Information Service, and Research Information Sharing Service were searched for Korean language articles using the terms "smartphone," "mobile phone," "SMS," "application," and "app." Given the sensitivity and specificity of the search in these databases, terms were not cross-searched with "hypertension," "myocardial ischemia," or "heart muscle ischemia," and no limits were set. All of the identified articles were extracted manually.

Study Selection

Data collection and screening were conducted independently by two researchers with over 3 years of clinical experience each. When their opinions conflicted, a third researcher joined the discussion until a consensus was reached.

Quality Assessment

Quality evaluations were performed on randomized controlled trials (RCTs) and nonrandomized controlled trials (NRCTs) using the SIGN study design and methodology algorithm (Shea et al., 2007). The other studies were evaluated by the U.S. National Institutes of Health quality tools (National Institutes of Health, 2018). Two researchers performed this evaluation, and their results were compared, with disagreements resolved via discussion (Shea et al., 2007; SIGN, 2018). Interventions and data collection conducted via an app (without direct contact with researchers) were considered blind, even when blinding was not described.

Results

Of the 3,570 articles (international: 574, Korean: 2,996) retrieved, 1,356 were excluded as duplicates, and a further 2,110 were excluded for not meeting the inclusion criteria. After reviewing the full texts of the remaining 104 articles, 87 were excluded for not meeting the eligibility criteria (Figure 1).

Study Characteristics

Seventeen articles were analyzed, nine of which were RCTs. The SIGN quality assessment revealed that 12 articles were acceptable (rating of at least 1+; Table 1). In terms of the National

Figure 1
Flow Diagram of the Study

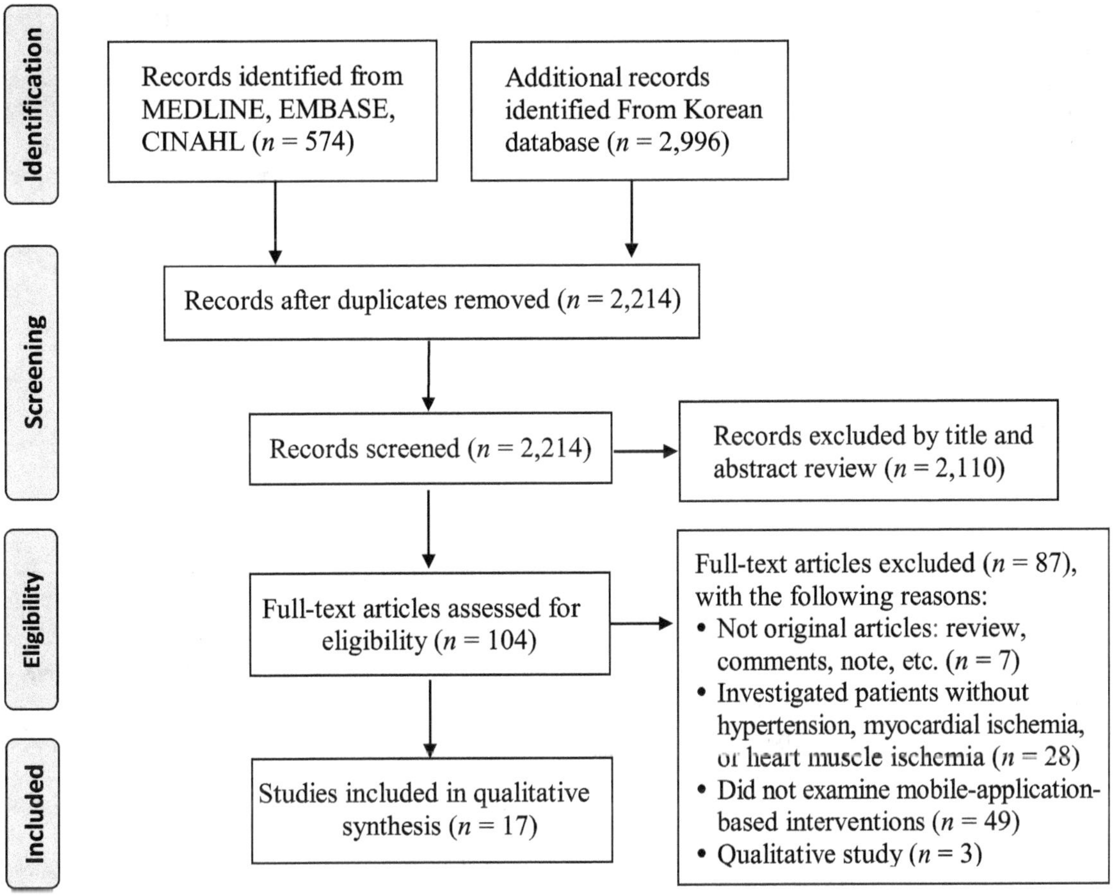

Institutes of Health quality assessment, one article was identified as of fair quality and four articles were identified as of poor quality (see Table 2). Eight of the articles examined patients with hypertension (only hypertension, n = 4; hypertension and other disorders, n = 4), and nine examined patients with IHD (only IHD, n = 7; IHD and others, n = 2). The mean age of the participants in these articles ranged between 47.5 and 73.8 years.

App Interventions

Interventions were classified by actual application, intervention duration, and app function as "monitoring," "education," and "reminders" (Table 3). The apps monitored physiological measurements, symptoms, and performance status; delivered educational content; and provided reminders for medication and physiological measurements. Interventions ranged from 3 weeks to 12 months, with six articles using an intervention duration of 6 months and five articles using an intervention duration of 3 months (Table 3).

Monitoring

The apps used various methods of data sharing and feedback, depending on the data input method and level of HCP involvement in monitoring. The data input methods were manual or automatic, and input data included BP, heart rate, body weight, blood glucose, step count, physical activity, medication intake, symptoms, QoL, stress, smoking status, diet, and laboratory data. The scope of data sharing included the patient, HCP, data centers (platforms or portals), and family members. The feedback types included no feedback, automatic feedback generated by app or data center algorithms, and HCP feedback. In one article, data were selectively transferred to the HCP via either an algorithm or a central data center. HCP feedback could be delivered via SMS, telephone, or face-to-face (Table 3).

Education

The educational content included information on the disease, BP measurement methods, medications, diet, exercise, smoking cessation, weight control, and overall lifestyle patterns. This content was delivered mainly in written form. Most apps had some educational content. One app even provided tailored educational content based on user-inputted data and delivered it via SMS (Table 3).

Reminders

Reminders usually focused on medication, monitoring, or lifestyle modification and were delivered via the app, SMS, e-mail, or phone call (Table 3).

Table 1

Methodological Quality Parameters of RCTs and NRCTs

Author (Year)/Country	Study Design	Level of Evidence	Random Sequence Generation (Selection Bias)	Allocation Concealment (Selection Bias)
Blasco et al. (2012)/ Spain	RCT	1+	Yes	Cannot say
Lee et al. (2013)/ South Korea	NRCT	1+	Cannot say	Cannot say
Davidson et al. (2015)/ United States	RCT	1+	Cannot say	No
Karhula et al. (2015)/ Finland	RCT	2+	Yes	Yes
Martin et al. (2015)/ United States	RCT	2+	Yes	Yes
Albini et al. (2016)/ Italy	NRCT	1+	No	Cannot say
Bloss et al. (2016)/ United States	RCT	1+	Cannot say	No
Johnston et al. (2016)/ Sweden	RCT	1+	Cannot say	No
Mertens et al. (2016)/ Germany	RCT	1+	Cannot say	Cannot say
Or & Tao (2016)/ Hong Kong	RCT	2+	Yes	Yes
Wolf et al. (2016)/ Sweden	NRCT	1+	No	Cannot say
Widmer et al. (2017)/ United States	RCT	2+	Yes	Yes

Note. RCT = randomized controlled trial; NRCT = nonrandomized controlled trial; Cannot say = mentioned but not clear.

Effectiveness of App Interventions

The effectiveness of the intervention was evaluated in terms of physiological factors, cognitive and behavioral factors, and psychological factors. Studies also measured user satisfaction and acceptance of the app/device (Tables 4 and 5).

Physiological Factors

BP

Thirteen articles (seven RCTs, two NRCTs, and four before/after studies) measured BP. Seven and six focused on patients with hypertension and IHD, respectively. Of the former, five (two RCTs, one NRCT, two before/after studies) had positive effects on BP. One RCT reported that the mean change in systolic BP (SBP) and diastolic BP (DBP) decreased significantly more in the intervention group than the control group from baseline to 1 month (SBP −16.7 mm Hg, $p < .001$; DBP −8.0 mm Hg, $p < .001$), 2 months (SBP −10.3 mm Hg; DBP −6.6 mm Hg, $p = .028$), and 3 months (SBP −13.0 mm Hg, $p = .043$; DBP −5.7 mm Hg) after the intervention (Or & Tao, 2016). The other RCT reported significantly reduced mean SBP and DBP in the intervention group compared with controls across all time points ($p < .001$), and the proportion of intervention participants that reached the BP target (<140/90 mm Hg) was significantly greater compared with controls after 1 month (70.6% vs. 15.8%; $p = .001$), 3 months (94.4% vs. 55.0%, $p = .009$), and 6 months (94.4% vs. 41.2%, $p = .003$; Davidson et al., 2015). One NRCT reported significant changes in BP compared with controls and an increase in the proportion of participants that reached the BP target (<149/90 mm Hg) after 6 months (72.3% vs. 40.0%, $p < .0001$; Albini et al., 2016). Two before/after studies reported significant changes in mean SBP from baseline to 1 month (preintervention −7 mm Hg, $p = .031$), 4 months (after intervention −8 mm Hg, $p = .004$), and 7 months (follow-up −9 mm Hg, $p = .006$; Patel et al., 2013) as well as decreased mean SBP and DBP between baseline and 8 weeks (SBP −7 mm Hg, $p = .008$ and DBP −4.9 mm Hg, $p = .002$; Bengtsson et al., 2016). In these studies, the users were able to immediately identify trends in BP (Albini et al., 2016; Bengtsson et al., 2016; Davidson et al., 2015; Or & Tao, 2016) or medication adherence (Patel et al., 2013). Two articles with apps that were designed to enable participants to immediately identify BP trends (Bloss et al., 2016) or medication adherence (Anglada-Martinez et al., 2016) did not identify a positive impact on BP.

Of the six articles (four RCTs, one NRCT, one before/after study) that focused on patients with IHD, two (one RCT, one NRCT) reported positive changes in submaximal rate pressure product (exercise capacity) after 12 weeks (−28.24 vs. −16.21, $p = .03$; Y. H. Lee et al., 2013) and the proportion of participants that reached a BP target (<149/90 mm Hg) after 12 months (62.1% vs. 42.9%, $p < .012$; Blasco et al., 2012). However, these studies reported no group differences in SBP or DBP changes. Both of these studies included interventions featuring monitoring feedback from HCPs. However, another article that used this feedback did not identify a positive impact on BP (Karhula et al., 2015).

BMI

BMI was assessed in three RCTs (Blasco et al., 2012; Johnston et al., 2016; Widmer et al., 2017). In the two RCTs that focused on IHD, BMI decreased significantly more in patients than in controls after 3 months (1.6 vs. 0.3, $p = .01$; Widmer et al.,

Blinding of Participants (Performance Bias)	Blinding of Personnel (Performance Bias)	Blinding of Outcome Assessors to Therapy (Detection Bias)	Intra- and/or Interrater Reliability Outcomes	Dropout Rate (%)	Intention to Treat Analysis
Cannot say	Yes	Yes	Yes	18.1	Yes
Cannot say	Cannot say	Cannot say	Yes	No comment	Cannot say
No	No	Yes	Yes	No comment	Does not apply
Cannot say	No	Yes	Yes	9.2	Yes
No	Cannot say	Yes	Yes	0	Yes
Cannot say	Cannot say	Cannot say	Yes	12.9	No
Yes	No	No	Yes	No comment	No
No	Yes	Yes	Yes	6.8	No
No	No	No	Yes	No comment	Does not apply
No	Cannot say	Yes	Yes	12.1	Yes
Cannot say	Cannot say	Cannot say	Yes	0	Does not apply
No	Yes	Yes	Yes	8.7	No

2017) and 12 months (−0.37 vs. 0.38, $p = .022$; Blasco et al., 2012). One RCT reported a nonsignificant increase in BMI after 6 months compared with controls (−0.6 vs. −0.5, $p = .366$; Johnston et al., 2016). Participant age, intervention duration, and app components were not shown to affect these results.

LDL

One RCT found a decrease in LDL cholesterol, with LDL cholesterol decreasing significantly more in the app-based intervention group than the e-diary group (−1.8 vs. −1.0, $p = .004$) after 6 months (Johnston et al., 2016). In two other RCTs, LDL cholesterol and/or triglycerides either decreased in both the intervention and control groups or were not compared between these groups (Blasco et al., 2012; Karhula et al., 2015). These interventions lasted for 8 weeks (Karhula et al., 2015), 6 months (Johnston et al., 2016), or 12 months (Blasco et al., 2012).

Cognitive and Behavioral Factors

Medication adherence

Seven articles examined medication adherence. Five of these reported a significant change and provided medication reminders (Anglada-Martinez et al., 2016; Johnston et al., 2016; Mertens et al., 2016; Moorhead et al., 2017; Patel et al., 2013). In one RCT, patients receiving SMS reminders and tailored education showed a lower nonadherence rate compared to patients receiving only SMS reminders (16.6 vs. 22.8, $p = .025$; Johnston et al., 2016). Another RCT showed that the use of acoustic pill reminders led to a greater increase in medication adherence during the intervention period than the use of paper diaries ($p < .001$; Mertens et al., 2016). In one before/after study, reminders and weekly motivational messages decreased missed medication days (vs. before the intervention; 3.5 vs. 0.4, $p = .018$) and increased medication adherence (36.5% vs. 55.9%, $p < .001$; Anglada-Martinez et al., 2016). One article reported that the mean (*SD*) medication adherence for antihypertensive drugs increased significantly while using app (0.58 [0.20]) both compared with baseline (0.54 [0.27]) and after the intervention (0.46 [0.31]; $F = 6.4$, $df = 2$, $p = .003$; Patel et al., 2013). One study that examined an app for monitoring ingestion of sensor-enabled medicines found that medication adherence was higher when patients saw a reminder than when they did not (75% [$SD = 18\%$] vs. 59% [$SD = 24\%$]) and that this effect was more pronounced in participants with lower medication adherence (Moorhead et al., 2017). HCP recommendations were found to have no effect on medication adherence (Blasco et al., 2012).

BP monitoring

Two RCTs examined self-monitoring frequency, including BP measurement. In one RCT, participants who input daily BP data into the app and received medication reminders showed significantly greater adherence to daily BP monitoring compared to participants who recorded data on paper ($p = .033$). Moreover, patients with hypertension showed stronger adherence than patients with other diseases ($p = .036$; Mertens et al., 2016). In the other RCT, BP monitoring frequency was similar in the intervention group (used an app that automatically recorded BP) and the control group (used paper; $p = .460$; Or & Tao, 2016). Finally, a before/after study revealed that BP monitoring decreased to 86% in the first intervention period and 77% in the second (Ammenwerth et al., 2015).

Table 2

Methodological Quality Parameters of Single-Arm Studies

Criteria	Patel et al. (2013)	Ammenwerth et al. (2015)	Bengtsson et al. (2016)	Anglada-Martinez et al. (2016)	Moorhead et al. (2017)
1. Was the study question or objective clearly stated?	Yes	Yes	Yes	Yes	Yes
2. Were eligibility/selection criteria for the study population clearly described?	Yes	Yes	Yes	Yes	Yes
3. Were the participants in the study representative of clinical population of interest?	Yes	Yes	Yes	CD	CD
4. Were all eligible participants enrolled?	Yes	CD	Yes	No	CD
5. Was the sample size sufficiently large?	Yes	No	Yes	No	CD
6. Was the intervention clearly described?	Yes	Yes	Yes	Yes	CD
7. Were the outcome measures clearly defined, valid, and reliable?	CD	CD	Yes	CD	Yes
8. Were the outcome assessors blinded to the participants' exposures/interventions?	CD	NR	CD	NR	Yes
9. Was the loss to follow-up after baseline 20% or less?	Yes	Yes	Yes	No	NA
10. Did the statistical methods examine changes in outcome measures from before to after the intervention? Were statistical tests done that provided *p* values for the pre-to-post changes?	Yes	CD	Yes	Yes	Yes
11. Were outcome measures of interest taken multiple times before the intervention and multiple times after the intervention?	No	Yes	No	No	Yes
12. If the intervention was conducted at a group level, did the statistical analysis take into account the use of individual-level data to determine effects at the group level?	NA	NA	NA	NA	NA
Quality rating (good, fair, or poor)	Fair	Poor	Poor[a]	Poor	Poor[b]

Note. CD = cannot determine; NR = not reported; NA = not applicable.
[a]White coat effect: Pretest blood pressure check was performed at clinic by physician or nurse, and posttest blood pressure check was performed at home.
[b]The definition of seeing the reminder used in this study was imprecise.

Physical activity

Five studies (four RCTs, one before/after study) assessed step counts (Ammenwerth et al., 2015; Martin et al., 2015) and physical activity (Blasco et al., 2012; Johnston et al., 2016; Widmer et al., 2017). In one RCT, the intervention group (provided a visible activity tracker and coaching messages informed by real-time activity) showed an increase in number of daily steps compared to those provided with a visible activity tracker only ($p < .001$) and those provided with nothing ($p < .001$; Martin et al., 2015). Three RCTs using, respectively, interventions with individualized automatic feedback (Johnston et al., 2016), automatic feedback for patient-entered values (Widmer et al., 2017), and feedback from HCP reviews (Blasco et al., 2012) reported no group differences in activity change. In addition, in one before/after study, the rate of achieving 3,000 steps per day decreased to 86% in the first intervention period and 73% in the second (Ammenwerth et al., 2015).

Smoking cessation

Three RCTs assessed smoking status (Blasco et al., 2012; Johnston et al., 2016; Widmer et al., 2017). Two reported no difference between the intervention and control groups in terms of smoking cessation rate (80% vs. 81%, $p = .964$; Blasco et al., 2012) or in terms of the number of quitters among active smokers (16 of 22 vs. 5 of 12, $p = .139$; Johnston et al., 2016). The remaining RCT did not detail postintervention results (Widmer et al., 2017). All of these articles focused on patients with IHD and provided feedback.

Psychological Factors

QoL, self-efficacy, anxiety, and stress

Seven and two articles assessed QoL and self-efficacy, respectively. Two articles (one RCT, one NRCT) reported increased QoL in an intervention group compared to a standard treatment group (Y. H. Lee et al., 2013; Widmer et al., 2017), whereas one before/after study reported an increase in QoL compared to baseline ($p < .001$; Ammenwerth et al., 2015). In one NRCT, self-efficacy increased more in an intervention group than in a standard treatment group ($p = .011$; Wolf et al., 2016), whereas in one RCT, no group difference was found (Bloss et al., 2016). Anxiety and stress were assessed in two articles, but neither showed significant changes (Blasco et al., 2012; Widmer et al., 2017). These articles had no similarities in terms of the duration or components of their respective interventions.

Satisfaction With and Acceptance of the App

Ten of the articles assessed user satisfaction and acceptance of the app/device. Acceptance and satisfaction rates were over 70% in five of the articles (Ammenwerth et al., 2015; Blasco et al., 2012; Davidson et al., 2015; Johnston et al., 2016; Patel et al., 2013). Two articles reported mean (*SD*) app satisfaction scores of 7.2 (2.7) out of 10 (Anglada-Martinez et al., 2016), 4.0 out of 5.0 for an activity tracker, and 3.8 out of 5.0 for a text message (Martin et al., 2015). In one study, technical affinity (i.e., positive attitude, excitement, and trust toward technology) was higher after an app-based intervention than after a paper-diary intervention ($p = .002$; Mertens et al., 2016). However, the average app usage rate decreased over time (Anglada-Martinez et al., 2016; Wolf et al., 2016).

Discussion

The contents and effectiveness of mobile-app-based interventions for patients with hypertension or IHD were assessed in this article. The app functions included "monitoring," "education," and "reminders," which are similar to those suggested by HCPs ("data provision and education," "patient monitoring," and "time management"; Ventola, 2014). As management during the asymptomatic stages of hypertension and cardiovascular disease is critical, strategies employing medication reminders and BP monitoring have been emphasized (Barnason et al., 2017; Souffront et al., 2016). App data may be shared with patients, family members, central data centers, and HCPs. Sharing data with patients is useful in terms of improving patient motivation, whereas sharing data with HCPs helps them manage patient symptoms and make accurate clinical judgments (J. Lee et al., 2016; Reboussin et al., 2018; Ventola, 2014). Providing data to family members may enhance patient self-management capabilities by promoting emotional support (Shawler et al., 2018). Although SMS and telephones have been used in the self-management of other chronic diseases, patient-centric, personalized feedback has been shown to provide the strongest benefit to intervention effects (Davies et al., 2012; Fukuoka et al.2010; Maher et al., 2014). As feedback has shifted from being delivered primarily by HCPs to being generated by app algorithms, app developers have begun considering data sharing for HCPs and patients as an option for facilitating the economical use of these apps in early symptom management.

Physiological, cognitive–behavioral, and psychological factors as well as acceptance and satisfaction were the primary focuses of this study. App-based interventions were shown to reduce BP only in patients with hypertension. This finding may result from differences in the disease rather than the components or functions of the app-based intervention. Patients with hypertension primarily complain of increased BP, whereas patients with IHD primarily complain of chest pains. Hypertension is a risk factor that is present in the history of most patients with IHD and thus should be targeted for prevention (Agbor-Etang & Setaro, 2015). However, because of differences in interventions and research designs, the precise effects of these interventions are difficult to discern. However, in the articles that identified BP reductions in patients with hypertension, the apps focused on trends in either BP or medication adherence (Albini et al., 2016; Bengtsson et al., 2016; Davidson et al., 2015; Or & Tao, 2016; Patel et al., 2013). These findings are consistent with studies showing that the visualization of self-reported data motivates patients to adhere to treatment (Hallberg et al., 2015; Neubeck et al., 2015). However, Hallberg et al. (2015) suggested that treatment compliance varies with patient ability to understand graphs. This is supported by findings from two studies in which BP levels did not abate despite the use of graphically presented self-report data (Anglada-Martinez et al., 2016; Bloss et al., 2016). Therefore, to motivate patients to follow their treatments, graphs should be easy to understand. Furthermore, using graphs for counseling may improve patient adherence.

Feedback from HCPs was a common component in interventions that improved BP outcomes in patients with IHD (Blasco et al., 2012; Y. H. Lee et al., 2013). Thangada et al. (2018) found that a mobile-app-based intervention containing additional HCP feedback improved BP outcomes and suggested that HCP feedback may help patients understand data trends and promote self-management. Neubeck et al. (2015) further suggested that feedback, including personal goal setting and tailored information, is useful for symptom management. However, Karhula et al. (2015) found that this type of feedback did not have a positive impact on BP. They measured this in terms of BP change, whereas the previous two studies focused on exercise capacity using BP and the achievement rate of BP targets. Thus, researchers should develop tools that more accurately measure intervention effects in patients with IHD who desire to control rather than reduce their BP.

BMI was assessed in three of the studies on patients with IHD (Blasco et al., 2012; Johnston et al., 2016; Widmer et al., 2017). BMI decreased in two studies and remained the same in one study (Johnston et al., 2016). Effective weight control interventions should focus on diet, physical activity, behavior therapy, and emotional support (Ramage et al., 2014). Furthermore,

Table 3

Components of Mobile-Application-Based Interventions for Patients With Hypertension and Ischemic Heart Disease

No.	Authors (Year)	Disease	Application	Duration
1.	Blasco et al. (2012)	ACS	Wireless app	12 months
2.	Lee et al. (2013)	ACS	Wireless monitoring (HeartCall)	4–6 weeks
3.	Patel et al. (2013)	HTN	Pill phone application	10 months (activation phase: 3 months)
4.	Ammenwerth et al. (2015)	ACS	MyCor health diary app	4.5 months
5.	Davidson et al. (2015)	HTN	App, bluetooth-BP monitor	6 months
6.	Karhula et al. (2015)	DM, heart disease	Personal health record app	8 weeks
7.	Martin et al. (2015)	DM, CHD	Fitbug Orb	Phase I: 2–3 weeks Phase II: 4–5 weeks
8.	Albini et al. (2016)	HTN	Misuriamo platform/Eurohypertension app	3 months
9.	Anglada-Martinez et al. (2016)	HTN, dyslipidemia, HF, HIV	Medplan platform/mobile phone app	6 months
10.	Bengtsson et al. (2016)	HTN	Circadian questions	8 weeks
11.	Bloss et al. (2016)	HTN, DM, arrhythmia	Mobile devices+ HealthyCircles	6 months
12.	Johnston et al. (2016)	MI	Web-based app	6 months
13.	Mertens et al. (2016)	ACS or MI	Medication Plan app	3 and 6 months
14.	Or & Tao (2016)	DM, HTN	Tablet computer-based disease self-monitoring system	3 months
15.	Wolf et al. (2016)	ACS	eHealth diary, symptom-tracking tool	6 months
16.	Moorhead et al. (2017)	HTN, DM	App, provider portal	3 months
17.	Widmer et al. (2017)	ACS	App or Web-based portal	3 months

Note. ACS = acute coronary syndrome; app = application; BP = blood pressure; BW = body weight; HbA1c = hemoglobin A1c; HCP = healthcare professional; SMS = short message services; HR = heart rate; HTN = hypertension; Pts = patients; DM = diabetes mellitus; CHD = coronary heart disease; HF = heart failure; MI = myocardial infarction.

Monitoring			Education		Reminder	
Data Entry	Scope of Data Sharing	Type of Feedback	Contents	Method	Purpose	Delivery Type
Manual (BP, BW, cholesterol, glucose, HbA1c)	Provider portal/HCP	Feedback from HCP review	—	—	Recommendations	SMS
Automatic (HR)	Provider portal/HCP	Feedback from HCP review	Risk factors for heart disease, diet, exercise	Face to face	Counseling	Call (once weekly)
Manual (medication taking)	Pts	None	—	—	Medication	App message
Manual (BP, HR, BW, step count, drug intake, glucose)	Provider portal	Automatic feedback	Medication, lifestyle	—	Individual goals	App message (once weekly)
Automatic (BP)	Pts	Automatic feedback	—	—	Medication, BP monitor, motivation	SMS
Manual and (glucose, BW, step count) automatic (BP)	Pts/provider portal/HCP	Feedback from HCP review	Self-management guide	Text	—	—
Automatic (step count, activity time)	Pts	Automatic feedback	Habit formation	App	Positive reinforcement	SMS (3 times/day)
Manual (BP)	Pts/family/ provider portal/HCP	Feedback from HCP review	HTN management	Q&A	Medication/BP measurement	App alarm/e-mail
Manual (medication)	Pts or caregiver/ provider portal/HCP	Feedback from HCP review	Drug information/ lifestyle	App	Medication	App alarm/Weekly motivational messages
Automatic (BP, HR), manual (drug intake)	Pts/provider portal/HCP	Automatic feedback	Well-being, symptoms, lifestyle, medication	Questions	Lifestyle change	Weekly motivational messages
Manual (BP, glucose, arrhythmia)	Pts/HCP	Feedback from HCP review	Disease, health behavior	App	Monitoring schedule	e-mail
Manual (drug adherence e-diary)	Pts	Automatic feedback	Drug adherence, e-diary, exercise, BW, smoking	Text	Medication	SMS (twice/ day)
Manual (BP, medication intake)	Pts	None	—	—	Medication	App alarm
Automatic (glucose, BP)	Pts/family	None	Measurement of glucose and BP/ diet, exercise	Video	—	—
Manual (fatigue, symptom) and automatic (activity)	Pts	None	—	—	—	—
Automatic (medication, activity, rest)	Pts, provider portal	None	—	—	Medication	App message
Manual (BP, BW, lipid, glucose)	Pts	Automatic feedback	—	—	—	—

Table 4

The Effects of Mobile-Application-Based Interventions for Patients With Hypertension and Ischemic Heart Disease in RCTs and NRCTs

No.	Authors (Year)/ Country	Study Design	Population	Intervention	Comparator
1.	Blasco et al. (2012)/ Spain	RCT	ACS 203 EG: 102 (DM 30, 60.6 yr, M/F 83/19), CG: 101 (DM 26, 61 yr, M/F 80/21)	Structured questionnaire	Usual care
2.	Lee et al. (2013)/ Korea	NRCT	55 ACS undergoing PCI: EG 26 (54.3 yr, M/F 22/4), CG 29 (57.8 yr, M/F 22/7)	Wireless monitoring (HeartCall)	Usual care
5.	Davidson et al. (2015)/ United States	RCT	HTN EG 18 (47.5 ± 11.8 yr, M/F 7/11) CG 20 (48.5 ± 11.3 yr, M/F 8/12)	Software application, Bluetooth-accessible BP monitor	Standard care
6.	Karhula et al. (2015)/ Finland	RCT	Heart disease 246 (69.1 yr, M/F 178/269, CG/EG 79/190), DM 225 (66.2 yr, M/F 129/250, CG/EG 70/180)	Mobile personal health record app	Standard care
7.	Martin et al. (2015)/ United States	RCT	• Total 48 • Phase I (*n* = 48): unblind 32, blind 16 • Phase II: text 16 (55 ± 8 yr, M/F 8/8, DM 2, CHD 2), no text 16 (58 ± 8 yr, M/F 9/7, DM 5, CHD 5), blind 16	Fitbug Orb	No text
8.	Albiniet al. (2016)/ Italy	NRCT	HTN 691 EG 303 (57.9 ± 11.3 yr, M/F180/123), CG 298 (56.9 ± 11.5 yr, M/F 188/110)	Misuriamo platform/ Eurohypertension app	Educational modules

Outcome				
Measurement Method	Physiological	Cognitive and Behavioral	Psychosocial	Satisfaction and Acceptance of App
• Measurement: baseline, 12 mo • Outcome: BP, BMI, QoL, anxiety, achievement goal (smoking, LDL, HbA1c)	•BP: ND • Achievement for goal (<140/90 mm Hg) in EG vs. CG: in BP (62.1% vs. 42.9%, $p = .012$) • BMI: change of BMI in EG vs. in CG (−0.37 vs. 0.38, $p = .022$) • LDL: ND • Achievement for goal (HbA1c < 7%) (86.4% vs. 54.2%, $p = .018$) among DM	• Medication adherence: ND • Physical activity: ND • Achievement for smoking cessation: ND	• QoL, anxiety: ND	• Adherence to protocol: 89.2 ± 16.0%
• Measurement: baseline, 12 wk • Outcome: QoL, submaximal rate pressure product (RPPsubmax), submaximal rate of perceived exertion (RPEsubmax), metabolic equivalent of the tasks (METs), maximal exercise time (ETmax)	• Change in EG vs. CG: RPPsubmax (−28.24 vs. −16.21 bpm·mm Hg, $p = .013$), RPEsubmax ($p = .018$), METs ($p = .021$), ETmax ($p = .012$)		• QoL change: EG vs. CG (4.8 vs. 0.9, $p = .022$)	
• Measurement: baseline, 1, 3, 6 mo • Outcomes: SBP/DBP, feasibility (retention rates), medication adherence, BP adherence	• BP control: 70.6% of EG vs. 15.8% of CG (<140/90 mm Hg) at 1 mo ($p < .001$). 94.4% of EG vs. 41.2% of CG at 6 mo ($p < .003$)	• Medication adherence: 92 ± 0.09 in EG • BP Adherence (every 3 days): 86.2 ± 6% in EG		• Feasibility: 88.4% in 6 mo
• Measurement: baseline, 8 wk • Primary outcome: QoL, HbA1c among DM pts. • Clinical outcome: BP, BW, waist circumference, lipid • Adherence to the health coaching (duration of coaching call)	• Clinical outcome (SBP, DBP, LDL, BW, waist circumference) of heart disease: ND between EG and CG • Within EG: waist circumference ↓ ($p = .02$), SBP↓ ($p < .001$), LDL ↓ ($p < .001$) • Within CG: LDL↓ ($p < .001$), SBP ↓ ($p < .001$)		• QoL: ND	• Duration of coaching call: heart disease higher than DM ($p = .004$)
• Measurement: baseline, run-in (1 wk), Phase I (app, 2–3 wk), phase II (app + text or no text, 4–5 wk) • Clinical outcome: step count, attainment of goal (10 000 steps/day) • Activity outcome: changes in total daily activity and aerobic time • Satisfaction		Mean change of step count • Phase I: ND • Phase II: text higher than no text (2534, 95% CI [1318, 3750], $p < .001$), blind (3376, 95% CI [1951, 4801], $p < .001$)		• Satisfaction score: for activity tracker 4.0 of 5.0, for text messages 3.8 of 5.0
• Measurement: baseline, 3, 6 mo • Outcome: BP	• Office BP control: 40.0% in CG vs. 72.3% in EG at 6 mo F/U ($p < .0001$) • At same time Home BP control in EG: 87.5%			

(continues)

Table 4

The Effects of Mobile-Application-Based Interventions for Patients With Hypertension and Ischemic Heart Disease in RCTs and NRCTs, Continued

No.	Authors (Year)/ Country	Study Design	Population	Intervention	Comparator
11.	Bloss et al. (2016)/ United States	RCT	EG 75 (56 ± 9 yr, HTN 67, NIDDM 10, IDDM 10, arrhythmia 10) CG 85 (55 ± 9.8 yr, HTN 71, NIDDM 17, IDDM 10, arrhythmia 19)	Mobile devices (BP, blood glucose, ECG) + Healthy Circles	usual care
12.	Johnston et al. (2016)/ Sweden	RCT	MI 186 (58 yr, M/F 150/36) EG 85 (56.8 yr) CG 77 (58.4 yr)	Web-based app	Simplified e-diary without secondary education and medication reminder
13.	Mertens et al. (2016)/ Germany	RCT	ACS or MI 24 (73.8 yr, M/F 12/12)	Medication Plan app	Pen and paper diary
14.	Or & Tao (2016)/ Hong Kong	RCT	EG 33 (HTN 19, DM + HTN 14, 69.3 ± 9.7 yr, M/F 14/19) CG 30 (DM 2, HTN 19, DM + HTN 9,69.7 ± 10.2 yr, M/F 6/14)	Tablet computer-based disease self-monitoring system	Paper diary
15.	Wolf et al. (2016)/ Sweden	NRCT	ACS • CG 105 (61.3 ± 8.9 yr, M/F 72/32) • PCC + eHealth 37 (59.8 ± 10.1 yr, M/F 30/7) • PCC no eHealth 57 (60.9 ± 8.7 yr, M/F 41)	eHealth diary + symptom-tracking tool	Drug adherence e-diary without the secondary prevention
17.	Widmer et al. (2017)/ United States	RCT	ACS 71 EG (CG + DHI) 37 (62.5 ± 10.7 yr, M/F 29/8), CG 34 (63.6 ± 10.9 yr, M/F 29/10)	App or Web-based portal	Standard Phase II

Note. RCT = randomized controlled trial; NRCT = nonrandomized controlled trial; ACS = acute coronary syndrome; EG = intervention group; CG = control group; BP = blood pressure; BMI = body mass index; QoL = quality of life; LDL =low-density lipoprotein; HbA1c = hemoglobin A1c; ND = no differences; DM = diabetes mellitus; PCI = percutaneous coronary intervention; M = male; F = female; yr = year; wk = week; mo = month; SBP = systolic blood pressure; DBP = diastolic blood pressure; F/U = follow-up; HTN = hypertension; NIDDM=non-insulin-dependent diabetes mellitus; IDDM=insulin dependent diabetes mellitus; ER = emergency room; HI = health insurance; pt = patient; MI = myocardial infarction; FBS = fasting blood glucose; ↓ means decreased.

Outcome				
Measurement Method	**Physiological**	**Cognitive and Behavioral**	**Psychosocial**	**Satisfaction and Acceptance of App**
• Measurement: baseline, 3 mo, 6 mo • Outcomes: claims data ($) (office visits, ER visits, inpatient stays, all visits), healthcare resource utilization (HI claims, hospital visits), health self-management (Health Locus of Control, health self-efficacy, pts activation)	• SBP in HTN, HbA1c in DM: ND • DBP in HTN: 3.6 mm Hg in EG (p = .035), 6.1 mm Hg in CG (p = .004), ND between groups		• Self-efficacy or pts activation: ND	
• Measurement: 1st (baseline), 2nd (6–10 wk), 3rd (6 mo) visit • Outcome: Pt self-reported drug adherence in e-diary (nonadherence score), smoking, BMI, LDL, SBP, exercise, QoL, Self-reported device usability score, pts satisfaction (EG), medication adherence	• SBP, BMI: ND • LDL: EG lower than CG (−1.8 vs. −1.0, p = .004)	• Nonadherence score: EG lower than CG (16.6 vs. 22.8, p = .025) • Smoking, physical activity: ND	• QoL: ND	• Device usability score: EG higher than CG at end (87.3 vs. 78.1, p = .001) • pts satisfaction: 97.5% in EG
• Measurement: 3 visit (initial, intervention, pen and paper phase) • Outcome: medication adherence, vital sign monitoring adherence, affinity for technology (person's positive attitude, excitement, trust toward technology)		• Medication adherence: app than paper (F = 27.4, df = 1, p < .001) • Documentation of BP (app than paper; F = 361.3, df = 1, p = .033)		• Technical affinity: tablet vs. paper (p = .002)
• Measurement: baseline, 1 mo, 2 mo, 3 mo • Outcome: SBP, DBP, FBS, HbA1c, DM and HTN knowledge, frequency of self-monitoring (glucose, BP by app in EG, records in log book in CG)	• SBP in HTN, HTN + DM: ↓ from baseline to 1 mo (p < .001) to 3 mo (p = .043) • DBP in HTN, HTN + DM: ↓ from baseline to 1 mo (p < .001) to 2 mo (p = .028) to 3 mo (ND) • FBS, HbA1c in DM, HTN + DM: ND	• Frequency of self-monitoring: ND • HTN knowledge: ND		
• Measurement: baseline, 4 wk, 8 wk, 6 mo • Outcome: eHealth Tool Use Patterns, Self-efficacy			• Self-efficacy: PCC + eHealth higher than CG (p = .011)	• Use time of eHealth tool: 38 ± 33 times (range 1–118) during first 8 wk, 64 ± 104 times (range 1–597) over 6-mo period
• Measurement: baseline, 3 mo, 6 mo • Outcome (baseline, 3 mo): lab (FBS, lipid, glucose), BP, BW, health behavior (diet, physical activity, QoL, stress, smoking), major adverse cardiac event	• BW: −5.1 ± 6.5 vs. −0.8 ± 3.8 kg (EG vs. CG, p = .02) • BMI: −1.6 ± 1.9 vs. −0.3 ± 1.7(EG vs. CG, p = .01) • Waist circumference: −8.3 ± 3.1 vs. 1.1 ± 4.1 cm (EG vs. CG; p = .01) • SBP, DBP, glucose, lipids, major adverse cardiac event: ND	• Min of physical activity: ND • Smoking: cannot identify	• QoL: 7.2 ± 1.3 in EG vs. 2.4 ± 1.6 in CG (p = .03) • Stress: ND	

Table 5

The Effects of Mobile-Application-Based Interventions for Patients With Hypertension and Ischemic Heart Disease in Single-Arm Studies

No.	Authors (Year)/ Country	Study Design	Population	Intervention	Comparator
3.	Patel et al. (2013)/ United States	Before/after study	HTN 50 (53.0 ± 8.7 yr)	Pill Phone app	None
4.	Ammenwerth et al. (2015)/ Austria	Before/after study	ACS 25 (63 yr, M/F 25/1)	MyCor health diary app	None
9.	Anglada-Martínez et al. (2016)/ Spain	Before/after study	Total 42 (56 ± 8 yr, HTN 17, dyslipidemia 12, HTN + dyslipidemia 5, HIV 8)	Medplan platform/mobile phone app	None
10.	Bengtsson et al. (2016)/ Sweden	Before/after study	HTN 51 (59.5 yr, M/F 26/24)	Circadian Questions	None
16.	Moorhead et al. (2017)/ United States	Interrupted time series	HTN, DM dose reminder efficacy 57 (58 ± 10.5 yr, M/F 28/29) dose reminder safe 74 (57 ± 9.9 yr, M/F 34/40)	Digital Health	None

Note. HTN = hypertension; BP = blood pressure; pt = patient; SBP = systolic blood pressure; DBP = diastolic blood pressure; ND = no differences; ACS = acute coronary syndrome; yr = year; wk = week; mo = month; M = male; F = female; F/U = follow-up; BW = body weight; HR = heart rate; QoL = quality of life; TG = triglyceride; ↓ means decreased.

	Outcome			
Measurement Method	**Physiological**	**Cognitive and Behavioral**	**Psychosocial**	**Satisfaction and Acceptance of App**
• Measurement: baseline (Visit 1), pre-use (Visit 2), use (Visit 3), off (Visit 4) • Outcome: BP, adherence with HTN medication (pharmacy refill rate), adherence with HTN medication (questionnaire; app during intervention period, Visit 3), satisfaction, pt-specific usage of Pill Phone	• SBP compared with baseline ($F = 4.4$, $p = .007$): ↓ Visit 1 ($p = .031$), ↓ Visit 2 ($p = .004$), ↓ Visit 4 ($p = .006$) • DBP: ND	• Adherence (pharmacy refill rate): Visit 1 = 0.54 ± 0.27, Visit 3 = 0.58 ± 0.20, Visit 4 = 0.46 ± 0.31 ($F = 6.4$, $df = 2$, $p = .003$) • Adherence (questionnaire): Visit 4 higher than Visit 1 ($p < .001$)	-	• satisfaction of medication reminder app at final: 96% • Pt-specific Usage of Pill Phone: ND
• Measurement: baseline, Phase 1 (telemonitoring, 4 wk), 1st F/U (4 wk), Interim phase (12 wk), Phase 2 (Telemonitoring, 2 wk), 2nd F/U • Outcome: system quality, information quality, service quality, user satisfaction, intention to use, net benefit, health diary data (BW, BP, footsteps), QoL	• BP, HR: ND	• Adherence to daily measurements: 86% (Phase 1), 77% (Phase 2) • Step counts (3,000 steps per day): 86% (Phase 1), 73% (Phase 2)	• QoL: pre-5.5, post 6.3 ($p < .001$)	• Device satisfaction: 72% (very or partly confident)
• Measurement: baseline, 3 mo, 6 mo • Outcome: QoL, medication adherence (Simplified Medication Adherence Questionnaire, SMAQ), medication adherence, health outcomes (BP in HTN, cholesterol and TG in dyslipidemia), healthcare resources visit	• SBP/DBP in HTN, HTN+Dyslipidemia: ND • Cholesterol and TG in dyslipidemia: ND	• Adherence: Pharmacy refills: ND • SMAQ: pre 36.5%, post 55.9% ($p < .001$) • Number of days with missing doses: pre 3.5, post 0.4 ($p = .018$)	• QoL: ND	• Satisfaction: satisfaction score:7.2 ± 2.7 in pts, recommend app: 71.4%, wanted to continue: 88.1% • usability: registered in app: overall 58.4%, 4 mo 60.2%, 6 mo 56 6% ($p < .001$)
• Measurement: baseline, 8 wk • Outcome: BP	• Mean SBP/DBP between baseline and 8 wk: SBP 7 mm Hg ↓ ($p = .008$), DBP 4.9 mm Hg ↓ ($p = .002$)			
• Measurement: continuous • Outcome: sensor-enabled medicines ingestion, medication adherence (within 2 hours after the scheduled dose time), dose reminder safe (event of overdoses)		• Mean difference in medication adherence after seeing and not seeing the medication dose reminder: 15.6 ± 15.6% (75 ± 18% vs. 59 ± 24%) • Dose reminder safe: no event		

patients' general characteristics and diseases should be considered. However, some studies (Blasco et al., 2012; Widmer et al., 2017) included weight measurement without education, and even when education was included, the interventions were not multidisciplinary.

In asymptomatic patients with cardiovascular disease, medication is important for preventing disease progression (Kjeldsen et al., 2014). Acknowledging this, several of the articles in this systematic review assessed medication adherence. Five of the articles (Anglada-Martinez et al., 2016; Johnston et al., 2016; Mertens et al., 2016; Moorhead et al., 2017; Patel et al., 2013) investigated apps with medication reminders, and although different measurement methods were used, all five reported significant results. These results are consistent with a previous study (Thakkar et al., 2016). However, medication adherence was higher in patients with IHD than in patients with hypertension. This may be because IHD is more severe than hypertension, as medication adherence is influenced by patient characteristics, disease severity, medication regimen, HCP and healthcare system characteristics, and socioeconomic factors (S. Q. Lee et al., 2018). Although app-based medication reminders are more effective and user-friendly for medication adherence according to cognitive behavioral theory, there may be weakened adherence when used over longer durations, as was previously observed in relation to the acceptance rate of health-related apps (Hincapie et al., 2019). Medication nonadherence is associated with the health system, risk factors of cardiovascular complications, age, therapy complexity, length of medical history, and socioeconomic status (Ho et al., 2009; Bokhour et al., 2006). Thus, factors related to medication adherence should be considered when using reminders to improve adherence (Barnason et al., 2017; S. Q. Lee et al., 2018).

Increased physical activity was found in one of the articles (Martin et al., 2015). Patients in that study were provided with education on habit formation, and positive reinforcement based on the cognitive behavioral model was provided three times per week to help sustain positive behavioral changes. Self-awareness of the management of chronic asymptomatic diseases is generally low, causing physical activity or self-monitoring to decline over time (Ammenwerth et al., 2015; Campbell et al., 2018; Zhao et al., 2016). Thus, strategies and attractive apps must be developed to ensure long-term self-management in patients with hypertension and cardiovascular disease (Brzan et al., 2016; Fu et al., 2017).

Two RCTs for IHD identified no positive effect of app-based interventions on smoking cessation. These interventions lasted for 6 (Johnston et al., 2016) and 12 months (Blasco et al., 2012) and focused on participants with mean ages of 58 (Johnston et al., 2016) and 60.6 years (Blasco et al., 2012). In a previous systematic review, mobile-phone-based interventions may be effective in inducing smoking cessation only after 6 months (Whittaker et al., 2016). The lack of an effect found in this systemic review is likely due to participants being older and having smoked for longer periods of time than the participants of studies covered in the previous review (mean age range: 18.2–44.8 years). Intention to quit and nicotine dependence are strong predictors of successful cessation, and intention to quit among older adults is lower than among younger individuals (Siahpush et al., 2006). A qualitative study found that most elderly smokers, though aware of the health risks of smoking, believed that the damage had already been done and that little benefit would be gained from quitting (Kerr et al., 2006). Thus, smoking cessation strategies tailored to older patients with hypertension or IHD should be implemented.

As for the psychological factors, QoL increased in three of the studies on patients with IHD (Ammenwerth et al., 2015; Y. H. Lee et al., 2013; Widmer et al., 2017). The QoL questionnaires focused on the emotional, social, and physical domains (e.g., chest pain), indicating that physical symptoms as well as psychosocial factors improved over time. Thus, interventions should focus on total relief for patients with IHD and consider using holistic approaches that involve the emotional, social, and physical domains. QoL may be improved through self-management due to monitoring and behavioral change (Johnson et al., 2016; Zhao et al., 2016). Therefore, overall, mobile apps may be effective in improving psychological factors.

Some of the studies found that the acceptance rates of apps were higher than those of paper diaries, although app acceptance rates decreased over time (Anglada-Martinez et al., 2016; Wolf et al., 2016). The decline in app acceptance may reflect users' app-engagement experiences, app technical functionality, ease of app use, and/or app design features (Anderson et al., 2016; Suh et al., 2015). These results suggest that additional strategies to sustain the intervention effects must be developed (Brzan et al., 2016; Fu et al., 2017).

Before 2000, team-based interventions were frequently used to improve self-management (Whelton et al., 2002). Recently, online health communication has rapidly increased as a result of smartphones and the Internet (Innovatemedtec, 2018; Statista, 2019). The effect of interventions that use the Internet or apps may vary based on the reliability of the data and user characteristics (Paige et al., 2017). Therefore, to maintain self-management among patients with hypertension or IHD, apps may be designed to incorporate online meeting functions (based on the user's characteristics or needs), patient-to-patient encouragement or reinforcement, patient-to-HCP online communication, and more-reliable educational content.

This systematic review showed that mobile apps have inconsistent effects on self-management in patients with hypertension and IHD. Similar to studies evaluating mobile apps for other chronic diseases, this inconsistency may result from differences in content, attractiveness, user convenience, suitability of educational content, user characteristics (e.g., culture, age, gender), and intervention duration (Brzan et al., 2016; Fu et al., 2017; Machado et al., 2016; Stuckey et al., 2017; Zhao et al., 2016). Because most of the of app-based interventions revealed diminishing effects over time, strategies such as providing accurate information, attractive reminders, and individualized content are necessary to promote their sustained effectiveness (Brzan et al., 2016; Fu et al., 2017).

Strengths and Limitations

All of the articles in this systematic review study were published in English only. Moreover, some were low-quality, single-arm studies. However, by including all study types regardless of quality, this study offers a broader review of interventions. The findings of this study indicate that interventions should selectively apply app functions based on patient characteristics in order to improve app accessibility, reduce costs, and promote self-management.

Conclusions

Mobile apps may provide an effective means to self-manage hypertension and IHD. Apps may be designed to provide educational content and individualized reinforcement strategies, including self-monitoring, feedback, and reminder functions, to promote long-term self-management. HCPs may use app-collected data to improve the accuracy of decision-making and to promote early symptom management, which will benefit patients who cannot regularly visit the hospital or clinic. Apps may provide an effective tool to improve the self-management efficacy of patients with hypertension or IHD, which will reduce complications and improve survival and QoL.

Author Contributions

Study conception and design: All authors
Data collection: JYC, EJK
Data analysis and interpretation: All authors
Drafting of the article: JYC, EJK
Critical revision of the article: EJK

References

Agbor-Etang, B. B., & Setaro, J. F. (2015). Management of hypertension in patients with ischemic heart disease. *Current Cardiology Reports, 17*(12), 119. https://doi.org/10.1007/s11886-015-0662-0

Albini, F., Liu, X., Torlasco, C., Soranna, D., Faini, A., Ciminaghi, R., Celsi, A., Benedetti, M., Zambon, A., di Rienzo, M., & Parati, G. (2016). An ICT and mobile health integrated approach to optimize patients' education on hypertension and its management by physicians: The patients optimal strategy of treatment(POST) pilot study. *Annual International Conference of the IEEE Engineering in Medicine and Biology Society, 2016*, 517–520. https://doi.org/10.1109/EMBC.2016.7590753

Ammenwerth, E., Woess, S., Baumgartner, C., Fetz, B., van der Heidt, A., Kastner, P., Modre-Osprian, R., Welte, S., & Poelzl, G. (2015). Evaluation of an integrated telemonitoring surveillance system in patients with coronary heart disease. *Methods of Information in Medicine, 54*(5), 388–397. https://doi.org/10.3414/ME15-02-0002

Anderson, K., Burford, O., & Emmerton, L. (2016). Mobile health apps to facilitate self-care: A qualitative study of user experiences. *PLOS ONE, 11*(5), e0156164. https://doi.org/10.1371/journal.pone.0156164

Anglada-Martinez, H., Martin-Conde, M., Rovira-Illamola, M., Sotoca-Momblona, J. M., Sequeira, E., Aragunde, V., Moreno, M. A., Catalan, M., & Codina-Jane, C. (2016). Feasibility and preliminary outcomes of a web and smartphone-based medication self-management platform for chronically ill patients. *Journal of Medical Systems, 40*(4), 99. https://doi.org/10.1007/s10916-016-0456-y

Barnason, S., White-Williams, C., Rossi, L. P., Centeno, M., Crabbe, D. L., Lee, K. S., McCabe, N., Nauser, J., Schulz, P., Stamp, K., & Wood, K., American Heart Association Council on Cardiovascular and Stroke Nursing, Council on Cardiovascular Disease in the Young, Council on Clinical Cardiology, & Stroke Council (2017). Evidence for therapeutic patient education interventions to promote cardiovascular patient self-management: A scientific statement for healthcare professionals from the American Heart Association. *Circulation. Cardiovascular Quality and Outcomes, 10*(6), e000025. https://doi.org/10.1161/HCQ.0000000000000025

Bengtsson, U., Kjellgren, K., Hallberg, I., Lindwall, M., & Taft, C. (2016). Improved blood pressure control using an interactive mobile phone support system. *The Journal of Clinical Hypertension (Greenwich, Conn.), 18*(2), 101–108. https://doi.org/10.1111/jch.12682

Blasco, A., Carmona, M., Fernandez-Lozano, I., Salvador, C. H., Pascual, M., Sagredo, P. G., Somolinos, R., Muñoz, A., García-López, F., Escudier, J. M., Mingo, S., Toquero, J., Moñivas, V., González, M. A., Fragua, J. A., López-Rodríguez, F., Monteagudo, J. L., & Alonso-Pulpón, L. (2012). Evaluation of a telemedicine service for the secondary prevention of coronary artery disease. *Journal of Cardiopulmonary Rehabilitation and Prevention, 32*(1), 25–31. https://doi.org/10.1097/HCR.0b013e3182343aa7

Bloss, C. S., Wineinger, N. E., Peters, M., Boeldt, D. L., Ariniello, L., Kim, J. Y., Sheard, J., Komatireddy, R., Barrett, P., & Topol, E. J. (2016). A prospective randomized trial examining health care utilization in individuals using multiple smartphone-enabled biosensors. *PeerJ, 4*, e1554. https://doi.org/10.7717/peerj.1554

Bokhour, B. G., Berlowitz, D. R., Long, J. A., & Kressin, N. R. (2006). How do providers assess antihypertensive medication adherence in medical encounters? *Journal of General Internal Medicine, 21*, 577–583.

Brzan, P. P., Rotman, E., Pajnkihar, M., & Klanjsek, P. (2016). Mobile applications for control and self management of diabetes: A systematic review. *Journal of Medical Systems, 40*(9), 210. https://doi.org/10.1007/s10916-016-0564-8

Campbell, D. J., Coller, J. M., Gong, F. F., McGrady, M., Prior, D. L., Boffa, U., Shiel, L., Liew, D., Wolfe, R., Owen, A. J., Krum, H., Reid, C. M., & Reid, C. M. (2018). Risk factor management in a contemporary Australian population at increased cardiovascular disease risk. *Internal Medicine Journal, 48*(6), 688–698. https://doi.org/10.1111/imj.13678

Davidson, T. M., McGillicuddy, J., Mueller, M., Brunner-Jackson, B., Favella, A., Anderson, A., Torres, M., Ruggiero, K. J., Treiber, F. A., & Treiber, F. A. (2015). Evaluation of an mHealth medication regimen self-management program for African American and Hispanic uncontrolled hypertensives. *Journal of Personalized Medicine, 5*(4), 389–405. https://doi.org/10.3390/jpm5040389

Davies, C. A., Spence, J. C., Vandelanotte, C., Caperchione, C. M., & Mummery, W. K. (2012). Meta-analysis of internet-delivered interventions to increase physical activity levels. *The International Journal of Behavioral Nutrition and Physical Activity, 9*, 52. https://doi.org/10.1186/1479-5868-9-52

Fu, H., McMahon, S. K., Gross, C. R., Adam, T. J., & Wyman, J. F. (2017). Usability and clinical efficacy of diabetes mobile applications for adults with type 2 diabetes: A systematic review. *Diabetes Research and Clinical Practice, 131*, 70–81. https://doi.org/10.1016/j.diabres.2017.06.016

Fukuoka, Y., Vittinghoff, E., Jong, S. S., & Haskell, W. (2010). Innovation to motivation—Pilot study of a mobile phone intervention to increase physical activity among sedentary women. *Preventive Medicine, 51*(3–4), 287–289. https://doi.org/10.1016/j.ypmed.2010.06.006

Hallberg, I., Ranerup, A., & Kjellgren, K. (2015). Supporting the self-management of hypertension: Patients' experiences of using a mobile phone-based system. *Journal of Human Hypertension, 30*(2), 141–146. https://doi.org/10.1038/jhh.2015.37

Hincapie, A. L., Gupta, V., Brown, S. A., & Metzger, A. H. (2019). Exploring perceived barriers to medication adherence and the use of mobile technology in underserved patients with chronic conditions. *Journal of Pharmacy Practice, 32*(2), 147–153. https://doi.org/10.1177/0897190017744953

Ho, P. M., Bryson, C. L., & Rumsfeld, J. S. (2009). Medication adherence: Its importance in cardiovascular outcomes. *Circulation, 119*(23), 3028–3035. https://doi.org/10.1161/CIRCULATIONAHA.108.768986

Innovatemedtec. (2018). *Health and wellness apps*. https://innovatemedtec.com/digital-health/health-and-wellness-apps

Johnson, H. M., Warner, R. C., LaMantia, J. N., & Bowers, B. J. (2016). "I have to live like I'm old." Young adults' perspectives on managing hypertension: A multi-center qualitative study. *BMC Family Practice, 17*, Article number 31. https://doi.org/10.1186/s12875-016-0428-9

Johnston, N., Bodegard, J., Jerstrom, S., Akesson, J., Brorsson, H., Alfredsson, J., Albertsson, P. A., Karlsson, J. E., & Varenhorst, C. (2016). Effects of interactive patient smartphone support app on drug adherence and lifestyle changes in myocardial infarction patients: A randomized study. *American Heart Journal, 178*, 85–94. https://doi.org/10.1016/j.ahj.2016.05.005

Joseph, N., Chiranjeevi, M., Sen, S., Singh, P., Saini, M., & Beg, S. (2016). Awareness on hypertension and its self-management practices among hypertensive patients attending outreach clinics of a medical college in South India. *Kathmandu University Medical Journal, 14*(55), 202–209.

Karhula, T., Vuorinen, A. L., Rääpysjärvi, K., Pakanen, M., Itkonen, P., Tepponen, M., Junno, U.-M., Jokinen, T., van Gils, M., Lähteenmäki, J., Kohtamäki, K., & Saranummi, N. (2015). Telemonitoring and mobile phone-based health coaching among Finnish diabetic and heart disease patients: Randomized controlled trial. *Journal of Medical Internet Research, 17*(6), e153. https://doi.org/10.2196/jmir.4059

Kerr, S., Watson, H., Tolson, D., Lough, M., & Brown, M. (2006). Smoking after the age of 65 years: A qualitative exploration of older current and former smokers' views on smoking, stopping smoking, and smoking cessation resources and services. *Health & Social Care in the Community, 14*(6), 572–582. https://doi.org/10.1111/j.1365-2524.2006.00659.x

Kjeldsen, S., Feldman, R. D., Lisheng, L., Mourad, J. J., Chiang, C. E., Zhang, W., Wu, Z., Li, W., & Williams, B. (2014). Updated national and international hypertension guidelines: A review of current recommendations. *Drugs, 74*(17), 2033–2051. https://doi.org/10.1007/s40265-014-0306-5

Lee, J., Yoon, W., Cho, S.-i., & Cho, Y. (2016). A strategic consideration on chronic disease prevention and management through mHealth utilization. *The Korean Journal of Public Health, 53*(1), 7–16. https://doi.org/10.17262/KJPH.2016.03.53.1.7 (Original work published in Korean)

Lee, S. Q., Raamkumar, A. S., Li, J., Cao, Y., Witedwittayanusat, K., Chen, L., & Theng, Y. L. (2018). Reasons for primary medication nonadherence: A systematic review and metric analysis. *Journal of Managed Care & Specialty Pharmacy, 24*(8), 778–794. https://doi.org/10.18553/jmcp.2018.24.8.778

Lee, Y. H., Hur, S. H., Sohn, J., Lee, H. M., Park, N. H., Cho, Y. K., Park, H. S., Yoon, H. J., Kim, H., Nam, C. W., Kim, Y. N., & Kim, K. B. (2013). Impact of home-based exercise training with wireless monitoring on patients with acute coronary syndrome undergoing percutaneous coronary intervention. *Journal of Korean Medical Science, 28*(4), 564–568. https://doi.org/10.3346/jkms.2013.28.4.564

Machado, G. C., Pinheiro, M. B., Lee, H., Ahmed, O. H., Hendrick, P., Williams, C., & Kamper, S. J. (2016). Smartphone apps for the self-management of low back pain: A systematic review. *Best Practice & Research Clinical Rheumatology, 30*(6), 1098–1109. https://doi.org/10.1016/j.berh.2017.04.002

Maher, C. A., Lewis, L. K., Ferrar, K., Marshall, S., De Bourdeaudhuij, I., & Vandelanotte, C. (2014). Are health behavior change interventions that use online social networks effective? A systematic review. *Journal of Medical Internet Research, 16*(2), e40. https://doi.org/10.2196/jmir.2952

Martin, S. S., Feldman, D. I., Blumenthal, R. S., Jones, S. R., Post, W. S., McKibben, R. A., Michos, E. D., Ndumele, C. E., Ratchford, E. V., Coresh, J., & Blaha, M. J. (2015). mActive: A randomized clinical trial of an automated mHealth intervention for physical activity promotion. *Journal of the American Heart Association, 4*(11), e002239. https://doi.org/10.1161/jaha.115.002239

Mertens, A., Brandl, C., Miron-Shatz, T., Schlick, C., Neumann, T., Kribben, A., Meister, S., Diamantidis, C., Albrecht, U.-V., Horn, P., & Becker, S. (2016). A mobile application improves therapy-adherence rates in elderly patients undergoing rehabilitation: A crossover design study comparing documentation via iPad with paper-based control. *Medicine, 95*(36), e4446. https://doi.org/10.1097/MD.0000000000004446

Moorhead, P., Zavala, A., Kim, Y., & Virdi, N. S. (2017). Efficacy and safety of a medication dose reminder feature in a digital health offering with the use of sensor-enabled medicines. *Journal of the American Pharmacists Association, 57*(2), 155–161.e1. https://doi.org/10.1016/j.japh.2016.12.067

National Institutes of Health. (2018). *Study quality assessment tools*. https://www.nhlbi.nih.gov/health-topics/study-quality-assessment-tools

Neubeck, L., Lowres, N., Benjamin, E. J., Freedman, S. B., Coorey, G., & Redfern, J. (2015). The mobile revolution—Using smartphone apps to prevent cardiovascular disease. *Nature Reviews Cardiology, 12*, 350–360. https://doi.org/10.1038/nrcardio.2015.34

Or, C., & Tao, D. (2016). A 3-month randomized controlled pilot trial of a patient-centered, computer-based self-monitoring system for the care of type 2 diabetes mellitus and hypertension. *Journal of Medical Systems, 40*(4), 81. https://doi.org/10.1007/s10916-016-0437-1

Paige, S. R., Krieger, J. L., & Stellefson, M. L. (2017). The influence of eHealth literacy on perceived trust in online health communication channels and sources. *Journal of Health Communication, 22*(1), 53–65. https://doi.org/10.1080/10810730.2016.1250846

Patel, S., Jacobus-Kantor, L., Marshall, L., Ritchie, C., Kaplinski, M., Khurana, P. S., & Katz, R. J. (2013). Mobilizing your medications: An automated medication reminder application for mobile phones and hypertension medication adherence in a high-risk urban population. *Journal of Diabetes Science and Technology, 7*(3), 630–639. https://doi.org/10.1177/193229681300700307

Ramage, S., Farmer, A., Eccles, K. A., & McCargar, L. (2014). Healthy strategies for successful weight loss and weight maintenance: A systematic review. *Applied Physiology, Nutrition, and Metabolism, 39*(1), 1–20. https://doi.org/10.1139/apnm-2013-0026

Reboussin, D. M., Allen, N. B., Griswold, M. E., Guallar, E., Hong, Y., Lackland, D. T., Miller, E. R. III, Polonsky, T., Thompson-Paul, A. M., & Vupputuri, S. (2018). Systematic review for the 2017 ACC/AHA/AAPA/ABC/ACPM/AGS/APhA/ASH/ASPC/NMA/PCNA guideline for the prevention, detection, evaluation, and management of high blood pressure in adults: A report of the American college of cardiology/American Heart Association task force on clinical practice guidelines. *Journal of the American College of Cardiology, 71*(19), 2176–2198. https://doi.org/10.1016/j.jacc.2017.11.004

Scottish Intercollegiate Guideline Network. (2018). *Methodology.* https://www.sign.ac.uk/methodology.html

Shawler, C., Edward, J., Ling, J., Crawford, T. N., & Rayens, M. K. (2018). Impact of mother-daughter relationship on hypertension self-management and quality of life: Testing dyadic dynamics using the actor-partner interdependence model. *The Journal of Cardiovascular Nursing, 33*(3), 232–238. https://doi.org/10.1097/jcn.0000000000000448

Shea, B. J., Grimshaw, J. M., Wells, G. A., Boers, M., Andersson, N., Hamel, C., Porter, A. C., Tugwell, P., Moher, D., & Bouter, L. M. (2007). Development of AMSTAR: A measurement tool to assess the methodological quality of systematic reviews. *BMC Medical Research Methodology, 7*(1), 10. https://doi.org/10.1186/1471-2288-7-10

Siahpush, M., McNeill, A., Borland, R., & Fong, G. T. (2006). Socioeconomic variations in nicotine dependence, self-efficacy, and intention to quit across four countries: Findings from the international tobacco control (ITC) four country survey. *Tobacco Control, 15*(3, Suppl.), iii71–iii75. https://doi.org/10.1136/tc.2004.008763

Souffront, K., Gestal, C., Melkus, G. D., & Richardson, L. (2016). Recognition of asymptomatic hypertension in an urban emergency department: Where are we now? *Advanced Emergency Nursing Journal, 38*(4), 320–326. https://doi.org/10.1097/TME.0000000000000118

Statista (2019). *Number of smartphone users worldwide from 2016 to 2021 (in billions).* https://www.statista.com/statistics/330695/number-of-smartphone-users-worldwide/

Stuckey, M. I., Carter, S. W., & Knight, E. (2017). The role of smartphones in encouraging physical activity in adults. *International Journal of General Medicine, 10,* 293–303. https://doi.org/10.2147/ijgm.s134095

Suh, H., Hong, H., Kim, M., Yoon, W., Lee, T., Jung, J., Hwang, S., & Cho, Y. (2015). Mhealth apps: The current status of usage and the factors of continuous use. *Journal of the HCI Society of Korea, 10*(1), 19–27. https://doi.org/10.17210/jhsk.2015.05.10.1.19 (Original work published in Korean)

Thakkar, J., Kurup, R., Laba, T., Santo, K., Thiagalingam, A., Rodgers, A., Woodward, M., Redfern, J., & Chow, C. K. (2016). Mobile telephone text messaging for medication adherence in chronic disease: A meta-analysis. *JAMA Internal Medicine, 176*(3), 340–349. https://doi.org/10.1001/jamainternmed.2015.7667

Thangada, N. D., Garg, N., Pandy, A., & Kumar, N. (2018). The emerging role of mobile-health applications in the management of hypertension. *Current Cardiology Reports, 20*(9), 78. https://doi.org/10.1007/s11886-018-1022-7

Ventola, C. L. (2014). Mobile devices and apps for health care professionals: Uses and benefits. *P & T : A Peer-reviewed Journal for Formulary Management, 39*(5), 356–364.

Whelton, P. K., He, J., Appel, L. J., Cutler, J. A., Havas, S., Kotchen, T. A., Roccella, E. J., Stout, R., Vallbona, C., Winston, M. C., & Karimbakas, J., National High Blood Pressure Education Program Coordinating Committee. (2002). Primary prevention of hypertension: Clinical and public health advisory from the national high blood pressure education program. *Journal of the American Medical Association, 288*(15), 1882–1888. https://doi.org/10.1001/jama.288.15.1882

Whittaker, R., McRobbie, H., Bullen, C., Rodgers, A., & Gu, Y. (2016). Mobile phone-based interventions for smoking cessation. *Cochrane Database of Systematic Reviews, 4,* CD006611. https://doi.org/10.1002/14651858.CD006611.pub4

Widmer, R. J., Allison, T. G., Lennon, R., Lopez-Jimenez, F., Lerman, L. O., & Lerman, A. (2017). Digital health intervention during cardiac rehabilitation: A randomized controlled trial. *American Heart Journal, 188,* 65–72. https://doi.org/10.1016/j.ahj.2017.02.016

Wolf, A., Fors, A., Ulin, K., Thorn, J., Swedberg, K., & Ekman, I. (2016). An eHealth diary and symptom-tracking tool combined with person-centered care for improving self-efficacy after a diagnosis of acute coronary syndrome: A substudy of a randomized controlled trial. *Journal of Medical Internet Research, 18*(2), e40. https://doi.org/10.2196/jmir.4890

World Health Organization. (2017). *Cardiovascular diseases (CVDs).* http://www.who.int/news-room/fact-sheets/detail/cardiovascular-diseases-(cvds)

Xie, B., Su, Z., Zhang, W., & Cai, R. (2017). Chinese cardiovascular disease mobile apps' information types, information quality, and interactive functions for self-management: Systematic review. *JMIR mHealth and uHealth, 5*(12), e195. https://doi.org/10.2196/mhealth.8549

Zhao, J., Freeman, B., & Li, M. (2016). Can mobile phone apps influence people's health behavior change? An evidence review. *Journal of Medical Internet Research, 18*(11), e287. https://doi.org/10.2196/jmir.5692

11

Predicting the Development of Surgery-Related Pressure Injury Using a Machine Learning Algorithm Model

Ji-Yu CAI[1] • Man-Li ZHA[1] • Yi-Ping SONG[1] • Hong-Lin CHEN[2*]

ABSTRACT

Background: Surgery-related pressure injury (SRPI) is a serious problem in patients who undergo cardiovascular surgery. Identifying patients at a high risk of SRPI is important for clinicians to recognize and prevent it expeditiously. Machine learning (ML) has been widely used in the field of healthcare and is well suited to predictive analysis.

Purpose: The aim of this study was to develop an ML-based predictive model for SRPI in patients undergoing cardiovascular surgery.

Methods: This secondary analysis of data was based on a single-center, prospective cohort analysis of 149 patients who underwent cardiovascular surgery. Data were collected from a 1,000-bed university-affiliated hospital. We developed the ML model using the XGBoost algorithm for SRPI prediction in patients undergoing cardiovascular surgery based on major potential risk factors. Model performance was tested using a receiver operating characteristic curve and the C-index.

Results: Of the sample of 149 patients, SRPI developed in 37, an incidence rate of 24.8%. The five most important predictors included duration of surgery, patient weight, duration of the cardiopulmonary bypass procedure, patient age, and disease category. The ML model had an area under the receiver operating characteristic curve of 0.806, which indicates that the ML model has a moderate prediction value for SRPI.

Conclusions: Applying ML to clinical data may be a reliable approach to the assessment of the risk of SRPI in patients undergoing cardiovascular surgical procedures. Future studies may deploy the ML model in the clinic and focus on applying targeted interventions for SRPI and related diseases.

KEY WORDS:
surgery-related pressure injury, machine learning, risk assessment, cardiovascular surgery.

Introduction

Pressure injury is generally defined as localized damage to the skin and underlying soft tissue, usually because of the location of the skin and tissue over a bony prominence or of the use of a medical or other device (Xiong et al., 2019). During surgery, patients are affected by procedure-related factors such as perioperative fasting, liquid fasting, postanesthesia compulsive position, and disinfectant-induced damp skin (Gao et al., 2018). Therefore, patients face an elevated risk of experiencing a surgery-related pressure injury (SRPI). A meta-analysis reported a general prevalence of SRPI of 18.96% (95% CI [15.3, 22.6]) among patients (Shafipour et al., 2016). An incidence rate of SRPI ranging from 0.3% to 57.4% and 18% among patients who underwent cardiovascular surgery was identified in a systematic review (95% CI [14.0, 22.0]; Chen et al., 2012). Pressure injury is an important safety indicator in healthcare systems. Pressure injuries not only adversely affect quality of life but also drain resources from healthcare systems worldwide (Girouard et al., 2008; Liao et al., 2018).

Commonly identified risk factors for SRPI include surgical positioning, type of anesthesia, duration of surgery, extracorporeal circulation, and pressure from internal retractors or from operating room staff (Campbell, 1989; Papantonio et al., 1994; J. Walsh, 1993). Evidence from clinical trials suggests that pressure injury is preventable in today's modern healthcare environment (Thomson & Brooks, 1999). Assessing the risk of pressure injury is recommended in clinical nursing care. Unfortunately, although some risk assessment tools for SRPI have been developed, they have limitations. Although the Braden Scale is a validated and widely used instrument for assessing pressure injury risk, this scale was developed for use in other care settings. The validity and reliability of using the Braden Scale to assess pressure injury development have been established in a variety of patient care settings. However, the results of a meta-analysis revealed that the Braden Scale had a low predictive value for SPRI development in patients who underwent surgery (He et al., 2012). Alternatively, the modified Norton scale has been used frequently in German hospitals. However, the sensitivity and specificity of this scale are 41% and 88%, respectively

[1]*BSN, Graduate Student, School of Nursing, Nantong University, Nantong City, Jiangsu, People's Republic of China* • [2]*MS, Associate Professor, School of Nursing, Nantong University, Nantong City, Jiangsu, People's Republic of China.*

(Feuchtinger et al., 2007). The Waterlow score is another widely used instrument for predicting pressure injury development. The studies indicated that this scale, although suitable for predicting postoperative morbidity and mortality in surgical patients, did not predict the likelihood of SRPI formation (Thorn et al., 2013). These traditional risk assessment scales are based on clinical experience dating from the 1970s and 1980s and lack sufficient data and evidence-based support.

Machine learning (ML), a recently developed field of smart technology, is increasingly being applied in the construction of predictive models. Incorporating ML improves the performance of predictive models and does not require explicit programming or manual guidance (Ethem, 2004; Marsland, 2009). Thus, ML is now widely recognized as an effective resource in medicine and healthcare. In a previous study, an ML-based predictive model constructed for urinary tract infections in the emergency department was superior to existing predictive models (Taylor et al., 2018). Another ML algorithm, XGBoost, was used to construct a risk prediction model for incident essential hypertension and achieved satisfactory predictive accuracy (Ye et al., 2018). Applying ML to longitudinal clinical data has provided a scalable tool for expanding screening for risk of nonfatal suicide attempts in adolescents (C. G. Walsh et al., 2018). Furthermore, ML techniques effectively and efficiently use large amounts of clinical data and are well suited for use in predicting SRPI.

The aims of this study were to integrate ML information with clinical information to predict SRPI risk among patients and to validate the validity of the developed ML predictive model as a reference for future studies.

Methods

Sample

This study adopted a secondary analysis approach using data from a prospective study of patients who had consecutive cardiac surgeries that was conducted to predict the incidence of SRPI using ML (Lu et al., 2017). The sample consisted of data on patients who underwent cardiac surgery and aortic surgery at a teaching hospital between January 2015 and December 2015. The inclusion criteria included all patients, regardless of age, with a pressure injury at the time of admission and before surgery. This study was approved by the ethics committee of the School of Nursing, Nantong University (Approval No. 2018056) in China.

Data Collection

Data for each patient were obtained from the original health records. A wide range of relevant predictors noted in prior studies, including demographic characteristics, SRPI information, and corticosteroid information, among others, were considered. Demographic characteristics included age, gender, weight, and disease category; SRPI information included number of ulcers, ulcer severity as determined using the National Pressure Ulcer Advisory Panel classification (Choi et al., 2016), anatomical location, and outcome; corticosteroid information included administration, type of drug used, drug dosage, and frequency of drug administration; and risk factors included use of vasoactive drugs, experiencing hypotensive periods, hemoglobin level, albumin level, and use of corticosteroids (Feuchtinger et al., 2005).

Model Construction

Models were constructed using all of the variables collected, and descriptive statistics were used to compare the baseline characteristics and outcomes. Univariate chi-square tests and *t* tests were used to compare categorical variables and continuous variables, respectively. *P* values ($< .10$) were deemed significant. The prospective data were used to construct the prediction model. XGBoost, an algorithm in ML, was used to generate predictive estimates on the basis of features retained in the univariate analysis (Plagnol et al., 2012). XGBoost is a novel, sparsity-aware algorithm used in conditions of sparse data and weighted quantile sketch for approximate tree learning. It is designed to improve the speed and performance of gradient-boosted decision trees. The final predictive estimate is calculated by summing the scores in the corresponding leaves of each tree (Ye et al., 2018). XGBoost adds an estimator to provide a better approximation. At each iteration, a new prediction model is built, and each model learns to correct the previous stage model. XGBoost does not require linear features or linear interactions between features and thus is a significantly better classifier than other algorithms. The model usually refers to the mathematical structure of how to make prediction-dependent variables given the independent variables. This algorithm has been recognized as having good accuracy, flexibility, and speed.

Model Evaluation

The performance of the model was evaluated based on the mixture matrix. The primary indicator of this prediction model was the area under the curve (AUC) of the receiver operating characteristic. The secondary indicators were sensitivity and accuracy with 95% CI. Most classification models have an AUC between 0.5 and 1, a random classifier has an AUC of 0.5, and a perfect classifier has an AUC of 1 (Qiao et al., 2018). The definition of sensitivity is the proportion of positive results out of the number of samples that were positive and the proportion of negative results out of the number of samples that were negative (Taylor et al., 2018).

Results

Patient Characteristics

This study included data from 149 patients, with ages ranging from 4 to 77 years. Seventy-nine patients were male, and 70 were female. In terms of disease category, 35 of the patients had congenital heart disease, 85 had valvular heart disease, 20 had coronary heart disease, and nine had macrovascular disease. Selected patient characteristics stratified by cardiovascular surgical patients are shown in Table 1.

Model Performance

The ML tool XGBoost was selected to construct the SRPI prediction model. The outcome evaluation index was the occurrence of SRPI. A score of 1 would be assigned to patients who developed SRPI, and a score of 0 would be assigned otherwise. We evaluated the SRPI prediction model in the form of confusion matrices, with sensitivity, specificity, and the Youden Index. In the prediction model, three patients were correctly predicted as positive for SRPI, and 34 were erroneously predicted as negative. One hundred twelve patients with no SRPI were correctly predicted as negative. The values of sensitivity and specificity were, respectively, 8.11% and 100%. The Youden Index was derived using the threshold at which the sum of sensitivity and specificity achieves the highest value. The value of Youden Index was calculated as 0.081.

Table 1

Baseline Patient Characteristics (N = 149)

Characteristic	Without SRPI (n = 112)		With SRPI (n = 37)		
	n	%	n	%	p
Gender					.815
Male	60	53.6	19	51.4	
Female	52	46.4	18	48.6	
Disease category					.074
Congenital heart disease	32	28.6	3	8.1	
Valvular heart disease	61	54.5	24	64.9	
Coronary artery disease	13	11.6	7	18.9	
Thoracic aortic aneurysms	6	5.4	3	8.1	
Vasoactive agents intraoperatively					.768
Yes	30	26.8	9	24.3	
No	82	73.2	28	75.7	
Vasoactive agents postoperatively					.737
Yes	76	67.9	24	64.9	
No	36	32.1	13	35.1	
Corticosteroids perioperative					.018
Yes	5	4.5	6	16.2	
No	107	95.5	31	83.8	
	M	SD	M	SD	p
Age (years)	48.2	18.3	54.7	15.0	.053
Weight (kilograms)	59.8	15.3	59.1	15.4	.805
Surgery duration (minutes)	221.7	85.8	263.6	93.0	.013
CPB duration (minutes)	48.9	23.1	48.9	23.1	.996

Note. SRPI = surgery-related pressure injury; CPB = cardiopulmonary bypass.

Figure 1

Receiver Operating Characteristic Curve for Surgical-Related Pressure Injuries by Machine Learning Model Versus Logistic Regression

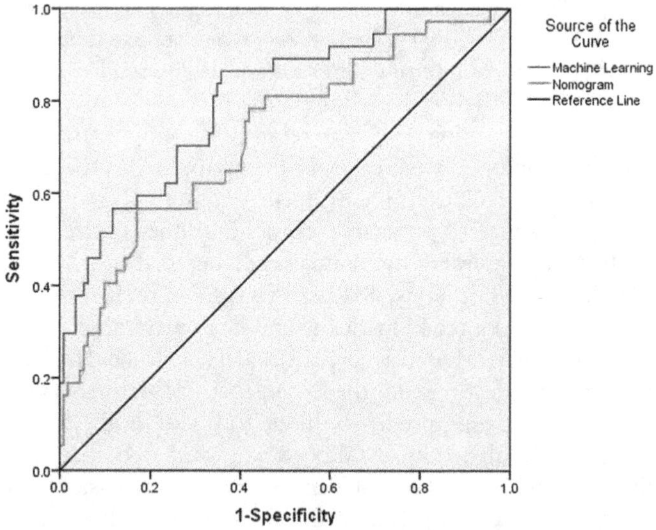

Positive predictive value and negative predictive value were used to describe the performance of the SRPI prediction model. The positive predictive value was 100%, indicating that 100% of patients who developed SRPI were predicted to do so. The negative predictive value was 76.71%, indicating that 76.71% of patients with no SRPI were predicted to do so.

By adopting the ML tool XGBoost, the developed pressure injury prediction model performed at an AUC value of 0.806. Figure 1 shows the receiver operating characteristic curve of the ML prediction model.

Predictor Importance

Nine predictors entered the ML model. These predictors were patient age, gender, disease category, weight, duration of surgery, duration of cardiopulmonary bypass procedure, perioperative corticosteroid administration, use of intraoperative vasoactive agents, and use of postoperative vasoactive agents.

Finally, the importance metrics were aggregated to summarize the five predictors that were important in this ML model. These included, in rank order of decreasing importance, (a) duration of surgery (in minutes), (b) weight (in kilograms), (c) duration of cardiopulmonary bypass procedure (in minutes), (d) age (in years), and (e) disease category (e.g., congenital heart disease). The importance of these five risk factors in predicting SPRI was 0.426, 0.193, 0.131, 0.126, and 0.124, respectively. Findings indicate that duration of surgery was the most important risk factor for SRPI. The proportional importance of each input variable is shown in Figure 2. Risk factors of insignificant importance, including gender, perioperative corticosteroid administration, use of

Figure 2

Relative Importance of Studied Variables to Surgical-Related Pressure Injuries

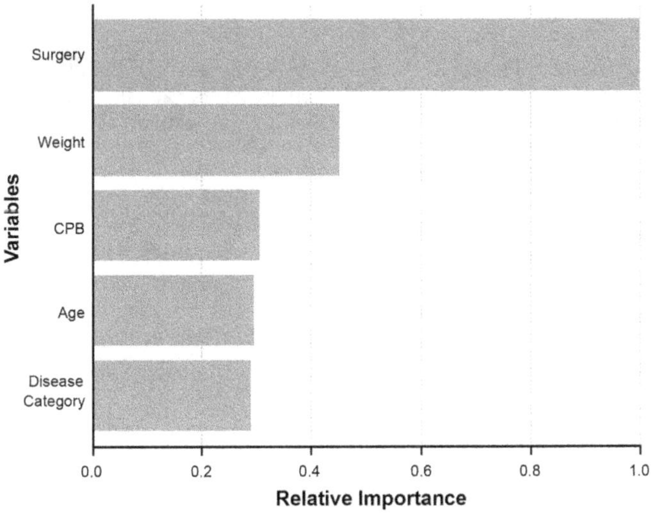

Note. CPB = cardiopulmonary bypass

intraoperative vasoactive agents, and use of postoperative vasoactive agents, are not shown.

Discussion

In this prospective observational study of surgical patients, we constructed a risk prediction model of SRPI development. The prediction model achieved an AUC of 0.806, indicating that this model has moderate predictive accuracy for SRPI in patients undergoing cardiovascular surgery.

In this study, an ML algorithm called XGBoost was adopted for feature selection and model construction. XGBoost is a nonparametric algorithm that does not assume a functional relationship between outcome and features, as is required for linear regression models (Jensen et al., 2012). As a result, this supervised ML method is a robust approach for handling correlated features. The resulting ML prediction model captured potentially powerful predictors of the development of SRPI. In this study, the highest risk of SRPI was borne by patients with longer surgery and cardiopulmonary bypass procedure durations, lower body weight, older age, and congenital heart disease.

Predictive models for SRPI have been developed previously. In a prior study conducted by the authors of this study, a nomogram score was constructed on the basis of logistic regression to predict the development of SRPI (Lu et al., 2017). The constructed logistic regression model contained four independent risk factors: duration of surgery, weight, disease category, and perioperative corticosteroid administration. The three risk factors duration of surgery, weight, and disease category were consistent with the ML model developed in this study. Moreover, age and duration of cardiopulmonary bypass procedure were also considered as important factors in the ML model. The logistic regression model was shown to have moderate power for predicting SRPI, with an AUC of 0.725, an outcome that was similar to this study. However, the ML model has more accurate discrimination power than the nomogram score. ML has been proposed by several authors as an approach to wound-tissue recognition. Kosmopoulos and Tzevelekou used ML for pressure injury diagnosis and presented some exploratory results (Kosmopoulos & Tzevelekou, 2007). Kaewprag et al. used the Bayesian network algorithm in ML to explore risk factors for pressure injuries in patients in intensive care units. That study indicated that the sensitivity of the ML predictive model was nearly three times higher than the logistic regression model, with no decline in overall accuracy (Kaewprag et al., 2017). Therefore, similar to logistic regression, ML may also be used as a technique along with data mining to improve assessment of risk of the development of SRPI.

The five most important variables based on the mean decrease in SRPI accuracy were, in descending order, duration of surgery, body weight, duration of cardiopulmonary bypass procedure, age, and disease category. A previous study (Chen et al., 2018) built an artificial neural network model to investigate the independent risk factors for SRPI in patients undergoing cardiovascular surgery. The factors identified included disease category, perioperative corticosteroid administration, age, and duration of surgery, and the importance of these factors to predicting SRPI was 0.268, 0.136, 0.237, and 0.360, respectively. In this study, two new risk factors, namely, weight and duration of cardiopulmonary bypass procedure, were identified. Duration of surgery is recognized as a high-risk factor for the development of SRPI. Extended duration of procedures leads to increased duration of hypoperfusion, ischemia of local compressed tissues, and decreasing temperature of the compressed position skin, which increase the risk of SRPI (Chen et al., 2017; O'Connell, 2106; Shen et al., 2015). According to a previous study, every 1-hour extension in surgery duration increases the risk of SRPI by 96% (Gao et al., 2018). In a meta-analysis of the association between duration of surgery and SRPI risk, the point estimates for surgery duration at 300 and 600 minutes, respectively, increased the SRPI risk by 3.653 and 13.344 times that of the risk at 60 minutes (Chen et al., 2017).

Weight was identified in this study as an important variable affecting SRPI risk. Although previous studies have shown that poor nutritional status is a common risk factor for pressure injury, only one previous study reported finding a correlation between higher risk of pressure injury and lower body mass in surgical patients (Gao et al., 2018). Most previous studies have cited body mass index as a potential risk factor and showed low body mass index as a significant predictor of SRPI (Alderden et al., 2018; Aloweni et al., 2019). In this study, we did not include body mass index, because it is not clear whether it is an independent risk factor for SRPI. Future studies may further confirm the predictive effect of body mass on SRPI.

The impact of cardiopulmonary bypass procedure duration was not adequately explored in a previous systematic review

(Rao et al., 2016). In this study, duration of cardiopulmonary bypass procedure was deemed as one of the most significant of the examined variables. Our finding that patients who undergo cardiopulmonary bypass are more likely to develop SRPI agrees with other previous studies (Alderden et al., 2018; Gao et al., 2018). Moreover, SRPI experienced after cardiopulmonary bypass may be related to poor peripheral circulation perfusion caused by intraoperative hypothermia, utilization of a warming blanket after cardiopulmonary bypass, and/or lack of subcutaneous tissue protection at heel (Gao et al., 2018). Further studies should pay attention to the effective prevention of heel-related SRPI.

The variables that were found to have no significant predictive effect are also informative for future research. Corticosteroid is a common variable associated with SRPI in cardiovascular surgical patients, as the use of corticosteroid decreases the levels of growth factor, which is deemed as an important factor for pressure injury development (Feuchtinger et al., 2005; Wicke et al., 2000; Yang et al., 2013). However, in this study, corticosteroid administration was not found to be an important risk factor. Future researchers may take into account these factors and multidisciplinary wound care.

Limitations

This study had limitations. First, the data were from a single healthcare institution within a confined geographic region. Thus, the generalizability of our findings may be limited. Second, not collecting data prospectively may affect the performance of the ML prediction model developed in this study. Third, the severity of all SRPI instances in this study were Stage 1.

Conclusion

An ML model for predicting SRPI risk in cardiovascular surgical patients was constructed in this study. Integrating predictive analysis into clinical care holds the potential to better identify high-risk patients and provide appropriate predictive intervention. Future studies may build on these findings to develop a potentially more robust and sensitive ML model for predicting SRPI risk.

Acknowledgments

This study was supported by the Postgraduate Research & Practice Innovation Program of Jiangsu Province (KYCX18_2430). We thank all of the people who participated in this study.

Author Contributions

Study conception and design: JYC, HLC
Data collection: JYC, MLZ, YPS
Data analysis and interpretation: JYC, MLZ, YPS
Drafting of the article: JYC
Critical revision of the article: HLC

References

Alderden, J., Pepper, G. A., Wilson, A., Whitney, J. D., Richardson, S., Butcher, R., Jo, Y., & Cummins, M. R. (2018). Predicting pressure injury in critical care patients: A machine-learning model. *American Journal of Critical Care, 27*(6), 461–468. https://doi.org/10.4037/ajcc2018525

Aloweni, F., Ang, S., Fook-Chong, S., Agus, N., Yong, P., Goh, M., Yong, P., Goh, M., Tucker-Kellogg, L., & Soh, R. C. (2019). A prediction tool for hospital-acquired pressure ulcers among surgical patients: Surgical pressure ulcer risk score. *International Wound Journal, 16*(1), 164–175. https://doi.org/10.1111/iwj.13007

Campbell, K. (1989). Pressure point measures in the operating room. *Journal of Enterostomal Therapy 16*(3), 119–124.

Chen, H. L., Chen, X. Y., & Wu, J. (2012). The incidence of pressure ulcers in surgical patients of the last 5 years: A systematic review. *Wounds 24*(9), 234–241.

Chen, H. L., Shen, W. Q., Liu, P., & Liu, K. (2017). Length of surgery and pressure ulcers risk in cardiovascular surgical patients: A dose–response meta-analysis. *International Wound Journal, 14*(5), 864 869. https://doi.org/10.1111/iwj.12722

Chen, H. L., Yu, S. J., Xu, Y., Yu, S. Q., Zhang, J. Q., Zhao, J. Y., Liu, P., & Zhu, B. (2018). Artificial neural network: A method for prediction of surgery-related pressure injury in cardiovascular surgical patients. *Journal of Wound, Ostomy, and Continence Nursing, 45*(1), 26–30. https://doi.org/10.1097/won.0000000000000388

Choi, E. P. H., Chin, W. Y., Wan, E. Y. F., & Lam, C. L. K. (2016). Evaluation of the internal and external responsiveness of the Pressure Ulcer Scale for Healing (PUSH) tool for assessing acute and chronic wounds. *Journal of Advanced Nursing, 72*(5), 1134–1143. https://doi.org/10.1111/jan.12898

Ethem, A. (2004). *Introduction to machine learning.* MIT Press.

Feuchtinger, J., Halfens, R., & Dassen, T. (2007). Pressure ulcer risk assessment immediately after cardiac surgery—Does it make a difference? A comparison of three pressure ulcer risk assessment instruments within a cardiac surgery population. *Nursing in Critical Care, 12*(1), 42–49. https://doi.org/10.1111/j.1478-5153.2006.00198.x

Feuchtinger, J., Halfens, R. J., & Dassen, T. (2005). Pressure ulcer risk factors in cardiac surgery: A review of the research literature. *Heart & Lung, 34*(6), 375–385. https://doi.org/10.1016/j.hrtlng.2005.04.004

Gao, L., Yang, L., Li, X., Chen, J., Du, J., Bai, X., & Yang, X. (2018). The use of a logistic regression model to develop a risk assessment of intraoperatively acquired pressure ulcer. *Journal of Clinical Nursing, 27*(15–16), 2984–2992. https://doi.org/10.1111/jocn.14491

Girouard, K., Harrison, M. B., & VanDenkerkof, E. (2008). The symptom of pain with pressure ulcers: A review of the literature. *Ostomy Wound Management, 54*(5), 30–40.

He, W., Liu, P., & Chen, H. L. (2012). The Braden Scale cannot be used alone for assessing pressure ulcer risk in surgical patients: A meta-analysis. *Ostomy Wound Management, 58*(2), 34–40.

Jensen, P. B., Jensen, L. J., & Brunak, S. (2012). Mining electronic health records: Towards better research applications and clinical care. *Nature Reviews Genetics, 13*(6), 395–405. https://doi.org/10.1038/nrg3208

Kaewprag, P., Newton, C., Vermillion, B., Hyun, S., Huang, K., & Machiraju, R. (2017). Predictive models for pressure ulcers from intensive care unit electronic health records using Bayesian networks. *BMC Medical Informatics & Decision Making, 17*(2, Suppl.), Article No. 65. https://doi.org/10.1186/s12911-017-0471-z

Kosmopoulos, D. I., & Tzevelekou, F. L. (2007). Automated pressure ulcer lesion diagnosis for telemedicine systems. *Engineering in Medicine & Biology Magazine IEEE, 26*(5), 18–22. https://doi.org/10.1109/EMB.2007.901786

Liao, Y., Gao, G., & Mo, L. (2018). Predictive accuracy of the Braden Q Scale in risk assessment for paediatric pressure ulcer: A meta-analysis. *International Journal of Nursing Sciences, 5*(4), 419–426.

Lu, C. X., Chen, H. L., Shen, W. Q., & Feng, L. P. (2017). A new nomogram score for predicting surgery-related pressure ulcers in cardiovascular surgical patients. *International Wound Journal, 14*(1), 226–232. https://doi.org/10.1111/iwj.12593

Marsland, S. (2009). *Machine learning: An algorithmic perspective* (1st ed.). Chapman & Hall/CRC.

O'Connell, M. P. (2006). Positioning impact on the surgical patient. *Nursing Clinics of North America, 41*(2), 173–192. https://doi.org/10.1016/j.cnur.2006.01.010

Papantonio, C. T., Wallop, J. M., & Kolodner, K. B. (1994). Sacral ulcers following cardiac surgery: Incidence and risks. *Advances in Wound Care, 7*(2), 24–36.

Plagnol, V., Curtis, J., Epstein, M., Mok, K. Y., Stebbings, E., Grigoriadou, S., Wood, N. W., Hambleton, S., Burns, S. O., Thrasher, A. J., Krummararatne, D., Doffinger, R., & Nejentsev, S. (2012). A robust model for read count data in exome sequencing experiments and implications for copy number variant calling. *Bioinformatics, 28*(21), 2747–2754. https://doi.org/10.1093/bioinformatics/bts526

Qiao, Z., Sun, N., Li, X., Xia, E., Zhao, S., & Qin, Y. (2018). Using machine learning approaches for emergency room visit prediction based on electronic health record data. *Studies in Health Technology & Informatics, 247*, 111–115.

Rao, A. D., Preston, A. M., Strauss, R., Stamm, R., & Zalman, D. C. (2016). Risk factors associated with pressure ulcer formation in critically ill cardiac surgery patients: A systematic review. *Journal of Wound Ostomy & Continence Nursing, 43*(3), 242–247. https://doi.org/10.1097/WON.0000000000000224

Shafipour, V., Ramezanpour, E., Gorji, M. A., & Moosazadeh, M. (2016). Prevalence of postoperative pressure ulcer: A systematic review and meta-analysis. *Electronic Physician, 8*(11), 3170–3176. https://doi.org/10.19082/3170

Shen, W. Q., Chen, H. L., Xu, Y. H., Zhang, Q., & Wu, J. (2015). The relationship between length of surgery and the incidence of pressure ulcers in cardiovascular surgical patients: A retrospective study. *Advances in Skin & Wound Care, 28*(10), 444–450. https://doi.org/10.1097/01.ASW.0000466365.90534.b0

Taylor, R. A., Moore, C. L., Cheung, K. H., & Brandt, C. (2018). Predicting urinary tract infections in the emergency department with machine learning. *PLOS ONE, 13*(3), Article e0194085. https://doi.org/10.1371/journal.pone.0194085

Thomson, J. S., & Brooks, R. G. (1999). The economics of preventing and treating pressure ulcers: A pilot study. *Journal of Wound Care, 8*(6), 312–316. https://doi.org/10.12968/jowc.1999.8.6.25879

Thorn, C. C., Smith, M., Aziz, O., & Holme, T. C. (2013). The Waterlow score for risk assessment in surgical patients. *Annals of the Royal College of Surgeons of England, 95*(1), 52–56. https://doi.org/10.1308/003588413X13511609954770

Walsh, C. G., Ribeiro, J. D., & Franklin, J. C. (2018). Predicting suicide attempts in adolescents with longitudinal clinical data and machine learning. *The Journal of Child Psychology and Psychiatry, 59*(12), 1261–1270. https://doi.org/10.1111/jcpp.12916

Walsh, J. (1993). Postop effects of OR positioning. *RN, 56*(2), 50–57

Wicke, C., Halliday, B., Allen, D., Roche, N. S., Scheuenstuhl, H., Spencer, M. M., Roberts, A. B., & Hunt, T. K. (2000). Effects of steroids and retinoids on wound healing. *Archives of Surgery, 135*(11), 1265–1270. https://doi.org/10.1001/archsurg.135.11.1265

Xiong, C., Gao, X., Ma, Q., Yang, Y., Wang, Z., Yu, W., & Yu, L. (2019). Risk factors for intraoperative pressure injuries in patients undergoing digestive surgery: A retrospective study. *Journal of Clinical Nursing, 28*(7–8), 1148–1155. https://doi.org/10.1111/jocn.14712

Yang, J. J., Wang, X. L., Shi, B. W., & Huang, F. (2013). The angiogenic peptide vascular endothelial growth factor-basic fibroblast growth factor signaling is up-regulated in a rat pressure ulcer model. *The Anatomical Record, 296*(8), 1161–1168.

Ye, C., Fu, T., Hao, S., Zhang, Y., Wang, O., Jin, B., Xia, M., Liu, M., Zhou, X., Wu, Q., Guo, Y., Zhu, C., Li, Y. M., Culver, D. S., Alfreds, S. T., Stearns, F., Sylvester, K. G., Widen, E., McElhinney, D., & Ling, X. (2018). Prediction of incident hypertension within the next year: Prospective study using statewide electronic health records and machine learning. *Journal of Medical Internet Research, 20*(1), Article e22. https://doi.org/10.2196/jmir.9268

The Effect of the Neuman Systems Model on Anxiety in Patients Undergoing Coronary Artery Bypass Graft

Elham AKHLAGHI[1] • Sima BABAEI[2]* • Abbas MARDANI[3] • Fatemeh ESKANDARI[4]

ABSTRACT

Background: Coronary artery bypass graft (CABG) surgery is the most commonly used surgical procedure for patients with coronary artery disease. Anxiety is a significant psychological problem associated with CABG surgery that may reduce related treatment outcomes.

Purpose: This study was designed to investigate the effect on anxiety of applying the Neuman Systems Model in patients awaiting and undergoing CABG surgery.

Methods: A single-blind, parallel-group randomized controlled trial was conducted on patients scheduled to receive coronary artery bypass surgery in an urban area of Iran. Seventy participants were enrolled using a convenience sampling method and randomly assigned to either the intervention group ($n = 35$) or the control group ($n = 35$). Participants in the intervention group received intervention in accordance with the Neuman Systems Model format, including meetings held at three levels of prevention. Patients' anxiety was measured using the State Anxiety Inventory before the intervention, immediately after the intervention, and at discharge time. The chi-square test, Fisher's exact test, independent sample *t* test, one-way repeated measures analysis of variance test, and Fisher's least significant difference were used to analyze the data.

Results: No significant difference was found between the mean anxiety scores of the two groups before the intervention ($p = .48$, $t = 0.71$). However, the mean anxiety score of the intervention group was significantly lower than that of the control group immediately after the intervention ($p = .008$, $t = 2.73$) and at discharge time ($p = .007$, $t = 2.77$).

Conclusions: The Neuman-based program is an effective and low-cost intervention that may be applied to reduce anxiety in patients awaiting and undergoing CABG surgery. This program may be a good guide in providing healthcare services.

Key Words:
Neuman Systems Model, anxiety, coronary artery bypass graft surgery, coronary artery disease.

Introduction

Cardiovascular disease, already the most common noncommunicable disease in the Middle East, is continuing to increase in prevalence in the region, with Iran among those countries with the highest prevalence rates (Moazzeni et al., 2021). Despite advances in medical science and equipment, coronary artery bypass graft (CABG) surgery remains the standard strategy for the treatment of advanced coronary artery disease (Palmerini et al., 2017), accounting for 78.8% of all cardiac surgeries in Iran (Akhlaghi et al., 2020).

Anxiety is a major problem in patients scheduled for heart surgery and is more prevalent in heart surgery than other surgeries because proper heart functioning is critical to the continuance of an individual's life (Hinkle & Cheever, 2013). The results of a meta-analysis by Takagi et al. (2017) indicate that prolonged anxiety in patients scheduled for cardiac surgery may be associated with a higher risk of postoperative mortality. Preoperative anxiety may increase the risk of postsurgical lesions, including atrial fibrillation, acute myocardial infarction, increased disease and mortality, and increased use of healthcare. In addition to being a distressing state, anxiety is a common denominator of many physical and mental disorders. In fact, for most illnesses and physical and mental disorders, anxiety is considered a major discomfort. In addition, anxiety in patients experiencing chronic and prolonged disease may cause major destructive physiological changes (Alipoor et al.,

[1]RN, Doctoral Candidate, School of Nursing and Midwifery, Iran University of Medical Sciences, Tehran, Iran • [2]PhD, RN, Assistant Professor, Nursing and Midwifery Care Research Center, Faculty of Nursing and Midwifery, Isfahan University of Medical Science, Isfahan, Iran • [3]RN, Doctoral Candidate, Nursing Care Research Center, School of Nursing and Midwifery, Iran University of Medical Sciences, Tehran, Iran • [4]PhD, RN, Support Worker, Psychiatric/Mental Health Nursing, Mental Health Community Making Life Better, Sydney, Australia.

2014). Tully et al. (2015) found that patients with high levels of anxiety have a higher risk of death before CABG surgery. Moreover, Middel et al. (2014) showed a positive relationship between preoperative anxiety and postoperative anxiety after CABG surgery. In addition, they showed that identifying patients with high anxiety would help healthcare providers offer specific interventions to reduce their anxiety and improve their quality of life.

Helping patients adapt to anxiety is a major responsibility of nurses. Nurses play an important role in preparing patients emotionally and psychologically during the preoperative period of cardiac surgery. Therefore, nurses should always look for ways to improve the quality of nursing care (Ramesh, 2017). In this regard, applying nursing theories and models in the advanced practice area of nursing may be beneficial for patients (Reed, 1993).

One of these models is the Neuman Systems Model (NSM), which is an open model-based perspective that provides proper function in stressful situations or at the time of the patient's response, which is recognized as a priority in nursing (Meleis, 2011). The NSM is based on an individual's relationship with and response to stress. The three key concepts of this model are stress, homeostasis, and patient's perception. The role of the nurse is to focus on the factors influencing the individual's response to stress and protecting the patient from the relevant risk factors (Heffline, 1990). In this model, the main goal of nursing is to maximize patient well-being by using nursing care to reduce stress. The nurse creates a relationship among the patient, environment, and health to establish a sustainable system. It is necessary for the nurse to evaluate the patient's perceived stressors to improve patient stability. As the relationship between the nurse and patient develops and mutual understanding improves, differences in understanding may be eliminated. The outcome of this partnership is complementary within a joint care plan that may be implemented with a clear objective in mind (Parvan et al., 2012).

Under the NSM, nurses are considered to be active contributors (Smith & Parker, 2015), and prevention is pursued as one of the most important nursing interventions to protect the patient. In this model, the goal of nursing is to strengthen a patient's defenses, improve their health, and, ultimately, improve their ability to cope with health issues (Meleis, 2011; Parvan et al., 2012). The main point is the importance of providing nursing care in the form of prevention levels. Primary prevention aims to prevent tension agents from penetrating defensive lines by reducing stress and strengthening defense lines. Secondary prevention attempts to increase goodness, reduce stress, and reinforce coping by strengthening defense lines. In fact, the goal of secondary prevention is to maintain the level of coping (Fawcett & Garity, 2008; McEwen & Wills, 2017).

Nursing interventions seek to reduce the stressors and situations deemed to affect or potentially affect the patient's desirable factors. The distinction made between the prevention levels in nursing interventions designed to reduce stress is one of the benefits of the NSM. Another advantage is its focus on prevention levels that are more socially acceptable because the community is progressively aware of the significant role of nurses in the healthcare system. A further strength of this model is its flexibility as a stimulus–response systems model that considers the basis for development of the theory and evaluates the relationship between nursing theory and clinical research and practice (Sultan, 2018).

Nursing theories should be developed with the goal of promoting practical applications in clinical practice. Developing and reviewing theories have the potential to open up new approaches to quality care that may challenge the current care system (Wadensten & Carlsson, 2003). Nursing is not only a practical discipline but also a knowledge-based profession. Therefore, to create new practical approaches, having the foundation of knowledge is one of the requirements in this field (Aghebati et al., 2012). There is a gap between theory and practice in the nursing profession, and nurses focus more on the practical aspects of nursing than on nursing science and art (Mrayyan, 2006). Moreover, the need to reduce anxiety using holistic care models in patients undergoing CABG is addressed in this article. This is an issue that has been insufficiently addressed in the scientific literature, especially in non-Western countries. Therefore, the existing gaps encouraged the development of a research project aimed at evaluating the effect of applying the NSM for anxiety in patients scheduled for CABG surgery.

Methods

Design

This study was a single-center, single-blinded, two-armed, randomized controlled trial conducted in an urban area of Iran from October 2017 to August 2018.

Participants and Sampling

Participants' inclusion criteria for this study were as follows: being a candidate for CABG surgery, having full consciousness, admitted at least 1 day before surgery, willing to participate in the study, able to communicate in the Farsi language, and aged 30–70 years. This age range was selected based on the rare number of candidates below 30 years old and in accordance with the literature, which has shown a significantly negative correlation between age and anxiety, as patients older than 70 years have been found to report the lowest level of anxiety before and after CABG surgery (Krannich et al., 2007). The exclusion criteria were as follows: discontinuing the patient's participation at any phase of the study, an emergency condition that required giving medical care to the patient during the intervention, and any delay in surgery (e.g., because of financial problems, not providing consent for surgery, deteriorating health condition). The minimum sample size required was 32 participants in each group based on Nasiry Zarrin Ghabaee et al. (2015), which applied the NSM to reduce the level of anxiety in orthopedic patients before surgery. In this study, the required sample size was determined with a 95% confidence and 80% test power, and the mean standard deviation of anxiety score was estimated in both groups. The final, target sample size was determined to be 35 people in each group in this study, considering a potential dropout rate of 10%.

$$n = 2S^2\frac{(Z_1 + Z_2)^2}{d^2} = 2s^2\frac{(1.96 + 0.84)^2}{0.49s^2} = 32$$

Patients who were referred to the cardiology center and were waiting for surgery enrolled in the study using a convenience sampling method based on eligibility criteria. Of the 75 total potential participants, 70 were randomly assigned to either the intervention group (n = 35) or the control group (n = 35) using the following cards/envelope shuffling method (Kim & Shin, 2014). First, code "A" was assigned to the intervention group, and code "B" was assigned to the control group. Then, the researcher (first author) wrote letters A and B on cards and placed them in an envelope. Next, each of the enrolled participants was asked to take one of the envelopes. Those who took an envelope containing Card A were included in the intervention group, and those who took an envelope containing Card B were included in the control group (Figure 1). The researcher (first author) implemented the intervention and collected the data.

Data Collection

A sociodemographic data questionnaire, the Revised Cardiac Surgery Stressors Scale (RCSSS), and the State Anxiety Inventory were used for data collection.

The sociodemographic data questionnaire was designed by researchers using a review of the literature and either self-completed by the participants who were literate or completed during the interview by the researcher for participants who were illiterate.

The State Anxiety Inventory questionnaire contains 20 questions scored on a 4-point Likert scale. Reverse ratings were applied for negative items, and a total score was calculated, ranging from 20 to 80, with score ranges categorized as low anxiety (20–37), moderate anxiety (38–44), and high anxiety (45–80). This questionnaire has been translated into 30 languages and has been adapted to suit the Iranian cultural setting. In this study, Cronbach's alpha (α) was calculated to assess the internal consistency reliability of the translated instrument, with the result of .97 indicating sufficient internal consistency based on a recommended level of > .70 (Spielberger, 2010). This questionnaire was completed by/for all of the participants at three points in time: before the intervention, immediately after the intervention, and at discharge time.

The RCSSS includes 37 questions, and the second part includes RCSSS cases in three subgroups: intrapersonal stressors, including 11 phrases; interpersonal stressors, including nine phrases; and extrapersonal stressors, including 17 phrases.

Figure 1
The Study Process Based on the CONSORT Flow Diagram

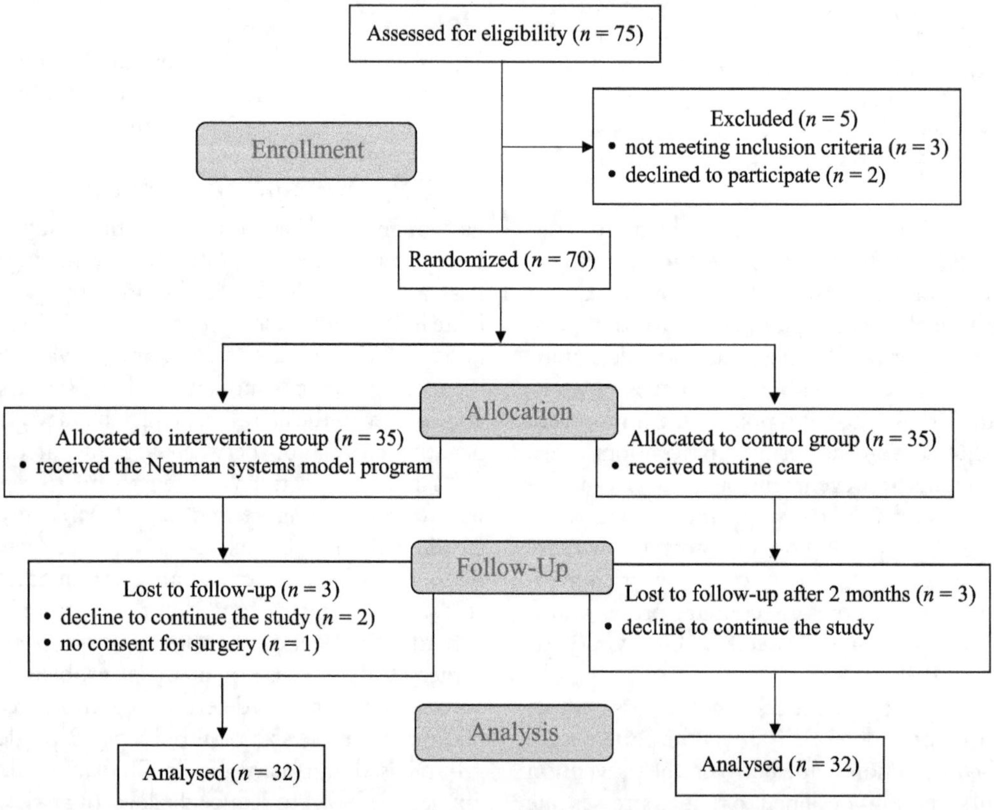

The items were ranked according to the level of concern of the participants on a Likert scale from 0 to 4, with 0 = *no worries*, 1 = *very low worries*, 2 = *low worries*, 3 = *moderate worries*, and 4 = *worries*. The lowest scale score of 0 indicates the absence of stressors, whereas the maximum score of 148 indicates the highest stressor factor, with ranges of 0–37 indicating very low stressors, 38–74 indicating low stressors, 75–110 indicating the presence of relatively stressful factors, and 111–148 indicating stressful factors. The reliability of this questionnaire was calculated using Cronbach's alpha coefficient (patient = .81; nurse = .93) in previous research in the Iranian context (Parvan et al., 2013). In this study, the reliability of the RCSSS calculated using Cronbach's alpha was shown to be adequate (patient = .82; nurse = .91). This scale was only used to categorize patients based on level of prevention.

Intervention

First, the potential and actual stressor factors for each patient, including intrapersonal, interpersonal, and extrapersonal, were evaluated using the RCSSS (patient part; Parvan et al., 2013). Second, appropriate goals and strategies for action were determined. If no actual stressors were found, interventions at the first level of prevention were carried out, and the influence of the stressors on the natural defense line was prevented by reducing the probability of exposure to stressors and strengthening the defense line. If stressors were identified based on the patient part of RCSSS, these factors were known as actual stressors, and the patient was placed in the second level of prevention. If different levels of stressors were identified, the RCSSS (nurse part; Parvan et al., 2012) was also completed by the responsible shift nurse to determine the patient stressor. The nurse's perception is considered as one of the steps of the NSM in relation to the patient's stress factors. On the basis of the study of the second level of prevention, the intervention was identified to reduce the stressors that caused damage to the natural and flexible defense line. The intervention was aimed at strengthening internal defense lines to reduce the reaction. In the presence of the stressors, the intervention continued at the third level of prevention after surgery using Benson's relaxation method. The main goal of the tertiary prevention component of the NSM is adaptability (Fawcett & Desanto-Madeya, 2012; Sahrakhil et al., 2017). To implement the Benson's relaxation procedure, patients were placed in a relaxed environment and in the most comfortable position. Then, they were asked to choose a calming word and take comfortable, deep breaths. They were asked to inhale through their nose and repeat their calming words during exhalation through their mouth. During this process, patients were asked to relax all of the muscles in their body from head to feet (Sahrakhil et al., 2017).

Prevention of the first and second levels was done in one or two 45- to 60-minute consecutive sessions before surgery. The first session was implemented on the day of admission in the morning or evening shift. The second session was implemented during the evening or night shift. The conversations were held individually at patient bedsides under conditions considered favorable by both patient and researcher. The contents of these conversations included a self-introduction, the purpose of the research, and a simple explanation about coronary artery anatomy, preoperative cardiac surgery, the operating room and intensive care unit, and postintensive care unit cardiac and postoperative orders and care (Table 1).

Table 1
Contents of Sessions, by Prevention Level

Session	Content
First	• In patients in the first prevention and at the time of admission • Introduce yourself and express the purpose of the research • An explanation of coronary anatomy, preoperative cardiac surgery, the operating room and ICU, post-ICU cardiac surgery, postoperative care and instructions (bathing, at home, diet, taking medication, and medicine intake), the role of proper nutrition in relieving stress and anxiety, and reassurance in the hospital environment and the operating room
Second	• In patients in the secondary prevention and in the second shift after admission • Discussion and clarification of issues • Intervention according to the needs and actual stressors detected by the patient and the nurse based on Neuman stressors • Intrapersonal (awareness of the rehabilitation phase, home care, routine care in the intensive care unit and other areas, surgery awareness, time back to section, duration of exercise, awareness of nutritional therapy) • Interpersonal (description of hospital therapy procedures, psychological support, relation with patients, and providing information about medications) • Extrapersonal (providing information on insurance and paying for expenses, talking to the healthcare sector and referring patients to charities, creating a quiet environment and reducing noise, staying in the ICU, injection instruction, training in connection with tubes and the patient's chest tube, and a tutorial on catheters showing the patient the connections)
Third	• In patients with the third prevention and in the postoperative stage • Promote relaxation responses by implementing Benson's relaxation method

Note. ICU = intensive care unit.

At the end of the first session, an educational booklet on the issues discussed was given to the intervention group. Moreover, the patient's companion in the intervention group received the care program from the researcher 1 day before the surgery based on the NSM. Of the 32 participants in the intervention group, 28 were assigned to the first and second levels of prevention and received the preoperative intervention. Only four received the third level of prevention. Preventive level assignments were determined based on the presence of stressors identified through the questionnaire on the revised cardiac surgery stressors (patient part). The participants assigned to the control group received usual care only.

Ethical Considerations

Ethical approval for this study was obtained from the Vice-Chancellor of Ethics of Research and Technology of Isfahan University of Medical Sciences (reference no: IR.MUI.REC.1396.3.838) and the Iranian Clinical Trial Center (reference no: IRCT2018011603897N1). The managers of the research settings were notified of the aim of this study and that participation would not result in any harm or difficulty. The participants were informed about the aim and procedure of this study and that data would be kept confidential. Finally, an informed consent form was signed by those who consented to participate.

Table 2

Demographic Characteristics and Patient Information by Group

Variable	Intervention Group		Control Group		*t*	*p*
	Mean	*SD*	Mean	*SD*		
Age (years)	60.72	8.14	57.23	11.14	1.40	.17
Number of previous hospitalizations	3.62	3.17	2.61	1.52	1.55	.13
Duration of the most recent hospitalization (days)	5.23	4.49	5.70	3.71	0.43	.67
Number of previous surgeries	1.68	1.06	1.53	0.72	0.51	.61
Variable	***n***	**%**	***n***	**%**	**z/χ^2**	***p***
Gender					χ^2 = 0.61	.43
Female	10	31.2	13	40.6		
Male	22	68.8	19	59.4		
Religion					–	.50
Shiite	31	96.9	32	100.0		
Sunni	1	3.1	0	0		
Marital status					χ^2 = 0.56	.76
Single	1	3.1	2	6.2		
Married	28	87.5	26	81.3		
Widowed	3	9.4	4	12.5		
Past cardiac catheterization in this hospital					χ^2 = 0.87	.35
Yes	24	75.0	27	84.4		
No	8	25.0	5	15.6		
Family history of cardiovascular disease surgery					–	.98
Yes	8	25.0	8	25.0		
No	24	75.0	24	75.0		
Family income					*z* = 0.77	.44
Less than living expenses	22	68.8	19	59.4		
More than living expenses	10	31.2	13	40.6		
Level of education					*z* = 0.62	.54
Illiterate	11	34.4	14	43.7		
Elementary school	9	28.1	8	25.0		
Secondary school	4	12.5	3	9.4		
High school	6	18.8	4	12.5		
University	2	6.2	3	9.4		
Date of previous hospitalization					*z* = 0.13	.89
Last 4 months	16	50.0	16	50.0		
Last 5–6 months	4	12.5	3	9.4		
Last 7–12 months	2	6.2	2	6.2		
More than the last 12 months	10	31.3	11	34.4		

Table 3
Comparison of RCSSS Scores Between the Intervention and Control Groups and Between Patient and Nurse Perspectives

Subgroup/Score	Intervention Group (n = 32)		Control Group (n = 32)		p	t
	Mean	*SD*	Mean	*SD*		
Intrapersonal	16.14	8.84	15.28	8.18	.73	0.34
Interpersonal	8.00	3.81	8.57	4.39	.77	0.30
Extrapersonal	23.08	9.50	22.93	12.95	.96	0.05
Total score	45.23	21.64	49.05	18.81	.59	0.54
Subgroup/Score	**Nurse**		**Patient**		p	t
	Mean	*SD*	Mean	*SD*		
Intrapersonal	26.04	4.58	16.14	8.84	< .001	5.63
Interpersonal	16.30	6.40	8.00	3.81	< .001	5.03
Extrapersonal	38.16	6.72	23.08	9.50	< .001	7.33
Total score	80.57	14.93	45.23	21.64	< .001	7.60

Note. RCSSS = Revised Cardiac Surgery Stressors Scale.

Data Analysis

SPSS software Version 22 (IBM, Inc., Armonk, NY, USA) was used for data analysis. Frequency and percentage for qualitative variables and mean and standard deviation for quantitative variables were applied using descriptive statistics to describe these variables. In addition, the chi-square test, Fisher's exact test, and an independent sample t test were conducted to find differences in sociodemographic variables between the two study groups. In addition, an independent sample t test was used to compare the mean anxiety scores between the intervention and control groups before the intervention, immediately after the intervention, and at discharge time. This test was also used to compare the mean RCSSS scores of patients and nurses. Moreover, the one-way repeated measures analysis of variance (ANOVA) test was applied to evaluate changes in mean anxiety scores over time in the two study groups and to compare mean anxiety over time in the intervention group. A p value < .05 was regarded as significant.

Results

As shown in Figure 1, of the 70 participants, three from each group were excluded from the final analysis because of exclusion criteria (n = 64). The mean age of participants in the intervention and control groups was 60.72 and 57.23 years, respectively. Most participants in the intervention (68.8%) and control (59.4%) groups were male. Other sociodemographic variables are listed in Table 2. There were no significant differences in sociodemographic variables between the two groups (Table 2).

As shown in Table 3, the results of RCSSS showed that no significant differences were present between the mean scores

Table 4
Comparison of Anxiety Scores Between the Intervention and Control Groups

Time	Intervention Group (n = 32)		Control Group (n = 32)		Independent t Test	
	Mean	*SD*	Mean	*SD*	t	p
Before intervention	44.27	11.04	42.40	9.83	0.71	.480
After intervention	37.66	8.28	43.75	9.53	2.73	.008
At discharge	36.46	8.60	42.69	9.36	2.77	.007
One-way repeated measures ANOVA						
F	11.34		1.79			
p	.001		.180			

Note. ANOVA = analysis of variance.

of the intervention and control groups ($p = .59, t = 0.54$). Regarding patients' and nurses' perspectives on RCSSS, the mean scores of the nurses were significantly higher than those of the participants ($p < .001, t = 7.60$; Table 3).

As shown in Table 4, no significant difference was found in preintervention mean anxiety scores between the two groups ($p = .48, t = 0.71$). The level of anxiety was moderate in the control group (42.40) and in the intervention group (44.27) before the intervention. However, the mean anxiety score in the intervention group was significantly lower immediately after the intervention ($p = .008, t = 2.73$) and at discharge time ($p = .007, t = 2.77$) than in the control group. Moreover, the one-way repeated measures ANOVA for each group revealed that the mean anxiety scores statistically significantly reduced over time in the intervention group ($p = .001, F = 11.34$) but not in the control group ($p = .18, F = 1.79$).

In the intervention group, the result of Fisher's least significant test after one-way repeated measures ANOVA showed that the mean anxiety score in the intervention group was significantly lower immediately after the intervention (mean difference [MD] = −6.61, $p = .001$) and at discharge time (MD = −7.81, $p < .001$) than before the intervention, with no significant difference found between immediately after the intervention and at discharge time (MD = 1.21, $p = .33$). On the basis of the results of the independent sample t test, at discharge time, no significant difference was identified in terms of anxiety scores between participants who received the first and second levels of prevention and those who received all three levels of prevention ($p = .34, t = 0.95$).

Discussion

The aim of this study was to investigate the effect of applying the NSM on anxiety in patients scheduled for CABG surgery. The findings revealed that using this care program based on this model had a significant effect on reducing anxiety in these patients.

Although there have been some discussions regarding the effect of nursing theories in practice, the value of using nursing theories for the advancement of the nursing profession has been supported in the literature (Bourdeanu & Dee, 2013). Theories and models of nursing provide a coherent and systematic framework to guide nursing assessments, planning, and interventions. In addition, theories and models can help generate more knowledge and differentiate what should be the basis of nursing practice (Polit & Beck, 2004). Furthermore, models can help nurses provide better care to patients (Huang et al., 2015). In this study, the NSM was used to provide care to patients.

The results of a previous study conducted on candidate patients for orthopedic surgery showed that using the NSM reduced the anxiety level in patients waiting for surgery (Nasiry Zarrin Ghabaee et al., 2015). Moreover, the finding of another study indicated that applying this model may reduce the level of stressors in patients scheduled for CABG surgery. In addition, providing care based on this model can effectively diminish the incidence of anxiety in patients with gastrointestinal malignancy, endometrial carcinoma, and lung cancer (Wang et al., 2019). The results of the reviewed studies are consistent with the results of this study.

In this study, patients reported a lower perception of stressors than nurses. This finding is consistent with the results of a previous study (Parvan et al., 2012). The misunderstanding of nurses may have an adverse effect on nursing care and induce stressful symptoms in patients during nurse–patient communication. Nurses should avoid applying their preconceptions in determining the severity of patient stressors (Parvan et al., 2012).

Studies have shown that the functional and psychological status of patients worsens when they are placed on the cardiac waiting list because they do not know what to expect (Guo, 2015; Rosenfeldt et al., 2011). At the same time, many nurses responsible for the care of candidate patients for heart surgery are not aware of the benefits to patients of preoperative interventions. Thus, they focus on postoperative interventions only (Alshvang, 2018). A substantial part of the NSM revolves around internal and external stressors, with an emphasis on patient education (Neuman & Fawcett, 2002). In this study, the intervention program was designed based on the NSM in the first and second levels of prevention. It was delivered to patients individually after identifying patient stressors during teaching sessions. Providing an educational booklet was also found to reduce anxiety level. In agreement with this study, a randomized controlled study by Guo et al. (2012) found that a preoperative educational intervention was effective in reducing anxiety in cardiac surgery patients. The results of another study showed nurse-initiated preoperational education and counseling to be associated with a reduced level of anxiety after CABG surgery (Zhang et al., 2012). However, according to the results of a recent systematic review, further research is required to investigate preoperative educational intervention effects in cardiac patients, especially in non-Western countries (Guo, 2015).

The NSM applies a holistic vision to discover the effects of stress on patients as well as to improve patient capabilities to adjust and rebalance (Verberk & Fawcett, 2017; Wang et al., 2019). Although the effect of this model has not been investigated in patients undergoing CABG surgery, the application of this model has been documented in the care of patients with various diseases. Ahmadi and Sadeghi (2017) suggested that this model be applied as a framework to assist nurses in the care of patients with multiple sclerosis. In addition, Wang et al. reported that the NSM is applicable to the care of patients with cirrhosis, patients with cancer, patients with hypertension, and patients with stroke.

The findings of this study show no difference in the intervention group at the time of discharge in terms of the level of anxiety between those who received the first and second levels of prevention and those who received all three levels of prevention. The aim of the first and second levels of prevention in the NSM is removing stressors, whereas the aim of the third level of the intervention is adapting to the stressors. Therefore, it should be considered that the stressors were still present in the participants who received the third level of prevention. This may be attributed to individual differences in terms of psychological or family status (Sedaghat et al., 2019). According to the findings in this study, adaptation using a relaxation method as the third level of prevention may be an effective intervention to reduce anxiety in patients scheduled for CABG surgery. However, the use and interpretation of our findings should be done with caution because these results may be attributable to the small number of participants who received all three levels of prevention.

Limitations

There were a number of limitations in this study. First, this study was performed at a single center using a small sample size. Second, although participants filled out the questionnaires in a low-stress environment, issues such as boredom and financial or family conflicts may still have occupied the thoughts of the participants and influenced their responses. Third, although the researchers tried to keep the participants in the two groups unaware of the identity of the intervention, participant ascertainment and observer bias may have still biased the results. Finally, individual cultural, social, religious, and spiritual factors may have influenced the participants' anxiety levels, which would decrease the generalizability of the results of this study to other countries.

Conclusions

The results of this study support that the NSM has the potential to significantly and positively reduce anxiety in patients scheduled for CABG surgery. This model may be easily used in practice as a guide for nurses to provide quality care to patients awaiting surgery. Therefore, the NSM may be a suitable theory to apply in reducing anxiety in patients scheduled for CABG surgery. The results of this study are applicable for nurses, nursing managers, and hospital managers to provide holistic care to patients in hospital and community settings.

Acknowledgments

The results of this research are part of a master's thesis in nursing that was approved by the Isfahan University of Medical Sciences (Grant No. 396838). We express our appreciation to the research deputy, patients, and nursing staff for their cooperation during this study.

Author Contributions

Study conception and design: EA, SB
Data collection: EA
Data analysis and interpretation: EA, SB, AM
Drafting of the article: All authors
Critical revision of the article: FE, AM

References

Aghebati, N., Mohammadi, E., & Ahmadi, F. (2012). The concept of nursing in holistic theories: An integrative review. *Evidence Based Care, 2*(2), 67–84. (Original work published in Persian)

Ahmadi, Z., & Sadeghi, T. (2017). Application of the Betty Neuman Systems Model in the nursing care of patients/clients with multiple sclerosis. *Multiple Sclerosis Journal—Experimental, Translational and Clinical, 3*(3), 1–8. https://doi.org/10.1177/2055217317726798

Akhlaghi, E., Babaei, S., & Abolhassani, S. (2020). Modifying stressors using Betty Neuman system modeling in coronary artery bypass graft: A randomized clinical trial. *Journal of Caring Sciences, 9*(1), 13–19. https://doi.org/10.34172/jcs.2020.003

Alipoor, A., Oraki, M., & Yazdian Sabet, M. (2014). Efficiency of brainwave entrainment by binaural beats in reducing anxiety. *Journal of Kermanshah University of Medical Sciences, 18*(1), Article e74271. https://doi.org/10.22110/jkums.v18i1.1385 (Original work published in Persian)

Alshvang, S. (2018). *Preoperative nurses' teaching for open heart surgery patients* [Doctorol dissertation]. Walden Dissertations and Doctoral Studies. https://scholarworks.waldenu.edu/cgi/viewcontent.cgi?article=5867&context=dissertations

Bourdeanu, L., & Doo, V. (2013). Assessment of chemotherapy-induced nausea and vomiting in women with breast cancer: A Neuman Systems Model framework. *Research and Theory for Nursing Practice, 27*(4), 296–304. https://doi.org/10.1891/1541-6577.27.4.296

Fawcett, J., & Desanto-Madeya, S. (2012). *Contemporary nursing knowledge: Analysis and evaluation of nursing models and theories.* F. A. Davis.

Fawcett, J., & Garity, J. (2008). *Evaluating research for evidence-based nursing practice.* F. A. Davis.

Guo, P. (2015). Preoperative education interventions to reduce anxiety and improve recovery among cardiac surgery patients: A review of randomised controlled trials. *Journal of Clinical Nursing, 24*(1–2), 34–46. https://doi.org/10.1111/jocn.12618

Guo, P., East, L., & Arthur, A. (2012). A preoperative education intervention to reduce anxiety and improve recovery among Chinese cardiac patients: A randomized controlled trial. *International Journal of Nursing Studies, 49*(2), 129–137. https://doi.org/10.1016/j.ijnurstu.2011.08.008

Heffline, M. S. (1990). Exploring nursing interventions for acute pain in the postanesthesia care unit. *Journal of Post Anesthesia Nursing, 5*(5), 321–328.

Hinkle, J. L., & Cheever, K. H. (2013). *Study guide for Brunner & Suddarth's textbook of medical-surgical nursing* (13th ed.). Lippincott Williams & Wilkins.

Huang, S., Xie, X., & Wu, S. (2015). Applying Roy Adaptation Model (RAM) in assessing health of patient with post-operative coronary artery bypass graft (CABG) surgery. *Hougner Protocols in Biomedical Sciences, 1*(2), 10–18.

Kim, J., & Shin, W. (2014). How to do random allocation (randomization). *Clinics in Orthopedic Surgery, 6*(1), 103–109. https://doi.org/10.4055/cios.2014.6.1.103

Krannich, J.-H. A., Weyers, P., Lueger, S., Herzog, M., Bohrer, T., & Elert, O. (2007). Presence of depression and anxiety before and after coronary artery bypass graft surgery and their relationship to age. *BMC Psychiatry, 7*(1), Article No. 47. https://doi.org/10.1186/1471-244X-7-47

McEwen, M., & Wills, E. M. (2017). *Theoretical basis for nursing* (5th ed.). Lippincott Williams & Wilkins.

Meleis, A. I. (2011). *Theoretical nursing: Development and progress* (5th ed.). Lippincott Williams & Wilkins.

Middel, B., El Baz, N., Pedersen, S. S., van Dijk, J. P., Wynia, K., & Reijneveld, S. A. (2014). Decline in health-related quality of life 6 months after coronary artery bypass graft surgery: The influence of anxiety, depression, and personality traits. *Journal of Cardiovascular Nursing, 29*(6), 544–554. https://doi.org/10.1097/JCN.0b013e3182a102ae

Moazzeni, S. S., Toreyhi, H., Asgari, S., Azizi, F., Tehrani, F. R., Hadaegh, F. R., & Hadaegh, F. (2021). Number of parity/live birth (s) and cardiovascular disease among Iranian women and men: Results of over 15 years of follow-up. *BMC Pregnancy and Childbirth, 21*, Article No. 28. https://doi.org/10.1186/s12884-020-03499-2

Mrayyan, M. (2006). Jordanian nurses' job satisfaction, patients' satisfaction and quality of nursing care. *International Nursing Review, 53*(3), 224–230. https://doi.org/10.1111/j.1466-7657.2006.00439.x

Nasiry Zarrin Ghabaee, D., Bagheri-Nesami, M., & Abbaspour, H. (2015). Application of Neuman Systems Model in nurse anesthetists to reduce patients' anxiety level: A randomized clinical trial. *Journal of Mazandaran University of Medical Sciences, 25*(126), 122–131.

Neuman, B. M., & Fawcett, J. (2002). *The Neuman Systems Model* (4th ed.). Prentice Hall.

Palmerini, T., Serruys, P., Kappetein, A. P., Genereux, P., Riva, D. D., Reggiani, L. B., Christiansen, E. H., Holm, N. R., Thuesen, L., Makikallio, T., Morice, M. C., Ahn, J. M., Park, S. J., Thiele, H., Boudriot, E., Sabatino, M., Romanello, M., Biondi-Zoccai, G., Cavalcante, R., ... Stone, G. W. (2017). Clinical outcomes with percutaneous coronary revascularization vs coronary artery bypass grafting surgery in patients with unprotected left main coronary artery disease: A meta-analysis of 6 randomized trials and 4,686 patients. *American Heart Journal, 190*, 54–63. https://doi.org/10.1016/j.ahj.2017.05.005

Parvan, K., Zamanzadeh, V., Dizaji, S. L., Shabestari, M. M., & Safaie, N. (2013). Patient's perception of stressors associated with coronary artery bypass surgery. *Journal of Cardiovascular and Thoracic Research, 5*(3), 113–117. https://doi.org/10.5681/jcvtr.2013.024

Parvan, K., Zamanzadeh, V., Lakdizaji, S., & Shabestari, M. M. (2012). Nurse's perception of stressors associated with coronary artery bypass surgery. *Journal of Caring Sciences, 4*(4), 237–243. https://doi.org/10.5681/jcs.2012.033

Polit, D. F., & Beck, C. T. (2004). *Nursing research: Principles and methods* (7th ed.). Lippincott Williams & Wilkins.

Ramesh, C. (2017). *Effectiveness of comprehensive nursing intervention programme (CNIP) on anxiety, fatigue, self-efficacy and quality of life among patients undergoing coronary artery bypass graft surgery in a tertiary care hospital—A randomized controlled trial* [Doctoral dissertation, Manipal College of Nursing, Manipal University]. http://hdl.handle.net/10603/180729

Reed, K. S. (1993). Adapting the Neuman Systems Model for family nursing. *Nursing Science Quarterly, 6*(2), 93–97. https://doi.org/10.1177/089431849300600209

Rosenfeldt, F., Braun, L., Spitzer, O., Bradley, S., Shepherd, J., Bailey, M., van der Merwe, J., Leong, J.-Y., & Esmore, D. (2011). Physical conditioning and mental stress reduction—A randomised trial in patients undergoing cardiac surgery. *BMC Complementary and Alternative Medicine, 11*(1), Article No. 20. https://doi.org/10.1186/1472-6882-11-20

Sahrakhil, M., Nasrabadi, T., & Ebrahimi Abyaneh, E. (2017). Effects of Benson's relaxation technique on comfort level of patients before coronary artery bypass grafting (a clinical trial). *Medical-Surgical Nursing Journal, 5*(4), 60–65.

Sedaghat, S., Rostami, S., Ebadi, A., & Fereidooni-Moghadam, M. (2019). Stressors in open-heart surgery patients: A qualitative study. *ARYA Atherosclerosis, 15*(4), 192–200. https://doi.org/10.22122/arya.v15i4.1840

Smith, M. C., & Parker, M. E. (2015). *Nursing theories and nursing practice*. F. A. Davis.

Spielberger, C. D. (2010). State-trait anxiety inventory. In I. B. Weiner & W. E. Crajghead (Eds.), *The Corsini Encyclopedia of Psychology*. Wiley Online Library. https://doi.org/10.1002/9780470479216.corpsy0943

Sultan, B. (2018). Application of Betty Neuman theory in care of stroke patient. *Annals of Nursing and Practice, 5*(1), Article 1092.

Takagi, H., Ando, T., Umemoto, T., & ALICE (All-Literature Investigation of Cardiovascular Evidence) Group. (2017). Perioperative depression or anxiety and postoperative mortality in cardiac surgery: A systematic review and meta-analysis. *Heart and Vessels, 32*(12), 1458–1468. https://doi.org/10.1007/s00380-017-1022-3

Tully, P. J., Winefield, H. R., Baker, R. A., Denollet, J., Pedersen, S. S., Wittert, G. A., & Turnbull, D. A. (2015). Depression, anxiety and major adverse cardiovascular and cerebrovascular events in patients following coronary artery bypass graft surgery: A five year longitudinal cohort study. *BioPsychoSocial Medicine, 9*(1), Article No. 14. https://doi.org/10.1186/s13030-015-0041-5

Verberk, F., & Fawcett, J. (2017). Thoughts about created environment: A Neuman systems model concept. *Nursing Science Quarterly, 30* (2), 179–181. https://doi.org/10.1177/0894318417693316

Wadensten, B., & Carlsson, M. (2003). Nursing theory views on how to support the process of ageing. *Journal of Advanced Nursing, 42*(2), 118–124. https://doi.org/10.1046/j.1365-2648.2003.02594.x

Wang, H.-P., Huang, Y.-Q., & Jin, C.-D. (2019). Betty Newman's systematic model and its application in clinical nursing. *TMR Integrative Nursing, 3*(4), 113–117. https://doi.org/10.12032/TMRIN20190429

Zhang, C. Y., Jiang, Y., Yin, Q. Y., Chen, F. J., Ma, L. L., & Wang, L. X. (2012). Impact of nurse-initiated preoperative education on postoperative anxiety symptoms and complications after coronary artery bypass grafting. *Journal of Cardiovascular Nursing, 27*(1), 84–88. https://doi.org/10.1097/JCN.0b013e3182189c4d

13

Factors Affecting Quality of Life Among the Elderly in Long-Term Care Hospitals

Hee-Kyung CHANG[1] • Cho-Rong GIL[2]* • Hye-Jin KIM[3] • Han-Ju BEA[4]

ABSTRACT

Background: There are challenges in sustaining person-centered care in aged care settings. Key related issues of concern such as quality of life among the older people in long-term care hospitals and interactions with nursing staff have been described previously.

Purpose: This study was designed to explore the factors affecting quality of life among older people living in long-term care hospitals in South Korea.

Methods: Older adult patients (N = 202) in three long-term care hospitals completed measures of cognitive functions, depression, care dependency, and interactions between nurse and patient and a quality-of-life assessment tool. Univariate analyses were used to examine the relationships among these variables, and a multiple linear regression analysis was used to explore the extent to which these variables predicted quality of life in these patients.

Results: The significant factors associated with quality of life were found to be cognitive functions (r = .373, p < .001), care dependency (r = .350, p < .001), and depression (r = −.504, p < .001). The regression model with depression and care dependency as predictor variables accounted for 25.7% of the variance in quality of life.

Conclusions/Implications for Practice: The correlation found in this study between quality of life and depression and care dependency provides additional evidentiary support for developing and applying nursing interventions that reduce depression and care dependency in older adult populations.

KEY WORDS:
depression, long-term care hospital, nurse–patient interaction, older people care, quality of life.

Introduction

The proportion of the population aged 65 years and above has increased annually, with this proportion (14.9%) surpassing the proportion of youths under 15 years old (12.4%) in 2019. By 2025, South Korea is expected to be a super-aged society, with a population of older people greater than 20% (National Statistical Office, 2019a). With this increase in the older adult population, the number of long-term care hospitals (LTCHs) in Korea increased to 1,577 in 2019, up 202.9% from 2009 (National Statistical Office, 2019b). LTCHs in Korea are medical institutions that provide medical treatment to patients who require care for geriatric or chronic diseases or those who are recovering after surgery or injury (Ministry of Health and Welfare, 2019). Those with health insurance may be admitted to an LTCH by personal request or at the recommendation of a doctor. LTCHs maintain one doctor for every 40 patients and one nurse for every six patients and provide rehabilitation services such as physical therapy and occupational therapy as well as medical services and care services (Song, 2012). As demand for LTCHs continues to increase steadily with population aging, factors such as the quality of life (QoL) of hospitalized older people are expected to become more important than the size or number of hospitals (McDermott et al., 2012).

QoL is a multidimensional concept that includes subjective well-being and happiness and considers personal characteristics as well as physical, psychological, and social aspects (Haas, 1999). QoL is widely considered as an indicator of individual health in explorations of daily living functions and well-being (Bowling, 1995). In particular, QoL in older people is very important, as it is closely related to happiness and the achievement of life goals.

Humans experience a variety of changes in old age such as physical changes because of illness or natural deterioration of physical functions, social changes because of the loss of roles in the home and society, a worsening economic situation, depression, solitude, and even suicidal impulses. Among these changes, the deterioration of physical functions because of aging affects brain function negatively and leads to decreased cognitive functioning, which causes memory problems, disorientation, diminished judgment, and poor comprehension (Gajewski & Falkenstein, 2016). It is known that older people

[1]PhD, RN, Associate Professor, College of Nursing, Gerontological Health Research Center in Institute of Health Sciences, Gyeongsang National University, Jinju, South Korea • [2]MSN, RN, Researcher, College of Nursing, Gerontological Health Research Center in Institute of Health Sciences, Gyeongsang National University, Jinju, South Korea • [3]MPH, RN, Assistant Professor and Researcher, Department of Nursing Science, Kyungsung University, Busan, South Korea • [4] MSN, RN, Assistant Professor, School of Nursing, Yeungnam University College, Nam-gu, Daegu, South Korea.

who are socially isolated because of reduced environmental stimulation often have reduced cognitive statuses (Coyle & Dugan, 2012). The decline in cognitive functions in older people makes it difficult for them to perform daily life activities independently, leading to depression and ultimately lowering their QoL (Svantesson et al., 2015).

Depression is one of the most prominent changes in the mental functioning of older people. It is known that older people in LTCHs have a relatively high level of depression because of their disconnection from familiar lifestyles and familiar social relationships (Olsen et al., 2016). However, it is important for older people to assess depression accurately because they often experience depression through physical symptoms such as headaches rather than through feeling depressed (Kamińska et al., 2015). Older people with decreased physical functions in terms of hearing, vision, and physical strength because of aging find it more difficult to perform activities such as eating, dressing, going to the bathroom, moving, and so on. Thus, they tend to rely on others for assistance and care (Meinerding et al., 2018). In consideration of this dependency, as well as the degradation of their human dignity and QoL, recent LTCHs have focused on providing nursing that reflects individual needs to maximize the use of the physical functions of older people and help them sustain an independent way of life (Brownie & Nancarrow, 2013). This suggests that older people's cognitive functions, depression, nursing dependency, and QoL are closely interrelated.

Person-centered care is a concept that has emerged as part of efforts to improve the QoL of older people living in LTCHs. Person-centered care refers to the recognition and practice of respecting the value and abilities of patients to protect their autonomy, self-esteem, and independence and meet their psychological needs (Flesner, 2009). Person-centered care may be effective in improving QoL in the physical, emotional, and social domains (Morgan & Yoder, 2012). Individualized nursing is essential for older people because each older person has unique physical, psychosocial, and mental problems and hence has different needs (Morgan & Yoder, 2012). It has been reported that person-centered care improves QoL and resolves psychological and social problems such as loneliness and depression, which are common in older people, by promoting communication between older people and medical staff (Brownie & Nancarrow, 2013). Therefore, understanding nurse–patient interactions is a prerequisite to providing person-centered care.

The Nurse–Patient Interaction Scale (NPIS), which is an appropriate instrument for understanding the communication and interactions between nurses and patients, includes factors such as having confidence in nurses, experiences of being respected and taken seriously, and satisfaction with communication (Haugan et al., 2012). However, because this scale has not been used in Korea, there is a need for studies and research to measure the interactions between nurses and patients using the NPIS to determine how nurses affect the lives of older people.

Previous studies related to factors affecting the QoL of older people have shown better physical functioning, which is associated with living in the community (De Vries et al., 2012), better cognitive function, and higher social activity (J. Kim et al., 2016), to be related to higher QoL. Older people in nursing homes with higher QoL were found to have lower levels of depression and better performance in activities of daily living (Barca et al., 2011). In South Korea, LTCHs provide not only medical treatment and care but also a place to live until death (Yi & Lee, 2015). In addition, as the cost burden is relatively low and the hospitalization procedure is simple, the number of older people hospitalized in LTCHs will likely continue to increase. However, there is insufficient research on the QoL of older people living in LTCHs.

Therefore, to study the QoL of older people who are hospitalized in LTCHs, it is necessary to adopt an integrated approach that includes physical factors such as care dependence, emotional factors such as depression, and social factors such as interactions. Therefore, this study was designed to identify the factors affecting the QoL of older people hospitalized in LTCHs as a reference for the development of nursing interventions that effectively improve the QoL of older LTCH residents.

Aims

The purpose of this study was to explore the QoL and related factors (cognitive functions, depression, care dependency, and nurse–patient interactions) of older people living in LTCHs and to provide necessary data for the development of nursing interventions to improve the QoL of people in this vulnerable population.

Methods

Design

This was a descriptive study of the QoL of older people hospitalized in LTCHs and related factors.

Settings and Sample

Ethical approval was received from the Gyeongsang University Research Board of Ethics (Approval No. GIRB-A18-Y-0030), and approval to access and use medical data containing personal information was obtained from the LTCHs in Suncheon, Gwangyang. To select the participants for this study, a nurse who was currently working at an LTCH recommended three LTCHs with capacities of over 200 patients each. Convenience sampling was used in this study. LTCHs A and B are located in Suncheon City, and LTCH C is located in Gwangyang City, with 245, 250, and 299 beds, respectively. They all received a first grade in the nursing grade evaluation conducted by the Ministry of Health and Welfare, which considers financial factors, programs, services, and resident rights.

The participants in this study ($N = 202$) were older people who had been admitted to one of the three participating LTCHs. All met the definition of an older person (> 65 years old) used by the United Nations and the Korean Welfare Law. First, to receive the approval of the institutions to collect data, we explained the purpose of the study to the administrators and obtained permission to proceed. Older people who were able to communicate and could respond to questions were recommended by the nurse working in LTCHs. After explaining the study purpose and obtaining informed consent, we collected information from the participants and their guardians. The inclusion criteria were as follows: (a) age of 65 years or older and were admitted to an LTCH, (b) ability to communicate sufficiently with the nurse, and (c) agreement to participate in the study and submit written consent (both participant and guardian). Those who had abused drugs or alcohol and those with severe intellectual disabilities who were unable to communicate were excluded.

The sample size was calculated using the G*Power 3.1.2 program. On the basis of an effect size of d = .15, a significance level of α = .05, and a power of $(1 - \beta)$ = .95, the number of samples required for a multiple regression analysis, including five independent variables, was estimated to be 138. Considering attrition because of mortality, a sample of 202 participants was recruited. Sixty-seven completed questionnaires were collected at LTCH A, 82 were collected at LTCH B, and 53 were collected at LTCH C.

Measures

Cognitive impairment was assessed using the Korean version of the Mini-Mental State Examination (MMSE-K; Kwon & Park, 1989). This tool was slightly modified from the original tool, the MMSE, based on the high rate of uneducated older people in South Korea. The MMSE-K consists of 12 questions: one item on time orientation (5 points), two items on location orientation (5 points), one item on memory registration (3 points), one item on memory recall (3 points), one item on focus and calculation (5 points), four items on language function (7 points), and one item on understanding and judgment (2 points), for 30 points in total. In cases in which a participant had no formal education, 3 additional points were allocated to the time orientation, attention, and language items. Those scoring between 24 and 30 points were categorized as having no cognitive impairment, those scoring between 18 and 23 points were categorized as having mild cognitive impairment, and those scoring 17 points or less were categorized as having severe cognitive impairment. MMSE-K is a tool with high reliability and validity, with a test–retest reliability of .89 and interscorer reliability of .82 at the time of development.

Depression was assessed using a Korean translation of the Short Geriatric Depression Scale developed by Sheikh and Yesavage (1986) as a simplified 15-item version of the Geriatric Depression Scale (GDS), which was developed by Cho et al. (1999). Answers take the form of "yes" or "no," and the total possible score is 15. The Short Geriatric Depression Scale showed satisfactory sensitivity and specificity when applied to the cutoff score of 8 in a study of neuropsychiatric ward patients (Cho et al., 1999). Therefore, the cutoff point used in the current study was 8, with a score of > 8 indicating depression. The Cronbach's α of this scale was .94 in Sheikh and Yesavage (1986) and Kuder–Richardson Formula 20 was .84 in this study.

Care dependency was assessed using the Korean version of the Care Dependency Scale (CDS-Korean version), which was modified in 2000 by Kim (E. J. Kim, 2000) from the original CDS-UK developed by Dijkstra et al. (2000). The CDS is a scale derived from observed behavior that is relatively easy for nurses and caregivers to measure. In this study, the surveyor observed the participants and filled out the questionnaire, which was previously confirmed by nurses who care for older people. The CDS consists of 15 items rated on a 5-point Likert scale, ranging from 1 (*completely dependent*) to 5 (*effectively independent*). Scale items address issues such as "eating/drinking," "communication," and "recreational activities." Total possible scores range from 15 to 70, with higher scores indicating lower care dependency. The Cronbach's α of this scale was .93 in the study of Kim and .96 in this study.

Interactions between nurses and patients were assessed using the NPIS, which was developed by Haugan et al. (2012). It consists of 14 items rated on a 10-point Likert scale, ranging from 1 (*not at all*) to 10 (*very much*). Total possible scores range from 14 to 140, with higher scores indicating better nurse–patient interaction. Scale items address statements such as "The nurses make all possible efforts to relieve my medical problems" and "I often am hurt or saddened by how the nurses interact with me." Although the NPIS has not been used in South Korea, this scale is widely used in Europe and the United States to describe interactions between patients and nursing staff in long-term care settings. The NPIS has shown good content validity and reliability among nursing home patients (Haugan et al., 2012). After approval from the tool's original developer and before data collection, the questionnaire was reviewed by an expert with years of practical experience in an LTCH and by a professor fluent in both English and Korean, who back-translated the NPIS into English and confirmed that no significant differences existed between the original English and Korean versions. The Cronbach's α of this scale was .92 in the study of Haugan et al. and was .92 in this study.

QoL was assessed using the Korean version of the Quality of Life-Alzheimer's Disease (KQoL-AD; Shin, 2006). The KQoL-AD was modified to fit the QoL-AD developed by Logsdon et al. (1999), which consists of 13 items rated on a 4-point Likert scale, ranging from 1 (*bad*) to 4 (*very good*). Total possible scores ranged from 13 to 52, with lower scores indicating worse QoL. Scale items address issues such as physical health, family, and ability to do things for fun. KQoL-AD is a tool for evaluating QoL in patients with dementia that has excellent content validity and test–retest reliability. As KQoL-AD is not affected by cognitive function or the dementia stage, this scale has been used on patients with non-dementia-related cognitive impairments as well as on patients with dementia (H. J. Kim et al., 2008). KQoL-AD may be used to evaluate the QoL in patients using self-reported data as well as using responses provided by caregivers. In this study, those participants who expressed experiencing difficulties in filling out this scale were permitted to have their legal agents complete the scale on their behalf. The Cronbach's α of the KQoL-AD was .88 in the study of Shin and was .88 in this study.

Data Collection

Data were collected for this study from July to August 2018. Two research assistants and three nurses trained in administering the survey for this study informed each of the participants and their legal guardians regarding the study purpose and explained that they could withdraw at any time. In addition, it was clearly stated in the questionnaire that all information from the survey would only be used for the purpose of this study and that all personal and medical information would be anonymized.

One-on-one interviews and observations with study participants were conducted by the research assistants. The research assistants read the questionnaire aloud and recorded the participant's responses. Four researchers were responsible for planning and overseeing the entire study. To minimize the influence of the researchers, the researchers informed the two research assistants, who were nursing students, about the study purpose, the precautions to take when collecting data, and measurement tool contents and methods. The goal of this precautionary activity was to maintain consistency in the methods and attitudes of the research assistants. After listening to all of the explanations, the participants and legal guardians who agreed to participate in the study were interviewed. General characteristics that were not definitively known by the participants (e.g., cost payer) were confirmed through legal guardians or medical records. The data collected through research assistant observations such as CDS were checked by three nurses who were trained in performing questionnaires. The survey took 20–30 minutes to complete, and the data were collected by four researchers on the same day. Two hundred two questionnaires were distributed, and all 202 were completed and used in the final analysis.

Data Analyses

SPSS Version 22.0 (IBM, Inc., Armonk, NY, USA) was used for statistical analyses. The characteristics, cognitive functions, depression, care dependency, nurse–patient interaction, and QoL of the participants were analyzed using descriptive analysis. Cronbach's alpha reliability analyses were conducted on data related to cognitive function, depression, care dependency, nurse–patient interaction, and QoL. The correlations between cognitive functions, depression, care dependency, nurse–patient interaction, and QoL were analyzed using correlation analyses and multiple regression analyses. The significance level was set at .05.

Results

Differences in the Mean Values of Quality of Life According to the Characteristics

The sample consisted of 202 participants, of whom 145 (71.8%) were female and 57 (28.2%) were male (Table 1). The age of participants ranged from 65 to 96 years, with a mean of 80.61 years. Slightly over half (56.4%) of the participants had no formal education, 71.8% of cost payers were the participants' children, 43.6% of the participants had lived in their current LTCH for over 2 years, and 18.3% of the participants were visited by family members less than once per month. Two thirds (66.3%) of the participants had severe cognitive impairment, and 63.9% had a GDS score over 8. Number of family visits ($F = 6.90, p < .001$), cognitive function ($F = 10.70, p < .001$), and depression tendencies ($t = 6.94, p < .001$) were found to have statistically significant impacts on the QoL of participants.

Descriptive Statistics of the Care Dependency Scale and Quality of Life

The average item score on the CDS was 3.26 ($SD = 0.84$), with the communication score (3.76 ± 1.13) earning the highest average score and the recreational activities score (2.85 ± 1.10) earning the lowest (Table 2). The average item score on the KQoL-AD was 2.10 ($SD = 0.03$), with the family relationship score (2.43 ± 0.68) earning the highest average score and the physical health score (1.90 ± 0.74) earning the lowest (Table 3).

Correlations Among Cognitive Functions, Depression, Care Dependency, Interaction Between Nurse and Patient, and Quality of Life

The correlations among cognitive function, depression, care dependency, interactions with nurses, and QoL were studied using correlation analysis (Table 4). The results indicate a positive correlation between cognitive functioning and QoL ($r = .373, p < .001$) and care dependency ($r = .350, p < .001$), respectively; a negative correlation between depression and QoL ($r = -.504, p < .001$); and a positive correlation between the NPIS and care dependency ($r = .235, p < .001$).

Factors Contributing to Quality of Life

The results of the multiple regression analysis on the factors affecting QoL in older people are shown in Table 5. GDS and CDS was found to be statistically significantly related to QoL ($F = 35.838, p < .001$) at a power of prediction of 26.5% ($R = .515, R^2 = .265$).

Discussion

In this study, the QoL of older people in LTCHs and related factors were explored to provide basic data on nursing interventions that may be used to develop interventions to improve QoL in this population.

As shown in Table 1, as women in South Korea have a longer life expectancy than men and as most older women do not have jobs, the risk of social isolation and poverty among older women whose husbands have passed away is high,

Table 1

Differences in Mean Values of Quality of Life, by Personal Characteristics (N = 202)

Characteristic	*n*	%	Quality of Life				
			Mean	*SD*	*t/F*	*p*	Scheffe
Gender					−0.98	.328	
Male	57	28.2	26.68	6.00			
Female	145	71.8	27.58	5.77			
Age (years; *M* and *SD*)	80.61	4.77			1.02	.385	
≤ 69	14	6.9	27.07	5.54			
70–79	75	37.1	28.00	5.44			
80–89	92	45.6	27.23	6.16			
> 89	21	10.4	25.52	5.89			
Education					0.49	.741	
Elementary school	69	34.2	27.81	6.11			
Middle school	8	4.0	28.88	10.41			
High school	9	4.4	28.22	6.36			
College or more	2	1.0	27.00	1.41			
No formal education	114	56.4	26.86	5.28			
Cost payer					2.22	.087	
Self	35	17.3	26.11	6.53			
Spouse	8	4.0	27.50	8.32			
Children	145	71.8	27.90	5.56			
Governmental subsidies	14	6.9	24.36	4.22			
Length of stay (years)					1.61	.203	
< 1	68	33.6	27.54	5.62			
1–2	46	22.8	28.43	5.75			
> 2	88	43.6	26.58	6.00			
Family visits (per month)					6.90	< .001	① > ③; ② > ③
① Usually (3 times and over)	81	40.1	28.47	6.09			
② Often (1–2 times)	84	41.6	27.55	4.99			
③ Seldom (< 1 time)	37	18.3	24.32	6.15			
MMSE-K					10.70	< .001	① > ③; ② > ③
① No cognitive impairment	32	15.9	30.38	4.92			
② Mild cognitive impairment	36	17.8	29.36	5.29			
③ Severe cognitive impairment	134	66.3	26.05	5.78			
GDS (score)					6.94	< .001	① > ②
① ≤ 8	96	36.1	30.02	5.94			
② > 8	106	63.9	24.89	4.53			

Note. MMSE-K = Korean version of the Mini-Mental State Examination for dementia screening; GDS = Geriatric Depression Scale.

leading to higher incidences of children taking joint responsibility for parental financial and psychological support (Shin & Park, 2018). Moreover, care by professional staff is required for older people with cognitive impairment. To resolve these problems, older people and their families in South Korea tend to choose LTCHs, which are cheaper than general hospitals and allow the integration of long-term hospitalization with daily life. However, it is believed that older people experience depression because they are disconnected from social support systems such as family and/or close friends, experience decreased social activity, and experience a monotonous daily life after moving into an LTCH.

The mean QoL score for participants in this study was 2.10 ± 0.03, which is slightly below median. This compares with the score of 31.82 ± 7.18 for community-dwelling older people registered at the Dementia Prevention Center (Park & Ahn, 2017). It is thought that the disconnection from support systems, the loss of social life, feelings of abandonment by their family, the stress of adapting to a new environment, and the monotonous daily life in LTCHs all affect QoL.

The mean care dependency score for participants in this study was 3.26 ± 0.84, which is higher than the mean 2.94 ± 0.82 score for 103 patients with stroke (I. Kim, 2018), indicating that older people in LTCHs are more independent than poststroke

Table 2

Care Dependency Scale (N = 202)

Item	Mean	*SD*
Eating/drinking	3.48	1.02
Incontinence	3.51	1.32
Body posture	3.40	1.12
Mobility	2.96	1.22
Day/night pattern	3.59	1.10
Getting (un)dressed	3.25	1.12
Body temperature	3.36	1.11
Hygiene	3.00	1.12
Avoidance of danger	3.16	1.01
Communication	3.76	1.13
Contact with others	3.26	1.13
Sense of rules/values	3.58	1.20
Daily activities	3.21	1.23
Recreational activities	2.85	1.10
Learning ability	2.86	1.13
Total score, mean and *SD*	49.23	13.71

Note. Range of each item score from 1 to 5.

patients. This is thought to be because of the relatively high severity of poststroke patients' conditions compared with older adults, who often require chronic disease or geriatric disease treatment/management. Unlike adolescents and adults in general, leisure and physical activities for older people are known to play an important role in maintaining health and energy in old age (Shimada et al., 2016). High levels of physical activity in older people have been shown to associate significantly with cognitive function in previous studies (Grimaud et al., 2017; Lin et al., 2012). In particular, after a 6-month aerobic exercise intervention, an increase in hippocampal volume was observed in older people with mild cognitive impairment (Ten Brinke et al., 2015). Therefore, it is possible to improve the independence of older people by applying pleasureful recreational activities and exercise together to stimulate cognitive function during leisure time (Tyndall et al., 2018).

The nurse–patient interaction score for older people in LTCHs was 7.55 ± 1.54. In Norway, the NPIS of nursing home patients without cognitive impairment was reported as 8.13 ± 1.63 (Haugan et al., 2016). The difference was considered to be because of the relatively low cognitive functioning of the participants in this study. It is known that improvements in

Table 3

Korean Version of the Quality of Life-Alzheimer's Disease Scale (N = 202)

Item	Mean	*SD*
Physical health	1.90	0.74
Energy	1.95	0.71
Mood	2.23	0.65
Living situation	2.34	0.67
Memory	2.05	0.74
Family	2.43	0.68
Marriage	2.21	0.74
Friends	2.31	0.72
Self	2.12	0.66
Ability to do chores	1.90	0.76
Ability to do things for fun	1.93	0.72
Money	1.93	0.65
Life as a whole	2.04	0.68
Total score, mean and *SD*	27.33	5.83

Note. Range of each item score: 1–4.

Table 4

Correlations Among MMSE-K, GDS, Care Dependency, NPIS, and Quality of Life (N = 202)

Variable	MMSE-K	GDS	CDS	NPIS	Quality of Life
MMSE-K	1				
GDS	−.273***	1			
CDS	.570***	−.265***	1		
NPIS	.019	−.019	.235***	1	
Quality of life	.373***	−.504***	.350***	.053	1

Note. MMSE-K = Korean version of the Mini-Mental State Examination for dementia screening; GDS = Geriatric Depression Scale; CDS = Care Dependency Scale; NPIS = Nurse–Patient Interaction Scale; Quality of life = Korean version of the Quality of Life-Alzheimer's Disease Scale.

***$p < .001$.

Table 5

Multiple Regression Analysis of Quality of Life With the Other Variables (N = 202)

Source Variance	*df*	*SS*	*MS*	*F*	*p*
Model 1 [a]					
Regression	1	7.857	7.857	48.192	< .001
Residual	200	32.607	0.163		
Total	201	40.464			
Model 2 [b]					
Regression	2	10.715	5.358	35.838	< .001
Residual	199	29.749	0.149		
Total	201	40.464			

Note. GDS = Geriatric Depression Scale; CDS = Care Dependency Scale.
[a]$R = .441$, $R^2 = .194$, $SE = .40378$. [b]$R = .515$, $R^2 = .265$, $SE = .38664$.

communication between older people and medical staff improve the former's QoL by helping them deal with problems common to older people such as loneliness and depression (Sagong & Lee, 2016). Thus, interventions based on interactions such as storytelling (Astell et al., 2010) should be implemented to help older people build healthy relationships with other older people or healthcare providers and experience high-quality interactions.

In this study, a significant difference in the QoL was found based on number of family visits ($F = 6.90, p < .001$), cognitive functions ($F = 10.70, p < .001$), and depression tendencies ($t = 6.94, p < .001$). This result supports the findings in previous studies that associated higher family visit frequencies with higher cognitive functioning and lower levels of depression with higher QoL (Barca et al., 2011; Gräske et al., 2015). Because of the traditional values of filial piety and familyism, it is common in South Korea for children to take care of their aging parents. For Korean older people, family is a basic requirement for successful aging as well as the most important source of support. Therefore, a nurse should assess the degree of family visitation together with the patient's perception of the level of family support and maintain close relationships via phone calls and messages. It is also necessary to create an institutional environment in which the family feels comfortable and is able to interact freely with their family member.

Decreased cognitive functioning affects sense of balance, making independent physical activity difficult and reducing QoL in older people (Shin et al., 2011). Physical activity is used as a helpful therapeutic care strategy to delay the loss of functional independence in older people. In particular, regular exercise is known to play an important role in increasing cerebral blood flow and neurotransmitter release, enhancing muscle flexibility and balance, and improving cognitive functioning (Gligoroska & Manchevska, 2012). Therefore, it is desirable to provide an exercise intervention program that maintains and enhances cognitive functioning and daily performance abilities in older people to improve QoL.

Depression in older people not only lowers physical functioning but, if neglected, may also cause cognitive dysfunction and dementia (Demnitz et al., 2016). Moreover, depression may threaten the health of older people because of its association with a higher risk of suicide. However, early detection of depression and proper medication or psychotherapy may help relieve symptoms and improve QoL. Therefore, active prevention, early detection, and appropriate treatment are very important. LTCH nurses are responsible to provide depression-related prevention education, early detection, and treatment. Thus, training in diagnosing depression should be provided to all healthcare providers who care for older people.

Depression and nursing dependence were found in this study to be predictor variables of QoL, explaining 26.5% of the variance in QoL. This is similar to a previous study that found depression, behavior, and degree of care needed for daily life to be related to the QoL of 181 people aged 65 years or older who were admitted to LTCHs (Ok & Lee, 2017). Therefore, we should pay attention to depression in older people hospitalized in LTCHs and try to improve their QoL using appropriate diagnosis and treatment. Furthermore, nurses should create an atmosphere in which older people may participate proactively in decision making and increase their independence and interactivity using health checks and daily living ability reinforcement programs.

This study adds to the scholarly knowledge by exploring the QoL of older people who were admitted to the unique environment of an LTCH, which is an institution midway between traditional hospital and nursing home settings. LTCHs provide care that addresses the physical, emotional, and social domains of patients. However, nurse–patient interactions, which were expected to relate significantly to QoL, were found to relate only insignificantly. Possibly because nurses submitted the surveys on behalf of the senior participants who had low cognitive functions. In a previous study (Haugan et al., 2012), the NPIS was related to QoL for nursing home patients with normal cognitive functioning. Thus, this issue should be reexamined and confirmed in future studies. Finally, the results of this study should be interpreted cautiously because of its use of a convenience sample of older people who were admitted to three LTCHs in two areas of South Korea.

Conclusions

QoL is a critical issue for the rising population of older adults living in LTCHs in South Korea. The purpose of this study was to investigate the effects of general characteristics, cognitive functioning, care dependency, depression, and nurse–patient interactions on the QoL of older people admitted to LTCHs and to suggest improvements. On the basis of the results of this study, the development and implementation of a nursing intervention method that lowers depression and care dependency in older people living in LTCHs may improve their QoL.

Acknowledgments

This study (No. 2018R1C1B6007828) was conducted with the support of the National Research Foundation of Korea and with funding from the Ministry of Science and Information and Communications Technologies.

Author Contributions

Study conception and design: HKC
Data collection: CRG, HJK, HJB
Data analysis and interpretation: All authors
Drafting of the article: All authors
Critical revision of the article: HKC, CRG

References

Astell, A. J., Ellis, M. P., Bernardi, L., Alm, N., Dye, R., Gowans, G., & Campbell, J. (2010). Using a touch screen computer to support relationships between people with dementia and caregivers. *Interacting with Computers, 22*(4), 267–275. https://doi.org/10.1016/j.intcom.2010.03.003

Barca, M. L., Engedal, K., Laks, J., & Selbæk, G. (2011). Quality of life among elderly patients with dementia in institutions. *Dementia and Geriatric Cognitive Disorders, 31*(6), 435–442. https://doi.org/10.1159/000328969

Bowling, A. (1995). What things are important in people's lives? A survey of the public's judgements to inform scales of health related quality of life. *Social Science & Medicine, 41*(10), 1447–1462. https://doi.org/10.1016/0277-9536(95)00113-L

Brownie, S., & Nancarrow, S. (2013). Effects of person-centered care on residents and staff in aged-care facilities: A systematic review. *Clinical Interventions in Aging, 8*, 1–10. https://doi.org/10.2147/CIA.S38589

Cho, M. J., Bae, J. N., Suh, G. H., Hahm, B. J., Kim, J. K., Lee, D. W., & Kang, M. H. (1999). Validation of Geriatric Depression Scale, Korean version (GDS) in the assessment of DSM-III-R major depression. *Journal of Korean Neuropsychiatric Association, 38*(1), 48–63 (Original work published in Korean)

Coyle, C. E., & Dugan, E. (2012). Social isolation, loneliness and health among older adults. *Journal of Aging and Health, 24*(8), 1346–1363. https://doi.org/10.1177/0898264312460275

De Vries, N. M., Van Ravensberg, C. D., Hobbelen, J. S. M., Rikkert, M. O., Staal, J. B., & Nijhuis-Van der Sanden, M. W. G. (2012). Effects of physical exercise therapy on mobility, physical functioning, physical activity and quality of life in community-dwelling older adults with impaired mobility, physical disability and/or multi-morbidity: A meta-analysis. *Ageing Research Reviews, 11*(1), 136–149. https://doi.org/10.1016/j.arr.2011.11.002

Demnitz, N., Esser, P., Dawes, H., Valkanova, V., Johansen-Berg, H., Ebmeier, K. P., & Sexton, C. (2016). A systematic review and meta-analysis of cross-sectional studies examining the relationship between mobility and cognition in healthy older adults. *Gait & Posture, 50*, 164–174. https://doi.org/10.1016/j.gaitpost.2016.08.028

Dijkstra, A., Brown, L., Havens, B., Romeren, T. I., Zanotti, R., Dassen, T., & Van Den Heuvel, W. (2000). An international psychometric testing of the care dependency scale. *Journal of Advanced Nursing, 31*(4), 944–952. https://doi.org/10.1046/j.1365-2648.2000.01354.x

Flesner, M. K. (2009). Person-centered care and organizational culture in long-term care. *Journal of Nursing Care Quality, 24*(4), 273–276. https://doi.org/10.1097/NCQ.0b013e3181b3e669

Gajewski, P. D., & Falkenstein, M. (2016). Physical activity and neurocognitive functioning in aging—A condensed updated review. *European Review of Aging and Physical Activity, 13*(1), 1–7. https://doi.org/10.1186/s11556-016-0161-3

Gligoroska, J. P., & Manchevska, S. (2012). The effect of physical activity on cognition–physiological mechanisms. *Materia Sociomedica, 24*(3), 198–202. https://doi.org/10.5455/msm.2012.24.198-202

Gräske, J., Meyer, S., Worch, A., & Wolf-Ostermann, K. (2015). Family visits in shared-housing arrangements for residents with dementia–A cross-sectional study on the impact on residents' quality of life. *BMC Geriatrics, 15*(1), Article 14. https://doi.org/10.1186/s12877-015-0012-5

Grimaud, E., Taconnat, L., & Clarys, D. (2017). Cognitive stimulation in healthy older adults: A cognitive stimulation program using leisure activities compared to a conventional cognitive stimulation program. *Geriatrie et Psychologie Neuropsychiatrie du Vieillissement, 15*(2), 214–223. https://doi.org/10.1684/pnv.2017.0669 (Original work published in French)

Haas, B. K. (1999). A multidisciplinary concept analysis of quality of life. *Western Journal of Nursing Research, 21*(6), 728–742. https://doi.org/10.1177/01939459922044153

Haugan, G., Moksnes, U. K., & Løhre, A. (2016). Intrapersonal self-transcendence, meaning-in-life and nurse–patient interaction: Powerful assets for quality of life in cognitively intact nursing-home patients. *Scandinavian Journal of Caring Sciences, 30*(4), 790–801. https://doi.org/10.1111/scs.12307

Haugan, G., Rannestad, T., Hanssen, B., & Espnes, G. A. (2012). Self-transcendence and nurse–patient interaction in cognitively intact nursing home patients. *Journal of Clinical Nursing, 21*(23–24), 3429–3441. https://doi.org/10.1111/j.1365-2702.2012.04217.x

Kamińska, M., Brodowski, J., & Karakiewicz, B. (2015). Fall risk factors in community-dwelling elderly depending on their physical function, cognitive status and symptoms of depression. *International Journal of Environmental Research and Public Health, 12*(4), 3406–3416. https://doi.org/10.3390/ijerph120403406

Kim, E. J. (2000). Psychometric testing of the care dependency scale for the institutionalized Korean demented patients. *Journal of Korean Academy of Psychiatric and Mental Health Nursing, 9*(3), 303–314. (Original work published in Korean)

Kim, H. J., Moon, S. Y., Kim, S. Y., & Han, S.-H. (2008). Assessment of the quality of life in patients with Alzheimer's disease. *Journal of the Korean Neurological Association, 26*(4), 308–313. (Original work published in Korean)

Kim, I. (2018). Care dependency of post-stroke patients and its affecting factors. *Korean Journal of Rehabilitation Nursing, 21*(2), 100–109. (Original work published in Korean)

Kim, J., Song, R., Kim, K. W., & Kim, J. L. (2016). Effect of cognitive function, social activity participation and social support on quality of life of community-dwelling elderly. *Journal of Korean Geriatric Psychiatry, 20*(1), 25–32. https://doi.org/10.0000/jkgp.2016.20.1.25 (Original work published in Korean)

Kwon, Y. C., & Park, J. H. (1989). Korean version of Mini-Mental State Examination (MMSE-K). *Journal of the Korean Neuropsychiatric Association, 28*(1), 125–135. (Original work published in Korean)

Lin, F., Friedman, E., Quinn, J., Chen, D. G. D., & Mapstone, M. (2012). Effect of leisure activities on inflammation and cognitive function in an aging sample. *Archives of Gerontology and Geriatrics, 54*(3), 398–404. https://doi.org/10.1016/j.archger.2012.02.002

Logsdon, R. G., Gibbons, L. E., McCurry, S. M., & Teri, L. (1999). Quality of life in Alzheimer's disease: Patient and caregiver reports. *Journal of Mental Health and Aging, 5*(1), 21–32.

McDermott, C., Coppin, R., Little, P., & Leydon, G. (2012). Hospital admissions from nursing homes: A qualitative study of GP decision making. *British Journal of General Practice, 62*(601), e538–e545. https://doi.org/10.3399/bjgp12X653589

Meinerding, M., DeFeis, B., Sunderaraman, P., Azar, M., Lawless, S., Perez-Vivaldo, C., Gu, Y., Stern, Y., & Cosentino, S. (2018). Assessing dependency in a multiethnic community cohort of individuals with Alzheimer's disease. *Innovation in Aging, 2*(1), 1–7. https://doi.org/10.1093/geroni/igy011

Ministry of Health and Welfare. (2019). *Medical law.* Retrieved November 23, 2019, from http://www.law.go.kr/%EB%B2%95%EB%A0%B9/%EC%9D%98%EB%A3%8C%EB%B2%95

Morgan, S., & Yoder, L. H. (2012). A concept analysis of person-centered care. *Journal of Holistic Nursing, 30*(1), 6–15. https://doi.org/10.1177/0898010111412189

National Statistical Office. (2019a). *2019 elderly statistics.* Retrieved September 28, 2020, from http://kostat.go.kr/portal/korea/kor_nw/1/6/1/index.board?bmode=read&bSeq=&aSeq=377701&pageNo=2&rowNum=10&navCount=10&currPg=&searchInfo=&sTarget=title&sTxt=

National Statistical Office. (2019b). *Hospital present conditions based on cities and provinces.* Retrieved September 28, 2020, from http://kosis.kr/statHtml/statHtml.do?orgId=354&tblId=DT_MIRE01#

Ok, E. M., & Lee, J. Y. (2017). A study on influential factors to the quality of life in geriatric hospital elderly inpatient. *Journal of Wholistic Nursing Science, 10*(1), 1–12. (Original work published in Korean)

Olsen, C., Pedersen, I., Bergland, A., Enders-Slegers, M. J., Patil, G., & Ihlebaek, C. (2016). Effect of animal-assisted interventions on depression, agitation and quality of life in nursing home residents suffering from cognitive impairment or dementia: A cluster randomized controlled trial. *International Journal of Geriatric Psychiatry, 31*(12), 1312–1321. https://doi.org/10.1002/gps.4436

Park, S. H., & Ahn, S. N. (2017). The effect of dual task program on reducing the risk of dementia in older adults. *Research Journal of Pharmacy and Technology, 10*(7), 2255–2259. https://doi.org/10.5958/0974-360X.2017.00399.7 (Original work published in Korean)

Sagong, H., & Lee, G. E. (2016). Person-centered care and nursing service quality of nurses in long-term care hospitals. *Journal of Korean Academy of Community Health Nursing, 27*(4), 309–318. http://dx.doi.org/10.12799/jkachn.2016.27.4.309

Sheikh, J. I., & Yesavage, J. A. (1986). Geriatric Depression Scale (GDS): Recent evidence and development of a shorter version. *Clinical Gerontologist: The Journal of Aging and Mental Health, 5*(1–2), 165–173. https://doi.org/10.1300/J018v05n01_09

Shimada, H., Makizako, H., Lee, S., Doi, T., Tsutsumimoto, K., Harada, K., Hotta, R., Bae, S., Harada, N. K., & Suzuki, T. (2016). Impact of cognitive frailty on daily activities in older persons. *The Journal of Nutrition, Health & Aging, 20*(7), 729–735. https://doi.org/10.1007/s12603-016-0685-2

Shin, B. M., Han, S. J., Jung, J. H., Kim, J. E., & Fregni, F. (2011). Effect of mild cognitive impairment on balance. *Journal of the Neurological Sciences, 305*(1-2), 121–125. (Original work published in Korean)

Shin, H. Y. (2006). A preliminary study on the Korean version of quality of life-Alzheimer's disease scale in community-dwelling elderly with dementia. *Journal of Preventive Medicine and Public Health, 39*(3), 243–248. (Original work published in Korean)

Shin, S. H., & Park, J. S. (2018). A structural equation model of quality of life in nursing home residents. *Journal of Korean Gerontological Nursing, 20*(3), 193–203. https://doi.org/10.17079/jkgn.2018.20.3.193 (Original work published in Korean)

Song, H. J. (2012). Long-term care hospital systems in developed countries and the implications for Korea. *Journal of the Korean Geriatrics Society, 16*(3), 114–120. (Original work published in Korean)

Svantesson, U., Jones, J., Wolbert, K., & Alricsson, M. (2015). Impact of physical activity on the self-perceived quality of life in non-frail older adults. *Journal of Clinical Medicine Research, 7*(8), 585–593. https://doi.org/10.14740/jocmr2021w

Ten Brinke, L. F., Bolandzadeh, N., Nagamatsu, L. S., Hsu, C. L., Davis, J. C., Miran-Khan, K., & Liu-Ambrose, T. (2015). Aerobic exercise increases hippocampal volume in older women with probable mild cognitive impairment: A 6-month randomised controlled trial. *British Journal of Sports Medicine, 49*(4), 248–254. https://doi.org/10.1136/bjsports-2013-093184

Tyndall, A. V., Clark, C. M., Anderson, T. J., Hogan, D. B., Hill, M. D., Longman, R. S., & Poulin, M. J. (2018). Protective effects of exercise on cognition and brain health in older adults. *Exercise and Sport Sciences Reviews, 46*(4), 215–223. https://doi.org/10.1249/JES.0000000000000161

Yi, M. J., & Lee, J. S. (2015). Nurse's experiences of the death of patients in geriatric hospitals. *Journal of Korean Academy of Nursing, 45*(4), 513–522. https://doi.org/10.4040/jkan.2015.45.4.513

14

Environment-Friendly Practices in Operating Rooms in Turkey

Yelda CANDAN DÖNMEZ[1] • Arzu ASLAN[2*] • Meryem YAVUZ VAN GIERSBERGEN[3]

ABSTRACT

Background: Environment-friendly practices refer to decreasing energy consumption, using resources carefully and sustainably, and reducing environmental pollution. An environment-friendly hospital is defined as a hospital where energy is saved, carbon emissions are decreased, and productivity and quality are increased. Operating rooms (ORs) account for most wastes generated daily by hospitals. Thus, adopting environment-friendly healthcare practices in ORs will have a positive impact on the environment.

Purpose: The aim of this study was to identify and recommend environment-friendly practices that are feasible for implementation in ORs in Turkey.

Methods: Data on the environment-friendly practices that are currently being practiced in the ORs of hospitals in Izmir Province were collected using face-to-face interviews with nurses who were in charge of ORs in Izmir Province. The interviews were conducted using an OR identification form and Greening the OR Checklist. The study population included all of the hospitals in Izmir Province, and the study sample included 18 ORs in the 11 hospitals that consented to take part in the research. Permission to conduct this research was obtained from the ethics committee of the nursing school as well as from the participating hospitals where the study was conducted.

Results: The hospitals included in the study had, on average, 7.44 ± 7.32 ORs, each of which employed an average of 16.83 ± 17.16 nurses. Four fifths (83.3%) of the ORs always monitored their wastes, and 88.9% gave their batteries to recyclers. In addition, 72.2% renewed their surgical sets to reduce excessive use of materials, and 72.2% preferred using reusable materials instead of single-use materials in their surgical sets. However, 66.7% of the ORs had no environmental team, 93% did not use an environmentally safe surface cleaner, 83.3% did not use sensor controls on lights, and 66.7% did not use LED lights.

Conclusions: Although most hospitals did not have a special team to recommend and enforce environment-friendly procedures, the OR nurses did their best to protect the environment.

KEY WORDS:
nursing, operating room, environment-friendly, greening, environmental health.

Introduction

Surgical and delivery rooms generate most of the daily waste volume of hospitals. Waste management is one of the most important issues faced by hospitals (Karayurt, Andıç, & Ceylan, 2014; Potera, 2012). For example, health institutions in the United States generate four million tons of waste annually, of which 15% is infectious (Kagoma, Stall, Rubinstein, & Naudie, 2012; Kwakye, Brat, & Makary, 2011). Despite their physically small footprint, operating rooms (ORs) generate about 20%–33% of the total waste of a hospital. A single surgical operation may generate more waste than an average family of four generates in a week. Waste reduction strategies hold the potential to reduce the environmental impact of hospitals without compromising the health of patients (Kagoma et al., 2012; Lee & Mears, 2012).

The inadequate management of waste causes environmental pollution and the multiplication of disease vectors such as insects, rodents, and worms and may lead to the transmission of diseases such as typhoid, cholera, hepatitis, and AIDS through injuries from contaminated syringes and needles (Karayurt et al., 2014; Terekli, Özkan, & Bayın, 2013). In addition to the health risks associated with poor management of medical waste, the environmental impact must also be considered, especially the risks of water, air, and soil pollution (Karayurt et al., 2014). Although the negative impacts of medical waste are continuing, implementing simple, environment-friendly practices holds the potential to reduce the adverse effects of this waste and reduce costs without compromising patient care (Karayurt et al., 2014; Kwakye et al., 2011; Potera, 2012).

Certain environment-friendly practices do not require any technical application, such as the segregation of OR wastes. OR wastes are solid, biologically hazardous wastes that require regular segregation. The cost of biologically hazardous waste disposal is eight times higher than that of normal solid waste disposal. Waste that is not properly segregated must be treated as biologically hazardous waste by default, which significantly increases overall disposal costs (Kagoma et al., 2012; Potera, 2012; Terekli et al., 2013). Most of the

[1]PhD RN, Assistant Professor, Faculty of Nursing, Department of Surgical Nursing, Ege University, Izmir, Turkey • [2]MSN, RN, Research Assistant, Faculty of Health Science, Department of Surgical Nursing, Manisa Celal Bayar University, Manisa, Turkey • [3]PhD, RN, Professor, Faculty of Nursing, Department of Surgical Nursing, Ege University, Izmir, Turkey.

waste that is generated in ORs is solid waste such as paper, cardboard, metal, and plastic. Waste in this category that is not contaminated by bodily fluids is typically easy to recycle (Karayurt et al., 2014; Potera, 2012).

Twelve liters of liquid waste may be generated during a single surgical operation, and an average OR generates around two tons of liquid waste every month (Kagoma et al., 2012). In ORs, liquids are collected in aspiration containers and must be treated as biologically hazardous waste. As wastewater has a tendency to splash and spray during manual disposal, health workers are exposed to infectious liquids, which constitute a professional threat (Huncke et al., 2012; Kagoma et al., 2012).

Healthcare professionals may take action to minimize waste by reducing waste production, conserving energy, using green or environment-friendly products, recycling, and reusing resources and materials in the OR (Kagoma et al., 2012; Kwakye et al., 2011).

Healthcare institutions should consider the impact of reusable and disposable products when purchasing supplies, equipment, and/or surgical instruments. Waste generation is directly related to the purchase and supply practices of each unit (Conrardy, Hillanbrand, Myers, & Nussbaum, 2010; Gadani & Vyas, 2011). To explore the opportunities to minimize waste, a critical analysis of purchasing practices, storage requirements, and the wastes that are generated during the process of purchasing supplies and equipment is required (Kagoma et al., 2012).

In selecting materials for ORs, it is important to consider waste management and the use of disposable materials. Disposable materials are preferred for infection prevention. The costs of labor and cleaning, including special materials and quality control systems, are eliminated when disposable products are used. Furthermore, the disinfectant solutions used to clean reusable materials may be toxic, and disposable instruments may be of poor quality and tend to accumulate, leading to garbage heaps that emit toxins into the atmosphere. For surgical interventions, materials that meet both low-cost and low-environmental-impact criteria should be identified (Huncke et al., 2012; Kagoma et al., 2012; Laustsen, 2010). Only 5%–20% of the anesthetic gasses given to patients are physically metabolized, with the remaining gasses, especially carbon dioxide, having 2,000 times greater potential of leading to global warming when released into the atmosphere. Preventing the emission of these gasses into the atmosphere may reduce environmental harm (Gadani & Vyas, 2011).

Implementing environment-friendly healthcare practices in ORs will positively impact the environment. Furthermore, these initiatives are easily implemented, generate results in the short term, and reduce expenses significantly (Hoeksema, 2010; Laustsen, 2010).

Purpose

This descriptive study was conducted to determine the environment-friendly practices of ORs located in Izmir Province, Turkey.

Research Questions

The following research questions were used for this study:

- What are the environment-friendly practices of OR nurses in Turkey?
- What are the environment-friendly practices of hospitals in Turkey?

Importance to Nursing

Leadership in Energy and Environmental Design for Healthcare, Green Guide for Health Care, American Society for Healthcare Engineering, Practice Greenhealth, and Health Care Without Harm are organizations that have established certification programs for green hospitals. The purpose of these and other similar programs is to generate alternatives to current resource-use practices; encourage the efficient use of energy, water, and materials; reduce all categories of waste; and create environment-friendly hospital buildings.

In terms of the current state of environment-friendly practices in Turkey, the "Regulations on Environmental Law Obtaining Permits and Licenses," published in the Official Gazette numbered 27214 on April 29, 2009, requires that health facilities of 20 beds or more must employ at least one environment official, establish an environmental management unit, or receive regular environmental counseling services from an authorized firm.

The Association of periOperative Registered Nurses (AORN) recommends that the OR support team implements and takes an active role in environment-friendly practices to maintain a safe and healthy environment (AORN, 2010). In addition, healthcare professionals should actively promote and participate in natural resource conservation strategies such as recycling and reprocessing supplies; improving energy efficiency; managing pharmacological waste (Kwakye et al., 2011; Laustsen, 2010); turning off lights and electronic devices (pumps and computers) when not in use; using occupancy sensors in public areas; using energy-efficient electrical equipment, lights, and appliances; and using waterless scrubs and solar film on windows where appropriate (Candan Dönmez, 2016; Kagoma et al., 2012; Kwakye et al., 2011).

Healthcare workers in ORs perform an important role in providing care that has a low environmental impact. Everyone has the responsibility to protect the environment by thinking globally and acting locally in their daily practice.

Literature Review

No studies related to environment-friendly practices in ORs have been published in Turkey. Thus, this article is important in highlighting this issue.

In April 2010, Practice Greenhealth launched the "Greening the OR" initiative, providing data, tools, and resources to support best practices for developing green ORs. Since April 2012, more than 200 healthcare facilities in the United States have endorsed the "Greening the OR" initiative (Kwakye et al., 2011; Practice Greenhealth, 2011).

After reviewing 43 studies on the environment-friendly practices in hospitals, the authors of "Green Surgical Practices for Health Care" convened a panel of experts who developed five practical strategies:

- Waste reduction and separation in ORs
- Reprocessing of single-use medical devices
- Purchasing environmentally friendly products
- Management of energy consumption
- Management of pharmaceutical waste (Kwakye et al., 2011).

Operational Definitions

Environment-friendly

Implementing environment-friendly processes reduces energy consumption, uses resources in sustainable and mindful ways, and decreases environmental pollution. An environment-friendly hospital is a productive and quality operation that uses energy efficiently and reduces carbon emissions. "P" and "3R," which focus on reinvention, reduction, reuse, and recycling, are strategies that are frequently adopted to achieve environment-friendly goals. The literature addresses environment-friendly implementations in six facets: reducing and separating waste, reusing disposable medical equipment, recycling waste, purchasing environment-friendly materials, managing energy consumption, and managing medical wastes (Karayurt et al., 2014; Terekli et al., 2013).

Green hospital

The "Green Hospital" concept has emerged from the efforts of hospitals to reduce and destroy toxic substances, provide a healthier environment, and adopt "green approaches" to healthcare (Practice Greenhealth, 2011). The primary topics that must be dealt with under this concept include architectural design and functionality, interior ventilation quality, energy management, water management, waste management, and connection with nature (Karayurt et al., 2014; Practice Greenhealth, 2011), among others.

Methods

Fifty-two hospitals were located in the target area (Izmir Province), including four university hospitals, 24 state hospitals, and 24 private hospitals. The research sample included 18 ORs from the 11 hospitals that agreed to participate in the study, including four state hospitals, three university hospitals, and four private hospitals.

Procedures for Protection of Participants' Rights

Written permission (no. 27344949-878) to conduct this study was obtained from the ethics committee of the nursing faculty as well as from Izmir Province, South and North Union General Secretariat of Public Hospitals, and the participating university and private hospitals. The purpose and methodology were explained to nurses and consented to by all participants.

Study Procedures and Methods

Data collection took place between February 24 and May 30, 2014. Eleven hospitals participated in the study. One university hospital had one OR in each department for a total of seven ORs, and the remaining participating hospitals had one OR each. Therefore, 18 ORs were included in the study. The 18 nurses who were in charge of these hospital ORs participated in face-to-face interviews, which gathered information on OR characteristics and environmental nursing practices in the OR.

Instruments, Including Reliability Measurement and Validity Evidence

Data were collected using the nine characteristics that define ORs, which were developed by the researchers based on a literature review, and using the Greening the OR Checklist designed by Practice Greenhealth (2011). The nine OR characteristics included name of the hospital, hospital type, bed capacity, type of OR, placement of the OR, total number of hallways, total number of nurses, number of nurses per shift, and number of surgeries per day. The Greening the OR Checklist contains 46 items that are categorized under four topics, including organizational development (three items), waste reduction and prevention in the OR (nine items), environmentally preferable purchasing in the OR (19 items), and built environment (15 items). This instrument was translated into Turkish and used after validation. Greening the OR Checklist was translated into Turkish by three specialists who are native speakers of the Turkish language and competent in the English language. Each item was first translated into Turkish, and then the Turkish text was back-translated into English by a specialist in English linguistics. A pilot study with OR nurses was conducted to test the linguistic accuracy and comprehensibility of the checklist. After verifying that the checklist could be fully understood and completed by the OR nurses, the translators evaluated the pilot study data to create the final version of the instrument. The Turkish-language version of this checklist was considered ready for use in Turkey after it had been adapted to the Turkish population and confirmed as equivalent to the original English-language version. Each item of the Greening the OR Checklist was assessed and quantified (number and percentage) based on the following four potential responses: "fully established," "implementation in progress," "not implemented," and "unaware of the program/process."

Results

Eleven hospitals participated in the research, of which 36.4% (n = 4) were state hospitals, 36.4% (n = 4) were private hospitals, and 27.3% (n = 3) were university hospitals. Eight (72.7%) of these hospitals had a central OR. The average number of rooms in the ORs was 7.44 ± 7.32, the average number of nurses employed was 16.83 ± 17.16, and the average number of surgeries conducted per day was 29.72 ± 35.55.

This study determined that 55.6% (n = 10) of the participating hospitals supported environment-friendly OR practices. However, 66.7% (n = 12) did not have a dedicated team, and 61.1% (n = 11) did not provide training related to environment-friendly ORs (see Table 1).

Moreover, this study found that 83.3% (n = 15) of these hospitals conducted waste audits, 88.9% (n = 16) segregated noninfectious wastes, 94.4% (n = 17) segregated domestic wastes, and 77.8% (n = 14) segregated liquid wastes. Sixteen ORs (88.9%) recycled batteries, and only 50.0% reused the containers used to collect spent sharps (Table 1).

In addition, 72.2% (n = 13) of the ORs rearranged OR kits to reduce excessive material use and preferred using reusable elements rather than disposables. Fifteen (83.3%) of the ORs preferred reusable metal materials for surgical instruments and reused pulse oximeter probes, whereas 66.7% (n = 12) did not reuse electrosurgical pads. Reusable surgical gowns were used by OR staff in 88.9% (n = 16) of the ORs (Table 1).

Furthermore, 83.3% (n = 15) of the ORs did not use lighting sensors, and 66.7% (n = 12) did not use a heating, ventilating, and air conditioning system to reduce air circulation in unoccupied rooms or use LED surgical lighting to save energy.

Finally, half of the ORs (50.0%) used an anesthetic gas capture system to remove waste anesthetic gasses and prevent venting, and 83.3% did not use an evacuation system for surgical smoke (Table 1).

Discussion

The following sections present the main findings of this study.

Organizational Development

This study revealed that ORs are deficient in creating and training environment-friendly teams. OR staffs are not educated on greening and safety benefits or opportunities for waste and cost reduction. It is important to educate health professionals on environment-friendly practices and on how to apply this knowledge in their clinical practice. Hospital administrators play a key role in increasing environmental training and awareness among staffs. Thus, hospital administrators should also receive environmental education (Weiss et al., 2016).

Waste Reduction and Prevention

The ORs in this study were fully capable of implementing waste reduction initiatives, with rates of accomplishment ranging from 77.8% to 94.4%. However, poor implementation of container systems for reusable sharps was found. Only the waste is destroyed when a reusable container is used, and the used container may be reutilized after being washed appropriately. Therefore, reusable containers produce greater environmental savings than recyclable or disposable containers. According to Stericycle report, one reusable container prevents 600 disposable sharps containers from being disposed in landfills. Reusing containers eliminates the need to manufacture new containers and helps conserve natural resources (Hubbard, Hayanga, Quinlan, Soltez, & Hayanga, 2017; Weiss et al., 2016).

Regarding waste segregation, noninfectious and biological wastes should be collected in discrete containers; radioactive and sharp wastes should be collected separately in disposable, clearly marked containers (Kwakye et al., 2011; Lee & Mears, 2012). By raising awareness among OR staff regarding the disposal of biologically hazardous waste and by providing access to waste containers, health institutions may better support the segregation of waste in ORs. One study found that 92% of the wastes deposited in biologically hazardous waste containers were not biologically hazardous and could be treated as nonhazardous waste (Huncke et al., 2012).

Closed liquid-collection systems reduce the risk of exposure during disposal. These systems collect liquids during their formation in the OR for discharge directly into sewage networks. Despite their high cost, these systems significantly reduce the amount of infectious waste, which would otherwise require a high-energy disposal process (Huncke et al., 2012; Kagoma et al., 2012).

In addition, the various batteries that are used in anesthesia and other medical equipment are recyclable. Programs to collect, transport, and remove environmentally hazardous, rechargeable batteries should be implemented and followed. Furthermore, all nickel–cadmium and lead–acid batteries should display the universal recycling symbol label and a warning that batteries should be recycled. Furthermore, all batteries should be easily dismountable for appropriate disposal, and the lead–acid batteries used in anesthesia machines and elsewhere should be recycled according to established protocols (Huncke et al., 2012). Purchasing reusable sharps and containers rather than disposables reduces waste and provides financial benefits (Kwakye et al., 2011).

Giving Preference to Environment-Friendly Purchasing in the Operating Room

This study showed that over 70% of the participating hospitals had programs to purchase environment-friendly materials. Managing hospital waste and implementing environment-friendly waste practices are important. Moreover, having an independent metals recycling unit in the hospital may increase the recycling of metal parts (Huncke et al., 2012).

Gaziantep University Hospital conducted a cost–benefit analysis of using disposable and reusable surgical gowns and drapes. The results revealed that using these disposable items was more useful despite their higher unit costs (Baykasoğlu, Dereli, & Yilankirkan, 2009).

TABLE 1.

Distribution of Environment-Friendly Practices in the OR (N = 18)

	Fully Established (> 1 Year)		Implementation in Progress		Not Implemented		Unaware of the Program/Process	
Item	*n*	%	*n*	%	*n*	%	*n*	%
Organizational development								
1. Endorse and participate in Practice Greenhealth's Greening the OR Initiative	10	55.6	2	11.1	3	16.7	3	16.7
2. Build a Green Team for surgical services/OR	1	5.6	2	11.1	12	66.7	3	16.7
3. Educate OR staffs on the benefits of greening, the opportunities for cost and waste reduction, and related safety benefits	3	16.7	1	5.6	11	61.1	3	16.7
Waste reduction and prevention in the OR								
1. Conduct a waste audit in surgical services/OR	15	83.3	2	11.1	1	5.6	–	–
2. Implement a process to divert preincision, nonpharmaceutical waste from regulated medical waste streams into a clear bag for noninfectious waste disposal	16	88.9	1	5.6	1	5.6	–	–
3. Implement a process to segregate noninfectious solid waste from the regulated medical waste stream during and after procedures	17	94.4	1	5.6	–	–	–	–
4. Utilize a fluid management system for capturing liquid waste from surgery in reusable containers that empty liquid directly into a sanitary sewer	14	77.8	1	5.6	2	11.1	1	5.6
5. Recycle batteries generated in the OR	16	88.9	–	–	1	5.6	1	5.6
6. Utilize a reusable sharps container system	8	44.4	–	–	9	50.0	1	5.6
Environmentally preferable purchasing in the OR								
1. Reformulate OR kits to reduce excess supplies and overage	13	72.2	3	16.7	2	11.1	–	–
2. Replace disposable items with reusable items in OR kits where demonstrated safe and economically viable	13	72.2	1	5.6	4	22.2	–	–
3. Utilize reusable hard cases for surgical instruments	15	83.3	3	16.7	–	–	–	–
4. Purchase reusable gowns for surgical staff and covers for mayo stands and back tables	16	88.9	–	–	2	11.1	–	–
5. Utilize mercury-free blood pressure devices	13	72.2	–	–	1	5.6	4	22.2
6. Use reusable pulse oximeter sensors/probes	15	83.3	–	–	2	11.1	1	5.6
7. Utilize reusable grounding pads	6	33.3	–	–	12	66.7	–	–
8. Utilize environmentally benign cleaners or disinfectants for hard surfaces in the OR	5	27.8	5	27.8	8	44.4	–	–
Built environment								
1. Utilize occupancy sensors for lighting to reduce energy use in unoccupied ORs	–	–	1	5.6	15	83.3	2	11.1
2. Program the HVAC system to reduce air changes when ORs are unoccupied to reduce energy use	1	5.6	–	–	12	66.7	5	27.8
3. Utilize LED surgical lighting to reduce energy use and increase thermal comfort	3	16.7	2	11.1	12	66.7	1	5.6
4. Use an anesthetic gas capture system to capture waste anesthetic gasses and prevent venting to the outside	9	50.0	2	11.1	7	38.9	–	–
5. Install a power boom with a laser smoke capture system	2	11.1	–	–	15	83.3	1	5.6

Note. OR = operating room; HVAC = heating, ventilating, and air conditioning; LED = light emitting diode.

However, another study that calculated the unit costs of reusable surgical drape sets and disposable surgical drape sets (Hekim, Durukan Köse, Bener, Gül, & Polat, 2015) determined that using disposable surgical drape sets was 33.74% cheaper than using reusable woven fabric surgical drapes.

The rate of using reusable electrosurgical pads and cleaning them with environmentally benign disinfectant products was still low in the participating ORs. A study conducted by Bektaş et al. (2013) tested the efficiency and safety of reusable and disposable electrosurgical pads on patients. Researchers found that reusable and disposable electrosurgical pads were more efficient and safe when devices were periodically checked and calibrated, users were trained, and patient plaques were used correctly.

The Built Environment

This study revealed that built environment implementations were performed at a lower rate in ORs than in other organizations. Most of the participating hospitals were in older facilities that were not up to current environment-friendly standards.

Color-forming diode bulbs (LED) are a new alternative for lighting ORs that decrease energy use by 49%. These light bulbs do not heat the environment and consequently reduce the amount of energy required for cooling. Using natural light is recommended. However, in conditions where natural lighting is insufficient, the use of motion sensors can save energy. Saving energy results in financial savings (Chapman & Chapman, 2011; Karayurt et al., 2014; Kwakye et al., 2011).

In ORs, smart heating and cooling systems should be used to gradually adjust the temperature in unoccupied rooms. Smart room heating and cooling systems provide energy savings of up to 25% of total energy consumption (Siemens, 2011).

Only 5%–20% of the anesthetic gasses given to patients are metabolized; the global warming potential of a halogenated anesthetic is up to 2,000 times greater than CO_2 when released into the atmosphere. Nitrous oxide and potent inhalable anesthetics are considered greenhouse gasses (Gadani & Vyas, 2011). The use of inhaled anesthetics has increased in the last 30 years, and desflurane, in particular, has a significantly greater impact on the environment than older alternative agents. A technical solution to the problem of disposal consists of separating anesthetic gasses such as isoflurane in the ORs (Gadani & Vyas, 2011; Huncke et al., 2012). According to research conducted by the University of Chicago, the health sector is responsible for 8% of total greenhouse gas emissions in the United States. Another study found that hospitals are a major contributor to carbon emissions. Preventing the emission of waste agents into the atmosphere may also reduce the environmental impact of hospitals, and systems for collecting and reusing anesthetic gasses are under development. According to a system currently in use in Canada, a canister with a filter is placed in the anesthesia scavenging system machine to absorb the anesthetic gasses. These canisters are collected, and the anesthetic is retrieved and purified at another facility (Candan Dönmez, 2016; Chung & Meltzer, 2009; Huncke et al., 2012).

Identifying the potential dangers of surgical smoke generated in the ORs and developing effective safety practices are important and necessary. The smoke generated during electrosurgical interventions and its particulates (toxic gasses, dead and living cell wastes, viruses, hair, etc.) cannot be removed from the OR using ordinary methods. They constitute respiratory, ophthalmic, dermatological, and mutagenic health risks for medical staffs and patients. ORs should use wall-mounted ultralow-penetration air filters, which are efficient in purifying air to 99.99%. In addition, proper safety protocols should be implemented to ensure that surgical smoke is evacuated properly (AORN, 2010; Conrardy et al., 2010).

Limitations

Although all of the hospitals in Izmir Province were part of the research scope, only a minority agreed to participate in this study and provided data.

Recommendations for Clinical Practice

The clinical recommendations supported by the findings of this study are discussed below.

Current efforts to build environment-friendly teams in the ORs are inadequate. An "environment-friendly team" should be created in each OR or surgical service. In addition, all hospital staffs should receive training on the benefits of environment-friendly hospitals.

Waste separation practices were found to be satisfactory in the participating hospitals. Waste supervision should be performed in the surgical units, and ORs should ensure that waste is collected and separated.

Battery recycling practices were also found to be satisfactory. The batteries used in the ORs should be recycled, OR sets should be reorganized to prevent wasting materials and to decrease surplus materials, and reusable materials should be given preference over disposable materials.

New hospitals should be built in compliance with environment-friendly objectives and practices. The OR unit should be located on the ground or middle floors, and heating requirements should be considered.

Recommendations for Future Research

Future studies should target larger numbers of hospitals and use larger sample sizes. Studies of environment-friendly practices may target all of the units of a hospital and not only ORs.

Conclusions

The purpose of this study was to identify the environment-friendly practices that are currently being practiced in ORs in Turkey. This study showed that OR nurses are committed to reducing waste to protect the environment. However, hospitals typically do not have special teams to implement environment-friendly procedures. The literature recommends that wastes be reduced and segregated, that disposable medical instruments be reused, and that wastes be recycled. The active participation of surgical nurses in environment-friendly practices will significantly and positively contribute to the protection and improvement of the environment.

References

Association of periOperative Registered Nurses. (2010). AORN guidance statement: Environmental responsibility. In AORN (Ed.), *Perioperative standards and recommended practices* (1st ed., pp. 533–540). Denver, CO: Author.

Baykasoğlu, A., Dereli, T., & Yilankirkan, N. (2009). Application of cost/benefit analysis for surgical gown and drape selection: A case study. *American Journal of Infection Control, 37*(3), 215–226. http://dx.doi.org/10.1016/j.ajic.2008.10.031

Bektaş, Z., Yılmaz, N., Yarenoğlu, A., Aldemir, G., Demir, S., & Özkan, M. (2013). Evaluation of re-usable and disposable cautery plates in the operation rooms. *İstanbul Medical Journal, 14,* 44–46. https://doi.org/10.5152/imj.2013.10 (Original work published in Turkish)

Candan Dönmez, Y. (2016). Environmentally friendly practices in the operating room. *Journal of Health, 24,* 10–12. (Original work published in Turkish)

Chapman, M., & Chapman, A. (2011). Greening critical care. *Critical Care, 15*(2), 302. https://doi.org/10.1186/cc9409

Chung, J. W., & Meltzer, D. O. (2009). Estimate of the carbon footprint of the US health care sector. *JAMA, 302*(18), 1970–1972. https://doi.org/10.1001/jama.2009.1610

Conrardy, J., Hillanbrand, M., Myers, S., & Nussbaum, G. F. (2010). Reducing medical waste. *AORN Journal, 91*(6), 711–721. https://doi.org/10.1016/j.aorn.2009.12.029

Gadani, H., & Vyas, A. (2011). Anesthetic gases and global warming: Potentials, prevention and future of anesthesia. *Anesthesia Essays and Researches, 5*(1), 5–10. https://doi.org/10.4103/0259-1162.84171

Hekim, S., Durukan Köse, S., Bener, S., Gül, A., & Polat, S. (2015). Cost analysis of reusable textile fabric surgical drape and disposable surgical drape. *Journal of Productivity, 3,* 87–102. (Original work published in Turkish)

Hoeksema, J. (2010). Taking steps to control costs in the OR. *AORN Journal, 92*(6), 632–641. https://doi.org/10.1016/j.aorn.2010.04.020

Hubbard, R. M., Hayanga, J. A., Quinlan, J. J., Soltez, A. K., & Hayanga, H. K. (2017). Optimizing anesthesia-related waste disposal in the operating room: A brief report. *Anesthesia & Analgesia, 125*(4), 1289–1291. https://doi.org/10.1213/ANE.0000000000001932

Huncke, T. K., Ryan, S., Hopf, H. W., Axelrof, D., Feldman, J. M., Torrillo, T., & Striker, A. B. (2012). *2012 greening the operating room: Reduce, reuse, recycle, and redesign.* Retrieved from https://www.kevinmd.com/blog/2012/04/greening-operating-room.html

Kagoma, Y., Stall, N., Rubinstein, E., & Naudie, D. (2012). People, planet and profits: The case for greening operating rooms. *CMAJ: Canadian Medical Association Journal, 184*(17), 1905–1911. https://doi.org/10.1503/cmaj.112139

Karayurt, Ö., Andıç, S., & Ceylan, H. (2014). Eco-Friendly practices in surgery clinic. *University School of Nursing Electronic Journal, 7*(4), 337–344. (Original work published in Turkish)

Kwakye, G., Brat, G. A., & Makary, M. A. (2011). Green surgical practices for health care. *Archives of Surgery, 146*(2), 131–136. https://doi.org/10.1001/archsurg.2010.343

Laustsen, G. (2010). Greening in healthcare. *Nursing Management, 41*(11), 26–31. https://doi.org/10.1097/01.NUMA.0000389012.82998.5d

Lee, R. J., & Mears, S. C. (2012). Greening of orthopedic surgery. *Orthopedics, 35*(6), e940–e944. https://doi.org/10.3928/01477447-20120525-39

Potera, C. (2012). Strategies for greener hospital operating rooms. *Environmental Health Perspectives, 120*(8), a306–a307. https://doi.org/10.1289/ehp.120-a306a

Practice Greenhealth. (2011). *Practice Greenhealth Greening the Operating Room Checklist.* Retrieved from https://practicegreenhealth.org/sites/default/files/upload-files/gor_checklist_r5_web.pdf

Regulations on Environmental Law Obtaining Permits and Licenses, Prime Ministry General Directorate of Legislative Development and Publication, Republic of Turkey, Official gazette numbered 27214. (2009, April 29; Original work published in Turkish).

Siemens. (2011). *ISH 2011: Siemens innovations make buildings more efficient.* Retrieved from http://www.siemens.com/press/pool/de/pressemitteilungen/2011/building_technologies/IBT201102007e.pdf

Terekli, G., Özkan, O., & Bayın, G. (2013). Environmental friendly hospitals: From the hospital to green hospital. *Ankara Journal of Health Services, 121*(2), 37–54.

Weiss, A., Hollandsworth, H. M., Alseidi, A., Scovel, L., French, C., Derrick, E. L., & Klaristenfeld, D. (2016). Environmentalism in surgical practice. *Current Problems in Surgery, 53*(4), 165–205. https://doi.org/10.1067/j.cpsurg.2016.02.001

15

Characterization of Metabolic Syndrome Risk Factors and Health-Related Behaviors in Korean Patients with Breast Cancer by Abdominal Obesity Status

Hye-Jin KIM[1] • Hee-Seung KIM[2]* • Hye-Ryoung KIM[3] • Yang-Sook YOO[2] • Byung Joo SONG[4]

ABSTRACT

Background: Breast cancer is the second most prevalent malignancy among Korean women. Changes in lifestyle during and after remission of breast cancer tend to increase abdominal visceral fat, leading to increased risks of metabolic syndrome and chronic diseases.

Purpose: This cross-sectional study examined the differences in metabolic syndrome risk factors and health-related behaviors between abdominally obese and nonabdominally obese groups of Korean patients with breast cancer.

Methods: The participants were assigned to nonabdominal obesity (waist circumference < 85 cm, n = 77) and abdominal obesity (waist circumference ≥ 85 cm, n = 59) groups, and a questionnaire was used to assess the prevalence of risk factors of metabolic syndrome and health-related behaviors in each. The chi-square test and t test were used to analyze the data.

Results: The average age was 54.2 years in the abdominal obesity group and 51.3 years in the nonabdominal obesity group. The average blood pressure and fasting blood glucose levels were higher in the abdominal obesity than the nonabdominal obesity group (117.3/76.3 vs. 108.9/70.4 mmHg, respectively [p = .001]; 96.9 and 90.1 mg/dl, respectively [p = .007]). High-density lipoprotein cholesterol was lower in the abdominal obesity than the nonabdominal obesity group (55.4 and 62.5 mg/dl, respectively [p = .005]), whereas triglycerides were higher in the abdominal obesity than the nonabdominal obesity group (151.6 and 111.3 mg/dl, respectively [p = .006]). The prevalence of metabolic syndrome in the abdominal obesity and nonabdominal obesity groups were 42.4% and 9.1%, respectively (p = .001). Moreover, eating habits differed between the two groups, with the frequency of vegetable consumption lower in the abdominal obesity than the nonabdominal obesity group (p = .040) and the frequencies of salty and sweet food consumption and of overeating higher in the abdominal obesity than the nonabdominal obesity group. The percentage of participants who exercised for 30 minutes three times per week was 52.5% in the abdominal obesity group and 71.4% in the nonabdominal obesity group (p = .024).

Conclusions/Implications for Practice: This observational study found more metabolic syndrome risk factors in the abdominal obesity group than the nonabdominal obesity group. Consumption of sweet foods and overeating were higher and the frequencies of vegetable intake and exercise were lower in the abdominal obesity group. These findings suggest that female abdominally obese patients with breast cancer exhibit health-related behaviors that require improvement and better management. Interventional programs should be developed based on the findings of this study to reduce cancer recurrence and mortality in patients with breast cancer.

KEY WORDS:
breast cancer, abdominal obesity, metabolic syndrome, dietary habits, exercise.

Introduction

The existing healthcare systems are being continuously challenged because of the rapidly increasing number of cancer survivors worldwide. Moreover, the current acute treatment and care-oriented healthcare models are being challenged by the different requirements of cancer survivors in different survivor phases (Lai, 2016).

On the basis of statistical data from 2012, breast cancer is the most prevalent cancer in women worldwide, with a rate of occurrence of 25.2% (Stewart & Wild, 2014). Breast cancer is the second most prevalent malignancy (after thyroid cancer) among Korean women, with approximately 45.7 per 100,000 Korean women diagnosed with breast cancer annually (Oh

[1]PhD, RN, Assistant Professor, Department of Nursing, University of Ulsan, Ulsan, ROK • [2]PhD, RN, Professor, College of Nursing, The Catholic University of Korea, Seoul, ROK • [3]PhD, RN, Assistant Professor, College of Nursing, Shinhan University, Dongducheon, ROK • [4]PhD, MD, Professor, Department of Surgery, College of Medicine, St. Mary's Hospital, The Catholic University of Korea, Bucheon, ROK.

et al., 2016). Although its etiology is not well understood, postmenopausal weight gain and obesity have been implicated (Cheraghi, Poorolajal, Hashem, Esmailnasab, & Doosti, 2012). According to U.S. National Institutes of Health data for 2008–2014, the 5-year survival rate of female patients with breast cancer in the United States is 89.7% (National Cancer Institute, 2015). The 5-year overall survival rate of Korean female patients with breast cancer is over 90% (Oh et al., 2016). Whereas the highest percentage of new breast cancer diagnoses occurs in women in their 60s in most countries, in Korea, the highest percentage occurs in women in their 40s (Park et al., 2017), which raises significant concerns related to posttherapeutic morbidities and quality-of-life issues (Maurea et al., 2010). Thus, actively managing the disease- and treatment-related health problems of patients with breast cancer is one of the goals of healthcare professionals (Kim, Chung, Kim, Byun, & Choi, 2013).

Antiestrogen therapy for patients with breast cancer is associated with the development of metabolic syndrome (Redig & Munshi, 2010), and chemotherapy in premenopausal patients with breast cancer may increase the incidence of metabolic syndrome (Li et al., 2018). Moreover, chemotherapy-associated pain, fatigue, and weakness may cause inactivity, leading to abdominal obesity (Demark-Wahnefried et al., 2001). Furthermore, an unhealthy diet and lack of exercise increase abdominal visceral fat, ultimately leading to metabolic syndrome and chronic diseases such as obesity, hypertension, and diabetes (Patterson et al., 2010). Central adiposity after the diagnosis of breast cancer may cause various diseases and adversely affects the prognosis of women with breast cancer (George et al., 2014). Asian women show more abdominal and visceral adiposity than White women with similar body mass index (BMI) levels (Lim et al., 2011). Previous studies have reported that the mortality rate associated with breast cancer increases as the waist–hip ratio of Asian American women increases (Kwan et al., 2014). The National Health and Nutritional Survey performed between 2007 and 2011 in Korea found that 44.7% of female patients with breast cancer exhibited abdominal obesity (waist circumference > 85 cm; Seo et al., 2014).

Metabolic syndrome refers to a cluster of metabolic conditions, including abdominal obesity caused by insulin resistance, hypertriglyceridemia, low-density hypercholesterolemia, hyperglycemia, or hypertension (O'Neill & O'Driscoll, 2015). The progression of three or more of these metabolic conditions increases the risk of cardiovascular diseases and mortality (Mottillo et al., 2010). Postmenopausal patients with breast cancer who are diagnosed with metabolic syndrome face a heightened risk of developing cardiovascular diseases or metabolic disorders (Healy et al., 2010). Moreover, these patients experience higher breast cancer recurrence, ultimately leading to a worse prognosis than patients with breast cancer and without metabolic syndrome (Berrino et al., 2014).

Although several Korean studies have investigated the associations between breast cancer and both obesity and metabolic syndrome (Kim, Cui, Shin, Kim, & Jung, 2014; Seo et al., 2014), the effects of abdominal obesity on metabolic syndrome risk factors and health-related behaviors in this patient population have rarely been addressed. Thus, examining the effects of abdominal obesity on the incidence of metabolic syndrome in patients with breast cancer and the health-related behaviors of these patients is important. Moreover, it is critical to improve lifestyle habits such as diet and exercise to inhibit the onset/exacerbation of abdominal obesity and metabolic syndrome (Dieli-Conwright et al., 2014).

This study investigated the differences between abdominally obese and nonabdominally obese patients with cancer in terms of the risk factors of metabolic syndrome and health-related behaviors in an attempt to provide fundamental data for the development of management programs for abdominal obesity in this vulnerable patient population. In this study, we hypothesized that obesity, blood pressure, blood sugar, and blood lipid levels would differ in patients with breast cancer according to their abdominal obesity status. In addition, we hypothesized that the incidence of metabolic syndrome and dietary and exercise habits would differ based on abdominal obesity status.

Methods

Study Design

This observational descriptive study was designed to investigate the differences in patient characteristics, metabolic syndrome risk factors, and health related behaviors between two groups of patients with breast cancer who were, respectively, abdominally obese and nonabdominally obese.

Participants

The participants were recruited from outpatient clinics of the Breast Center in Seoul St. Mary's Hospital and from among patients with breast cancer who attended a support group hosted by this hospital from August 2015 to April 2016.

The inclusion criteria were as follows: (a) women between 18 and 69 years old, (b) being diagnosed with breast cancer (between Grades 0 and III), and (c) currently or previously receiving anticancer therapy for breast cancer (surgery, chemotherapy, radiotherapy, or antihormone therapy).

The exclusion criteria were as follows: (a) currently participating in another clinical trial or (b) being diagnosed with a mental disorder or alcohol or drug addiction.

During recruitment, the author provided detailed explanations of the aims and procedures involved in the study to all patients. An initial sample of 200 participants was recruited, and 136 participated in the study. The reasons for participant withdrawal before study completion included being unable to visit the hospital for data collection and refusing to provide blood samples. This study was approved by the institutional review board of the Catholic University of Korea (IRB No. MC15ENSI0084), and informed consent was obtained from all of the participants.

Using the G*power program (Version 3.1.9.2, Heinrich-Heine-Universität Düsseldorf, Düsseldorf, Germany; Faul, Erdfelder, Lang, & Buchner, 2007), a sample size of 102 participants, with 51 in each group, was calculated as necessary to obtain a medium effect size of 0.50, a significance level of .05, and a power of 0.80 (Cohen, 1988). In this study, the effect size was estimated as "medium" because no similar studies are available to estimate the effect size (Nahm, 2015).

A previous study confirmed waist circumference as a stronger index for potential health risk than BMI (Zhu et al., 2002). Therefore, the final sample in this study was composed of 136 participants, with 77 in the nonabdominal obesity group and 59 in the abdominal obesity group. Abdominal obesity was determined based on a waist circumference of 85 cm or greater, in accordance with the obesity treatment guidelines developed by the Korean Society for the Study of Obesity (2012).

Outcomes Measured

Data collection was performed between September 2015 and April 2016. An experienced nurse with 6 years of nursing experience collected data between 7:30 and 8:30 a.m. on weekdays at the outpatient examination room in the Department of Endocrinology, Seoul St. Mary's Hospital. Blood pressure was measured after the participants had filled out a structured questionnaire. After measuring height, weight, and body fat, the investigator obtained 5 ml of venous blood.

Obesity index, blood pressure, fasting blood glucose, and lipid levels

Height and weight were measured using the automatic height and weight scale DS-102 (Jenix, Seoul, Korea). Skeletal muscle mass, body fat mass, and body fat percentage were measured using Inbody 720 (Biospace, Seoul, Korea). BMI was calculated by dividing weight (kilograms) by the square of the height (square meters). BMI cutoff values were as follows: 18.5–22.9 kg/m^2 was normal, 23.0–24.9 kg/m^2 was overweight, and > 25 kg/m^2 was obese (Kim, Lee, et al., 2014).

Waist and hip circumferences were measured using a tape measure (Hoechstmass Balzer GmbH, Hessen, Germany). In an examination room with private curtains, the same investigator asked each participant to lift up her shirt and made waist and hip circumference measurements. This investigator took two consecutive readings of each measurement to confirm the consistency of results and, if the results were not in agreement, performed an additional third measurement. Waist circumference was measured horizontally at the midpoint between the lowest rib and iliac crest in an upright position. Hip circumference was measured at the point of maximum protrusion of the hip in an upright position.

The patients were instructed to rest before measuring blood pressure, which was measured three consecutive times at 5-minute intervals using an automated blood pressure measuring device (TM2655P by A&D, Tokyo, Japan) in a seated position. The mean value of the second and third measurements was recorded and used in the data analysis.

The participants were instructed to fast for 8 hours before measuring fasting blood glucose and blood lipid levels. The investigator collected their blood samples from a peripheral vein and measured fasting blood glucose by the glucose oxidase method using a Hitachi 7600-110 (Roche, Basel, Switzerland). Insulin was measured using a Dream Gamma Counter-10 (Shinjin Medics, Goyangsi, Korea). High-density lipoprotein cholesterol (HDL-C), low-density lipoprotein cholesterol (LDL-C), and triglycerides were measured using a DDP Modular System Chemistry Analyzer (Roche, Basel, Switzerland).

Metabolic syndrome risk factors

Metabolic syndrome was diagnosed when a patient had at least three of the five risk factors suggested by the National Cholesterol Education Program Adult Treatment Panel III (2002), as follows:

1. Waist circumference ≥ 85 cm (Kim, Lee, et al., 2014)
2. Systolic blood pressure ≥ 130 mmHg or diastolic blood pressure ≥ 85 mmHg
3. Fasting blood glucose ≥ 100 mg/dl (Genuth et al., 2003)
4. HDL-C < 50 mg/dl
5. Triglyceride level ≥ 150 mg/dl

Health-related behaviors

The dietary habits and food intake frequency scale developed by Oh et al. (2008) and modified and adapted by Kim and Kim (2013) was used to analyze the dietary habits and food intake patterns of the participants. This 11-item scale comprises three items for dietary habits and eight items for food intake patterns. We surveyed the weekly frequencies of overeating, dining out, and eating breakfast to determine dietary habits and the weekly frequency of consuming major food categories (vegetables, fruits, dairy products, vegetable oils, high-fat and high-calorie snacks, and high-sodium and high-sugar foods) to determine food intake patterns. The response of participants to the question "Do you currently consume alcohol or smoke" was used to determine their alcohol and smoking statuses. The response of participants to whether they engaged in at least 30 minutes of moderate exercise (3–6 metabolic equivalents of energy expenditure) three times a week was used to determine their exercise habit status. Participants who performed walking exercises were instructed to write down the weekly frequency and length of each session.

Data Analysis

The collected data were analyzed using SPSS PASW Version 18 (IBM, Armonk, NY, USA). Continuous variables were expressed as mean ± standard deviation (*SD*). Percentage and mean differences in general characteristics, breast cancer features, and health-related behaviors between the two groups were analyzed using the chi-square test and *t* test. Mean differences in cardiometabolic risk factors were analyzed using the *t* test, and metabolic syndrome risk factors were analyzed using the chi-square test. Statistical significance was set at $p < .05$.

Results

Patient and Tumor-Related Characteristics

The mean ages of the abdominal obesity and nonabdominal obesity groups were 54.2 and 51.3 years, respectively. There was no difference in menopausal status between the two groups. A significantly higher percentage of patients in the abdominal obesity group than the nonabdominal obesity group (22.0% vs. 7.8%, $p = .018$) was taking hypertension medications. However, no significant intergroup differences were found in terms of taking diabetes or hyperlipidemia medications. The duration of breast cancer was significantly longer in the abdominal obesity group (mean = 4.7 years) than in the nonabdominal obesity group (mean = 3.2 years; $p = .036$). There were no differences in other breast cancer features between the two groups. With respect to clinical stage status, 15.3% were in Stage 0, 28.8% were in Stage I, 37.3% were in Stage II, and 18.6% were in Stage III in the abdominal obesity group, whereas 6.5% were in Stage 0, 36.4% were in Stage I, 44.2% were in Stage II, and 11.7% were in Stage III in the nonabdominal obesity group, showing no difference between the groups. About 20.3% of the abdominal obesity group and 13.0% of the nonabdominal obesity group reported a history of recurrence, with no significant intergroup difference. Around 27.1% of the abdominal obesity group and 24.7% of the nonabdominal obesity group were currently undergoing chemotherapy, with a respective 10.2% and 15.6% undergoing radiation therapy and a respective 30.5% and 28.6% undergoing hormone therapy, revealing no significant differences in treatment status between the two groups (Table 1).

TABLE 1.

Patient and Tumor-Related Characteristics

	Nonabdominal Obesity Group ($n = 77$)		Abdominal Obesity Group ($n = 59$)			
Characteristic	*n*	%	*n*	%	t/χ^2	*p*
Age (years; *M* and *SD*)	51.3	9.3	54.2	8.3	1.90	.059
Menopausal status					1.59	.208
Premenopausal	23	29.9	12	20.3		
Postmenopausal	54	70.1	47	79.7		
Age at menopause[a] (years; *M* and *SD*)	48.0	5.4	48.4	5.8	0.33	.746
Currently taking medication for						
Hypertension	6	7.8	13	22.0	5.64	.018
Diabetes	3	3.9	3	5.1		1.000[b]
Hyperlipidemia	10	13.0	11	18.6	0.82	.366
Tumor characteristics						
Time since diagnosis (years; *M* and *SD*)	3.2	3.3	4.7	4.8	2.12	.036
Range	0–6.5		0–9.5			
Clinical stage					5.31	.257
0	5	6.5	9	15.3		
I	28	36.4	17	28.8		
II	34	44.2	22	37.3		
III	10	12.9	11	18.6		
Breast cancer recurrence					1.33	.249
Yes	10	13.0	12	20.3		
No	67	87.0	47	79.7		
Time elapsed since last treatment (years; *M* and *SD*)	1.0	0.8	1.3	1.1	1.88	.063
Current treatment status						
Chemotherapy	19	24.7	16	27.1	0.10	.747
Radiation therapy	12	15.6	6	10.2	0.85	.356
Antihormone therapy	22	28.6	18	30.5	0.06	.806

Note. Abdominal obesity group: waist circumference ≥ 85 cm.
[a]Nonabdominal obesity group: $n = 54$; abdominal obesity group: $n = 47$.
[b]Fisher's exact test.

TABLE 2.
Obesity Index, Blood Pressure, Fasting Blood Glucose, and Lipid Levels

Variable	Nonabdominal Obesity Group (n = 77)		Abdominal Obesity Group (n = 59)			
	M	*SD*	*M*	*SD*	*t*	*p*
Height (cm)	157.4	5.6	158.5	5.1	1.20	.231
Weight (kg)	53.4	4.9	68.1	8.9	11.44	.001
Body mass index (kg/m^2)	21.6	1.9	27.2	3.2	11.81	.001
Skeletal muscle mass (kg)	20.0	2.4	22.4	2.5	5.74	.001
Body fat mass (kg)	16.2	4.2	26.6	6.3	10.98	.001
Percent body fat (%)	30.1	6.5	38.6	5.1	8.29	.001
Waist circumference (cm)	78.6	4.0	93.7	7.4	14.22	.001
Hip circumference (cm)	92.4	4.1	102.1	6.0	10.71	.001
Blood pressure (mmHg)						
Systolic	108.9	13.8	117.3	14.0	3.49	.001
Diastolic	70.4	10.9	76.3	8.7	3.40	.001
Fasting blood glucose (mg/dl)	90.1	13.5	96.9	15.1	2.76	.007
Insulin (μU/ml)	4.1	2.7	7.1	4.3	4.64	.001
Lipid profiles						
HDL-C (mg/dl)	62.5	14.5	55.4	13.8	2.86	.005
LDL-C (mg/dl)	123.8	42.6	122.4	30.0	0.22	.824
Triglycerides (mg/dl)	111.3	60.7	151.6	97.0	2.80	.006

Note. Abdominal obesity group: waist circumference ≥ 85 cm. HDL-C = high-density lipoprotein cholesterol; LDL-C = low-density lipoprotein cholesterol.

Obesity Index, Blood Pressure, Fasting Blood Glucose, and Lipid Levels

Body weight was higher in the abdominal obesity group (68.1 kg) than the nonabdominal obesity group (53.4 kg; p = .001). Consequently, BMI was also higher in the abdominal obesity group (27.2 kg/m^2) than the nonabdominal obesity group (21.6 kg/m^2; p = .001).

In addition, skeletal muscle mass was higher in the abdominal obesity group (22.4 kg) than in the nonabdominal obesity group (20.0 kg; p = .001), body fat mass and percentage values were higher in the abdominal obesity group (26.6 kg and 38.6%, respectively) than in the nonabdominal obesity group (16.2 kg and 30.1%, respectively; p = .001), and hip circumference was greater in the abdominal obesity group (102.1 cm) than in the nonabdominal obesity group (92.4 cm; p = .001).

Furthermore, blood pressure was higher in the abdominal obesity group (117.3/76.3 mmHg) than in the nonabdominal obesity group (108.9/70.4 mmHg; p = .001), and fasting blood glucose was higher in the abdominal obesity group (96.9 mg/dl) than in the nonabdominal obesity group (90.1 mg/dl; p = .007). With respect to lipid profiles, mean HDL-C levels were lower in the abdominal obesity group (55.4 mg/dl) than the nonabdominal obesity group (62.5 mg/dl; p = .005), whereas triglyceride levels were higher in the abdominal obesity group (151.6 mg/dl) than in the nonabdominal obesity group (111.3 mg/dl; p = .006; Table 2).

Metabolic Syndrome Risk Factors

The prevalence of metabolic syndrome was higher in the abdominal obesity group (42.4%) than in the nonabdominal obesity group (9.1%; p = .001).

With respect to specific metabolic syndrome risk factors, the proportion of participants with blood pressure higher than 130/85 mmHg and fasting blood glucose higher than 100 mg/dl was higher in the abdominal obesity group (39.0% and 28.8%, respectively) than in the nonabdominal obesity group (15.6% and 9.1%, respectively; $p < .05$ for both; Table 3).

Health-Related Behavior

The frequency of vegetable intake was lower in the abdominal obesity group (4.9 times/week) than in the nonabdominal obesity group (5.6 times/week; p = .040), the frequency of salty foods intake was higher in the abdominal obesity group (1.6 times/week) than in the nonabdominal obesity group (1.1 times/week; p = .033), and the frequency of sweet foods intake was higher in the abdominal obesity group (1.5 times/week) than in the nonabdominal obesity group (1.0 times/week; p = .022). Furthermore, the frequency of overeating

TABLE 3.
Metabolic Syndrome Risk Factors

Variable	Nonabdominal Obesity Group (n = 77) n	%	Abdominal Obesity Group (n = 59) n	%	χ^2	p
Metabolic syndrome						
Yes	7	9.1	25	42.4	20.56	.001
No	70	90.9	34	57.6		
Hypertension (BP ≥ 130/85 mmHg)						
Yes	12	15.6	23	39.0	9.57	.002
No	65	84.4	36	61.0		
Impaired fasting glucose (≥ 100 mg/dl)						
Yes	7	9.1	17	28.8	8.94	.003
No	70	90.9	42	71.2		
Low HDL-C (< 50 mg/dl)						
Yes	24	31.2	25	42.4	1.82	.177
No	53	68.8	34	57.6		
Hypertriglyceridemia (≥ 150 mg/dl)						
Yes	20	26.0	24	40.7	3.30	.069
No	57	74.0	35	59.3		

Note. Abdominal obesity group: waist circumference ≥ 85 cm. HDL-C = high-density lipoprotein cholesterol; BP = blood pressure.

was higher in the abdominal obesity group (1.8 times/week) than in the nonabdominal obesity group (1.2 times/week; p = .013). The proportion of participants who exercised at least three times a week for at least 30 minutes per session was lower in the abdominal obesity group (52.5%) than in the nonabdominal obesity group (71.4%; p = .024; Table 4).

TABLE 4.
Health-Related Behaviors

Variable	Nonabdominal Obesity Group (n = 77) M	SD	Abdominal Obesity Group (n = 59) M	SD	t/χ^2	p
Dietary habits						
Breakfast[a]	5.9	2.0	5.5	2.1	1.20	.234
Vegetable intake[a]	5.6	1.9	4.9	1.9	2.08	.040
Fruit intake[a]	5.9	1.7	5.6	1.7	1.21	.228
Dairy product intake[a]	3.4	2.2	3.1	2.2	0.96	.338
Vegetable oil intake[a]	4.6	2.0	4.4	2.1	0.56	.575
High-fat diet[a]	1.3	1.2	1.4	1.0	0.69	.492
High-calorie snacks intake[a]	1.0	1.2	1.2	1.3	0.94	.352
High-salt diet[a]	1.1	1.2	1.6	1.4	2.15	.033
Sweet foods intake[a]	1.0	1.2	1.5	1.5	2.31	.022
Overeating[a]	1.2	1.3	1.8	1.3	2.51	.013
Eating out[a]	2.0	1.4	1.9	1.5	0.40	.689
Drinking (n and %)	9	11.7	13	22.0	2.64	.104
Smoking (n and %)	0	0	0	0		
Physical activity						
Regular exercise[b] (n and %)	55	71.4	31	52.5	5.13	.024
Walking time (hours/week)	2.8	2.9	2.3	2.8	1.06	.291

Note. Abdominal obesity group: waist circumference ≥ 85 cm.
[a]Weekly frequency.
[b]More than 3 days per week.

Discussion

This study aimed to assess the differences in risk of metabolic syndrome and health-related behaviors between female breast cancer patients with abdominal obesity and those without abdominal obesity.

The results show that the abdominal obesity group exhibited higher mean weight, BMI, body fat mass, waist and hip circumferences, blood pressure, fasting blood sugar, triglyceride, and insulin levels and a lower mean HDL-C level than the nonabdominal obesity group. In terms of dietary habits, the abdominal obesity group consumed fewer vegetables and more sweet and salty foods and exhibited a greater frequency of excessive food consumption than the nonabdominal obesity group. Finally, the participants in the abdominal obesity group performed regular exercise less frequently than their nonabdominally obese counterparts.

The cohort in this study included 59 (43.4%) abdominally obese participants and 77 (56.6%) nonabdominally obese participants. These numbers are similar to previously reported proportions of Korean female abdominally obese patients with breast cancer (44.7%; Seo et al., 2014). The values for body weight, BMI, skeletal muscle mass, body fat percentage, waist circumference, and hip circumference were all consistently and significantly higher in the abdominal obesity group than in the nonabdominal obesity group. Moreover, the mean BMI, body fat percentage, and waist circumference values were higher (for the abdominal obesity group) and lower (for the nonabdominal obesity group) than the mean values for 125 breast cancer survivors in the 2011 National Health and Nutrition Survey (Seo et al., 2014; 24.8 kg/m^2, 34.9%, and 82.8 cm, respectively).

The results found that increased waist circumference increased the prevalence of obesity, indicating that abdominal obesity resulted in obese body compositions overall, rather than only an increase in waist circumference. Furthermore, as suggested in a study that showed a 1.18-fold higher cancer recurrence rate in patients with breast cancer with a waist circumference ≥ 85 cm (Berrino et al., 2014), abdominal obesity is also related to breast cancer recurrence. Thus, patients with breast cancer with concurrent abdominal obesity should take precautions against breast cancer relapse and against metabolic-syndrome-related cardiovascular diseases. Overall, obesity, as indicated by parameters such as BMI, should also be noted because postmenopausal obesity is strongly associated with the development of breast cancer (Lahmann et al., 2004). In fact, a previous study on Korean breast cancer survivors reported a high overall rate of obesity, with 48.4% obese survivors, 44.7% survivors with abdominal obesity, and 89.2% survivors having greater than 30% body fat (Seo et al., 2014). This is because breast cancer is more common in obese postmenopausal women than in normal-weight postmenopausal women and because obese patients with breast cancer face a heightened risk of recurrence.

Our results showed that the abdominal obesity group had higher fasting blood glucose and triglyceride levels but lower HDL-C levels than the nonabdominal obesity group, which is similar to the results of a previous study that found the odds ratios for fasting blood glucose (1.17), triglyceride (1.17), and LDL-C (1.10) levels to be high in the abdominal obesity group (Fan et al., 2016). This may be explained by the finding that waist circumference correlates positively with increased fasting blood glucose, triglyceride, and LDL-C levels but negatively with HDL-C levels (Bering, Mauricio, Silva, & Correia, 2015). The rate of breast cancer recurrence is 1.58 times higher in patients with a triglyceride level of > 150 mg/dl and 1.83 times higher in patients with HDL-C of < 50 mg/dl (Berrino et al., 2014), highlighting the importance of managing dyslipidemia in patients with breast cancer to reduce the risks of cardiovascular diseases and to prevent the recurrence of cancer.

A higher proportion of patients in the abdominal obesity group consumed hypertension medications and had higher blood pressure at the time of measurement than those in the nonabdominal obesity group. The higher morbidity rate for hypertension in the abdominal obesity group may be because of the role of obesity as a major cause of hypertension (Seo et al., 2014). Moreover, higher numbers of metabolic syndrome risk factors were associated with a higher risk of breast cancer recurrence. Indeed, patients who present three or more metabolic syndrome risk factors are 2.17 times more likely to experience a relapse (Berrino et al., 2014).

With respect to dietary habits, the abdominal obesity group consumed vegetables less frequently, ate salty and sweet foods, and overate more often than the nonabdominal obesity group. These findings are similar to those obtained in a previous analysis of the National Health and Nutrition Survey, wherein Korean obese women showed less diversity in food intake but more sodium intake than normal-weight Korean women (Bae, 2012). These findings also echo a previous report that correlated larger waist and hip circumferences with enjoying saltier seasonings (Chang, 2010). A previous study that analyzed the dietary habits of Korean survivors of breast cancer found that the participants consumed more carbohydrates and less fiber than the general population (Seo et al., 2014). As a diet high in vegetable, fruit, and fiber is recommended to patients with cancer (Rock et al., 2012) to reduce the risks of relapse and mortality (Kwan et al., 2009), it is critical to educate patients and provide interventions that promote appropriate dietary habits.

The proportion of participants who engaged in moderate-intensity exercises three times a week for at least 30 minutes each session was lower in the abdominal obesity group than in the nonabdominal obesity group. This was similar to a previous study that found a lower percentage of obese middle-aged women engaging in regular exercise compared with their normal-weight and overweight counterparts (Chang, 2010). The efficacy of regular exercise in reducing waist circumference has been well documented. For instance, extending moderate- to high-intensity exercise for 30 minutes was shown to reduce waist circumference by 2.22 cm (Boyle, Vallance, Buman, & Lynch, 2017), and the rate of abdominal obesity was found to be lower among older adults who engaged in more health-related behaviors (Bulló et al., 2011). Thus, education on and the promotion of consistent adherence to health-related behaviors such as increased vegetable intake, a low-fat diet, and regular moderate- to high-intensity exercise (Rock et al., 2012) should be directed to patients with breast cancer to improve their prognoses.

This study found that, compared with their peers in the nonabdominal obesity group, the abdominally obese participants had higher body weight, BMI, body fat mass, body fat percentage, waist circumference, hip circumference, blood pressure, fasting blood glucose, triglyceride, and insulin values as well as lower HDL-C levels. Furthermore, the abdominal obesity group ate vegetables and exercised less frequently as well as overate and consumed sweet and salty foods more frequently. This comparison of metabolic syndrome risk factors and health-related behaviors between patients with breast cancer with and without abdominal obesity has produced meaningful results that shed light on the perils of abdominal obesity and present an objective standard for achieving desired changes in lifestyle habits.

Limitations

This study is affected by several limitations. First, actual parallels and odds/hazard ratios could not be obtained because of the small number of participants. Moreover, the obese group could not be further distinguished into mediates and moderates for additional statistical analysis to assess the differences in variables because of the small cohort size. A larger sample should be examined in the future to confirm the prevalence of relevant lifestyle habits in patients with breast cancer of different abdominal obesity statuses.

Second, although a structured questionnaire was used in this study to investigate health-related behaviors, the self-report format introduced the risk of data bias. In particular, abdominally obese patients may underrate or overrate their diet patterns and exercise habits. Thus, in the future, instruments that are able to objectively measure health-related behaviors such as diet and exercise habits should be developed.

Third, this study used a cross-sectional approach. Thus, the strength of relationships between independent and dependent variables could not be determined. Furthermore, whether abdominal obesity occurred before or after the diagnosis of breast cancer remains unclear. Therefore, we suggest conducting further cohort studies that assess the health condition and behaviors of female patients with breast cancer based on their abdominal obesity status to further investigate potential associations.

Despite these limitations, this study is meaningful as it is the first to investigate the prevalence of metabolic syndrome risk factors and health-related behaviors in Korean patients with breast cancer of different abdominal obesity statuses. The results showed that the abdominal obesity group was affected by more metabolic syndrome risk factors than the nonabdominal obesity group. Therefore, abdominally obese patients with breast cancer face a greater need to improve their health-related behavior, calling for an effective intervention program, guided by these results, to reduce relapse and mortality.

Acknowledgments

This research was supported by a National Research Foundation of Korea grant funded by the Korea government (No. NRF-2015R1A2A2A01002514). We would like to thank all of the women who participated in this study.

Author Contributions

Study conception and design: HSK
Data collection: HJK, HRK, YSY, BJS
Data analysis and interpretation: HJK, HSK, HRK
Drafting of the article: All authors
Critical revision of the article: HJK, HSK

References

Bae, Y. J. (2012). Evaluation of nutrient and food intake status, and dietary quality in Korean female adults according to obesity: Based on 2007–2009 Korean National Health and Nutrition Examination Survey. *Korean Journal of Nutrition, 45*(2), 140–149. https://doi.org/10.4163/kjn.2012.45.2.140 (Original work published in Korean)

Bering, T., Mauricio, S. F., Silva, J. B., & Correia, M. I. (2015). Nutritional and metabolic status of breast cancer women. *Nutrición Hospitalaria, 31*(2), 751–758. https://doi.org/10.3305/nh.2015.31.2.8056

Berrino, F., Villarini, A., Traina, A., Bonanni, B., Panico, S., Mano, M. P., ... Pasanisi, P. (2014). Metabolic syndrome and breast cancer prognosis. *Breast Cancer Research and Treatment, 147*(1), 159–165. https://doi.org/10.1007/s10549-014-3076-6

Boyle, T., Vallance, J. K., Buman, M. P., & Lynch, B. M. (2017). Reallocating time to sleep, sedentary time, or physical activity: Associations with waist circumference and body mass index in breast cancer survivors. *Cancer Epidemiology, Biomarkers, & Prevention, 26*(2), 254–260. https://doi.org/10.1158/1055-9965.EPI-16-0545

Bulló, M., Garcia-Aloy, M., Martínez-González, M. A., Corella, D., Fernández-Ballart, J. D., Fiol, M., ... Salas-Salvadó, J. (2011). Association between a healthy lifestyle and general obesity and abdominal obesity in an elderly population at high cardiovascular risk. *Preventive Medicine, 53*(3), 155–161. https://doi.org/10.1016/j.ypmed.2011.06.008

Chang, H. S. (2010). A study on weight control behaviour, eating habits and health-related life habits according to obesity degree by body fat percentage among middle-aged women in Gunsan City. *Korean Journal of Community Nutrition, 15*(2), 227–239. https://doi.org/10.7318/KJFC/2015.30.1.105 (Original work published in Korean)

Cheraghi, Z., Poorolajal, J., Hashem, T., Esmailnasab, N., & Doosti, I. A. (2012). Effect of body mass index on breast cancer during premenopausal and postmenopausal periods: A meta-analysis. *PLoS ONE, 7*(12), e51446. https://doi.org/10.1371/journal.pone.0051446

Cohen, J. (1988). *Statistical power analysis for the behavioral sciences* (2nd ed.). Hillsdale, NJ: Lawrence Earlbaum Associates.

Demark-Wahnefried, W., Peterson, B. L., Winer, E. P., Marks, L., Aziz, N., Marcom, P. K., ... Rimer, B. K. (2001). Changes in weight, body composition, and factors influencing energy balance among premenopausal breast cancer patients receiving adjuvant chemotherapy. *Journal of Clinical Oncology, 19*(9), 2381–2389. https://doi.org/10.1200/JCO.2001.19.9.2381

Dieli-Conwright, C. M., Mortimer, J. E., Schroeder, E. T., Courneya, K., Demark-Wahnefried, W., Buchanan, T. A., ... Bernstein, L. (2014). Randomized controlled trial to evaluate the effects of combined progressive exercise on metabolic syndrome in breast cancer survivors: Rationale, design, and methods. *BMC Cancer, 14*, 238. https://doi.org/10.1186/1471-2407-14-238

Fan, H., Li, X., Zheng, L., Chen, X., lan, Q., Wu, H., ... Liu, Z. (2016). Abdominal obesity is strongly associated with cardiovascular disease and its risk factors in elderly and very elderly community-dwelling Chinese. *Scientific Reports, 6*, 21521. https://doi.org/10.1038/srep21521

Faul, F., Erdfelder, E., Lang, A. G., & Buchner, A. (2007). G*Power 3: A flexible statistical power analysis program for the social, behavioral, and biomedical sciences. *Behavior Research Methods, 39*(2), 175–191. https://doi.org/10.3758/BF03193146

Genuth, S., Alberti, K. G., Bennett, P., Buse, J., DeFronzo, R., Kahn, R., ... Expert Committee on the Diagnosis and Classification of Diabetes Mellitus. (2003). Follow-up report on the diagnosis of diabetes mellitus. *Diabetes Care, 26*(11), 3160–3168. https://doi.org/10.2337/diacare.26.11.3160

George, S. M., Bernstein, L., Smith, A. W., Neuhouser, M. L., Baumgartner, K. B., Baumgartner, R. N., & Ballard-Barbash, R. (2014). Central adiposity after breast cancer diagnosis is related to mortality in the health, eating, activity, and lifestyle study. *Breast Cancer Research and Treatment, 146*(3), 647–655. https://doi.org/10.1007/s10549-014-3048-x

Healy, L. A., Ryan, A. M., Carroll, P., Ennis, D., Crowley, V., Boyle, T., ... Reynolds, J. V. (2010). Metabolic syndrome, central obesity and insulin resistance are associated with adverse pathological features in postmenopausal breast cancer. *Clinical Oncology, 22*(4), 281–288. https://doi.org/10.1016/j.clon.2010.02.001

Kim, G. D., Chung, B. Y., Kim, K. H., Byun, H. S., & Choi, E. H. (2013). Comparison of climacteric symptoms and cognitive impairment in breast cancer survivors and healthy women. *Asian Oncology Nursing, 13*(1), 11–17. https://doi.org/10.5388/aon.2013.13.1.11 (Original work published in Korean)

Kim, H. S., & Kim, H. R. (2013). Comparison of the metabolic syndrome risk factors, physical activity, and diet habits between the fifties and sixties in postmenopausal women. *Journal of Korean Biological Nursing Science, 15*(3), 133–138. https://doi.org/10.7586/jkbns.2013.15.3.133 (Original work published in Korean)

Kim, J. Y., Cui, X. G., Shin, H. J., Kim, K. S., & Jung, Y. S. (2014). Body mass index and response to neoadjuvant chemotherapy in Korean breast cancer. *Journal of Breast Disease, 2*(1), 1–7. https://doi.org/10.14449/jbd.2014.2.1 (Original work published in Korean)

Kim, M. K., Lee, W. Y., Kang, J. H., Kang, J. H., Kim, B. T., Kim, S. M., ... Lee, K. Y. (2014). 2014 clinical practice guidelines for overweight and obesity in Korea. *Endocrinology and Metabolism, 29*(4), 405–409.

Korean Society for the Study of Obesity. (2012). *Obesity treatment guideline 2012.* Seoul, ROK: Author. (Original work published in Korean)

Kwan, M. L., John, E. M., Caan, B. J., Lee, V. S., Bernstein, L., Cheng, I., ... Wu, A. H. (2014). Obesity and mortality after breast cancer by race/ethnicity: The California breast cancer survivorship consortium. *American Journal of Epidemiology, 179*(1), 95–111. https://doi.org/10.1093/aje/kwt233

Kwan, M. L., Weltzien, E., Kushi, L. H., Castillo, A., Slattery, M. L., & Caan, B. J. (2009). Dietary patterns and breast cancer recurrence and survival among women with early-stage breast cancer. *Journal of Clinical Oncology, 27*(6), 919–926. https://doi.org/10.1200/JCO.2008.19.4035

Lahmann, P. H., Hoffmann, K., Allen, N., van Gils, C. H., Khaw, K. T., Tehard, B., ... Riboli, E. (2004). Body size and breast cancer risk: Findings from the European Prospective Investigation into Cancer and Nutrition (EPIC). *International Journal of Cancer, 111*(5), 762–771. https://doi.org/10.1002/ijc.20315

Lai, Y. H. (2016). Perspectives on cancer survivorship: Care and challenges. *The Journal of Nursing Research, 24*(2), 190–192. https://doi.org/10.1097/jnr.0000000000000163

Li, X., Liu, Z. L., Wu, Y. T., Wu, H., Dai, W., Arshad, B., ... Kong, L. Q. (2018). Status of lipid and lipoprotein in female breast cancer patients at initial diagnosis and during chemotherapy. *Lipids in Health and Disease, 17*(1), 91. https://doi.org/10.1186/s12944-018-0745-1.

Lim, U., Ernst, T., Buchthal, S., Latch, M., Albright, C. L., Wilkens, L. R., ... Marchand, L. L. (2011). Asian women have greater abdominal and visceral adiposity than Caucasian women with similar body mass index. *Nutrition & Diabetes, 1*(5), e6. https://doi.org/10.1038/nutd.2011.2

Maurea, N., Coppola, C., Ragone, G., Frasci, G., Bonelli, A., Romano, C., & Iaffaioli, R. V. (2010). Women survive breast cancer but fall victim to heart failure: The shadows and lights of targeted therapy. *Journal of Cardiovascular Medicine, 11*(12), 861–868. https://doi.org/10.2459/JCM.0b013e328336b4c1

Mottillo, S., Filion, K. B., Genest, J., Joseph, L., Pilote, L., Poirier, P., ... Eisenberg, M. J. (2010). The metabolic syndrome and cardiovascular risk a systematic review and meta-analysis. *Journal of the American College of Cardiology, 56*(14), 1113–1132. https://doi.org/10.1016/j.jacc.2010.05.034

Nahm, F. S. (2015). Understanding effect sizes. *Hanyang Medical Reviews, 35*(1), 40–43. https://doi.org/10.7599/hmr.2015.35.1.40 (Original work published in Korean)

National Cancer Institute. (2015). *Cancer stat facts: Female breast cancer.* Retrieved from https://seer.cancer.gov/statfacts/html/breast.html

National Cholesterol Education Program Adult Treatment Panel III. (2002). Third report of the National Cholesterol Education Program (NCEP) expert panel on detection, evaluation, and treatment of high blood cholesterol in adults (Adult Treatment Panel III) final report. *Circulation, 106*(25), 3143.

Oh, C. M., Won, Y. J., Jung, K. W., Kong, H. J., Cho, H., Lee, J. K., ... The Community of Population-Based Regional Cancer Registries. (2016). Cancer statistics in Korea: Incidence, mortality, survival, and prevalence in 2013. *Cancer Research and Treatment, 48*(2), 436–450. https://doi.org/10.4143/crt.2016.089

Oh, E. J., Joh, H. K., Lee, R., Do, H. J., Oh, S. W., Lym, Y. L., ... Cho, D. Y. (2008). Relations between the dietary habits and components of the metabolic syndrome in premenopausal women. *Journal of the Korean Academy of Family Medicine, 29*(10), 746–776. Original work published in Korean

O'Neill, S., & O'Driscoll, L. (2015). Metabolic syndrome: A closer look at the growing epidemic and its associated pathologies. *Obesity Reviews, 16*(1), 1–12. https://doi.org/10.1111/obr.12229

Park, E. H., Min, S. Y., Kim, Z., Yoon, C. S., Jung, K. W., Nam, S. J., ... Hur, M. H. (2017). Basic facts of breast cancer in Korea in 2014: The 10-year overall survival progress. *Journal of Breast Cancer, 20*(1), 1–11. https://doi.org/10.4048/jbc.2017.20.1.1

Patterson, R. E., Flatt, S. W., Saquib, N., Rock, C. L., Caan, B. J., Parker, B. A., ... Pierce, J. P. (2010). Medical comorbidities predict mortality in women with a history of early stage breast cancer. *Breast Cancer Research and Treatment, 122*(3), 859–865. https://doi.org/10.1007/s10549-010-0732-3

Redig, A. J., & Munshi, H. G. (2010). Care of the cancer survivor: Metabolic syndrome after hormone-modifying therapy. *The American Journal of Medicine, 123*(1), 87.e1–87.e6. https://doi.org/10.1016/j.amjmed.2009.06.022

Rock, C. L., Doyle, C., Demark-Wahnefried, W., Meyerhardt, J., Courneya, K. S., Schwartz, A. L., ... Gansler, T. (2012). Nutrition and physical activity guidelines for cancer survivors. *CA: a Cancer Journal for Clinicians, 62*, 243–274. https://doi.org/10.3322/caac.21142

Seo, J. S., Park, H. A., Kang, J. H., Kim, K. W., Cho, Y. G., Hur, Y. I., & Park, Y. R. (2014). Obesity and obesity-related lifestyles of Korean breast cancer survivors. *Korean Journal of Health Promotion, 14*(3), 93–102. https://doi.org/10.15384/kjhp.2014.14.3.93 (Original work published in Korean)

Stewart, B. W., & Wild, C. P. (2014). *World cancer report 2014*. Lyon, France: International Agency for Research on Cancer.

Zhu, S., Wang, Z., Heshka, S., Heo, M., Faith, M. S., & Heymsfield, S. B. (2002). Waist circumference and obesity-associated risk factors among whites in the third National Health and Nutrition Examination Survey: Clinical action thresholds. *The American Journal of Clinical Nutrition, 76*(4), 743–749. https://doi.org/10.1093/ajcn/76.4.743

16

Impacts of Fatigue, Stress and Perceived Health Status on Women with Rheumatic Diseases: A Comparison Study

Hsuan-Man HUNG[1]* • Ming-Fu CHEN[2] • Chung-Hey CHEN[3]

ABSTRACT

Background: Rheumatic conditions, which increase in prevalence as populations age, are a growing public health problem that disproportionately affects women. Understanding the influences of rheumatic diseases (RDs) on fatigue, stress, and perceived health status is deemed important to the improvement of physical and mental health for women with RDs.

Purpose: This study was designed to compare the fatigue, stress, and perceived physical and mental health status of women with RDs (RD group) with those of peers who did not have chronic illnesses (comparison group).

Methods: A cross-sectional, purposive sample and comparative design was used. Four hundred forty-three women with a mean age of 46.2 years participated in this study. Those with physician-diagnosed RDs (n = 212) were enrolled in the RD group, and those without chronic disease were enrolled in the comparison group (n = 231). Measures used included a demographic datasheet, Fatigue Severity Scale, Perceived Stress Scale, and Short Form-12 Items Health Survey. Analysis of covariance was used to examine the intergroup differences for major variables based on demographic covariates.

Results: The RD group reported significantly more fatigue and stress than the comparison group. Moreover, the RD group reported significantly poorer perceived physical health status, significantly poorer physical functioning and general health, and greater bodily pain compared with the comparison group. Conversely, the RD group reported significantly better perceived mental health status, significantly lower vitality, and better role emotional status than the comparison group.

Conclusions/Implications for Practice: The findings support the theory that RDs have a negative impact on perceived stress and fatigue in women. Physical function, bodily pain, and general health may be the most significantly affected domains of perceived physical health in women with RDs. Of note, with the exception of the vitality subscale, RDs did not adversely affect the perceived mental health of participants with RD in this study. Healthcare professionals should cooperate with clinical rheumatologists, psychologists, and physiotherapists to provide comprehensive care that includes long-term education to help patients with RD self-manage stress, restore vitality, relieve pain, and increase physical function.

KEY WORDS:
women's health, stress, fatigue, rheumatic diseases.

Introduction

Rheumatic diseases (RDs), a broad category of symptoms and disorders, are characterized by the presence of inflammation and autoimmune problems (such as rheumatoid arthritis [RA], systemic lupus erythematosus [SLE], and fibromyalgia [FM]; American College of Rheumatology, 2019). RDs are heterogeneous with respect to their clinical presentation and may affect joints, tendons, ligaments, bones, muscles, and organs, which may lead to a concomitant diagnosis of musculoskeletal disease, multimorbidities such as RA overlapping with FM and disability, rapidly increasing healthcare costs, and significantly more days away from work (World Health Organization, 2018; Yu, See, Kuo, Chou, & Chou, 2013). These conditions have a significant impact on both individuals and society and carry a high risk of mortality, especially for RDs that are caused by autoimmune system defects (Yu et al., 2013). Furthermore, RDs are painful and typically become chronic and have a high prevalence worldwide in adult populations (Li et al., 2012; Zeng et al., 2008). With populations aging, the prevalence of RDs is projected to increase and become a large public health problem that disproportionately affects women (Goldblatt & O'Neill, 2013; Jokar & Jokar, 2018). It has been estimated that one in 12 women will develop an RD during her lifetime (Crowson et al., 2011).

Fatigue is a major problem associated with multiple RDs; it is a contributing factor to disability and an important indicator of overall health status (Sandıkç & Özbalkan, 2015). An international study found that severe fatigue affects one of every two patients with RDs. However, the etiology of fatigue in RDs remains largely unknown and inadequately

[1]PhD, RN, Associate Professor, Department of Nursing, Fooyin University, Kaohsiung, Taiwan, ROC • [2]MD, Attending Physician, Department of Rheumatology, St. Joseph Hospital, Kaohsiung, Taiwan, ROC • [3]PhD, RN, Chair Professor, Department of Nursing, Hungkuang University, Taichung, and Adjunct Professor, Department of Nursing & Institute of Allied Health Sciences, National Cheng Kung University, Taiwan, ROC.

addressed in clinical practice (Overman, Kool, Da Silva, & Geenen, 2016). In addition to fatigue, stress plays a pivotal role in inducing RD-related symptoms. Stress increases inflammation in patients with RA and SLE (Davis et al., 2008; de Brouwer et al., 2013; Jacobs et al., 2001), disrupts sleep in patients with SLE (Palagini et al., 2016), and exacerbates the activity of RDs (Jacobs et al., 2001). Thus, improving the physical function of patients with RDs is important (Chen & Wang, 2007; Sok, Ryu, Park, & Seong, 2019). As fatigue and stress are known factors that contribute to physical inactivity and the reduced effectiveness of coping strategies (Rieger et al., 2018; Taylor & Dorn, 2006), identifying the influences of RDs on fatigue and stress in women should play a key role in planning nursing interventions. However, few studies have studied the comparative impacts of fatigue and stress on women with RD and their healthy peers.

Perceived health status includes physical and mental health. Prior research has found a significant correlation between better perceived health status and better perceived illness control in individuals with chronic illnesses (Lange & Piette, 2005). Moreover, as self-reported health status reflects physical, psychological, and social well-being dimensions, self-reported health status may be considered when assessing healthcare outcomes (Weinert, Cudney, & Spring, 2008). A review of 37 studies that was designed to assess the health burden of patients with FM using a subjective health questionnaire (Short-Form Health Survey-12 [SF-12] and Short-Form Health Survey-36 [SF-36]) found that the SF-12 comprises a broad range of health profiles and is applicable for comparisons across groups with different health conditions (Hoffman & Dukes, 2008). Eliciting the multidimensional perceived health status of women who experience RDs may identify the health domains that are most affected by RDs and suggest interventions that may significantly improve their health. Therefore, the purpose of this study was to compare fatigue, stress, and perceived physical and mental health statuses between a group of women with RDs (RD group) and a comparison group of women without chronic diseases.

Methods

Design and Participants

A cross-sectional, purposive sampling and comparative design was used. Potential subjects were approached in the rheumatology clinics of teaching hospitals and in residential communities in southern Taiwan. Eligible subjects were invited to participate in this study after hearing a detailed explanation of the study purpose and providing informed consent. Inclusion criteria were as follows: (a) at least 20 years old, (b) diagnosed by a physician either as having an RD (RD group) or as having no chronic disease (comparison group), and (c) able to communicate in Mandarin Chinese or Taiwanese. Otherwise-eligible subjects with any of the following criteria were excluded from participation: (a) currently pregnant, (b) disabled, or (c) diagnosed with a psychiatric disorder. The healthy (without chronic disease) women in the comparison group were enrolled from the community. G-Power 3.1.2 (Heinrich Heine Universitat, Dusseldorf, Germany) was used to estimate sample size based on a significance level of $\alpha < .05$ and a power of 0.8, with a medium ($f = .25$) effect size (Faul, Erdfelder, Lang, & Buchner, 2007); a minimum of 135 participants in each group would be necessary to detect mean intergroup differences. As the typical response rate for paper-and-pencil questionnaires is about 73% (Kongsved, Basnov, Holm-Christensen, & Hjollund, 2007), a minimum sample size of 184 participants in each group was suggested for this study. The period of data collection was April 2015 to March 2016. Permission from the institutional review board was obtained before study implementation (Approval No. 15-046-B1).

Measures

Demographic data were collected on age, educational level, marital status, employment status, and health habits.

Fatigue severity scale

The nine-item Fatigue Severity Scale, which was designed to assess the severity of fatigue in different situations, was used to measure fatigue in this study, with scores ranging from 1 = *strongly disagree* to 7 = *strongly agree* (Krupp, LaRocca, Muir-Nash, & Steinberg, 1989). The range of total possible scores was 9–63, with higher scores associated with greater fatigue severity. The Cronbach's alpha coefficient for this scale was .93 in this study.

Perceived stress scale

The 10-item Perceived Stress Scale (PSS) was used to measure stress in this study (Cohen, Kamarch, & Mermelstein, 1983). All of the items were scored on a 5-point scale ranging from 0 = *never* to 4 = *very often*, with a maximum possible score of 40 (Cohen et al., 1983), with higher scores associated with greater perceived stress. The Cronbach's alpha for the PSS in this study was .90.

Short-Form Health Survey-12

Perceived health status is a subjective assessment of health that was measured in this study using SF-12 Version 2 (V2), developed by Ware, Kosinski, and Keller in 1996. The SF-12 V2 uses 12 items in each of the eight subscales of the SF-36 (physical functioning, role physical, bodily pain, general health, vitality, social functioning, role emotional, and mental health) to calculate two summary scores (Physical Component Summary [PCS] and Mental Component Summary [MCS]). The possible scores for this scale range from 0 to 100, with higher scores indicating better perceived physical and mental health status. The Cronbach's alphas of the PCS-12 and MCS-12 in this study were .80 and .84, respectively.

Data Analysis

Data were analyzed using IBM SPSS Statistics Version 18.0 (IBM, Inc., Armonk, NY, USA). The demographic characteristics of the two groups were compared using an independent *t* test, a χ^2 test, and a Fisher exact test. Because employment status and alcohol consumption differed significantly between the groups, analysis of covariance was used to examine the intergroup differences for major variables.

Results

Four hundred forty-three of the 458 individuals who were invited to participate submitted valid questionnaires—a response rate of 96.7%. The 212 participants with physician-diagnosed RDs were enrolled in the RD group, and those without chronic disease were enrolled in the comparison group (n = 231). The average age of the participants in this study was 46.2 years (range: 21–80 years). Most (71.8%) were married, and half (51.0%) were educated to the high school level or less. The top three diagnoses among the participants in the RD group who had a single RD (n = 196, 92.5%) were RA (n = 139, 65.6%), SLE (n = 45, 21.2%), and Sjögren's syndrome (n = 40, 18.9%). The mean duration from the first physician diagnosis of RD was 6.4 years. Nearly all (n = 196, 92.5%) in the RD group received regular medical care, including prescribed oral drugs (90.6%) such as disease-modifying antirheumatic drugs, steroids, and analgesics; biologic therapies (17.9%); and traditional Chinese medicine (6.1%). Table 1, which compares the demographic characteristics of the two groups, highlights significant intergroup differences in employment status (p = .006) and alcohol consumption (p = .003). The RD group had a significantly higher rate of unemployment and a significantly lower level of alcohol consumption. Thus, employment status and alcohol consumption were identified as significant covariates. In addition, a borderline significant difference was identified in marital status between the groups (p = .052), with fewer married individuals in the RD group. Table 2 shows differences in stress, fatigue, perceived physical health status, and perceived mental health status. A significant difference in fatigue was found between the groups (p = .001), with the RD group self-reporting as experiencing significantly more fatigue. Mean (*SD*) PSS scores of 15.44 (6.86) for the RD

TABLE 1.
Basic Characteristics by Group (N = 443)

	RD Group (n = 212)		Comparison Group (n = 231)			
Characteristic	n	%	n	%	t/χ^2	p
Age (years, *M* and *SD*)	46.46	12.53	46.26	8.04	0.204	.839
Education					2.245	.297
Senior high school or lower	108	60.0	118	51.1		
College/university	94	44.3	94	40.7		
Graduate school or higher	10	4.7	19	8.2		
Marital status					3.764	.052
Married	143	67.5	175	75.8		
Single	69	32.5	56	24.2		
Living with					2.945	.225
Family members	192	90.6	211	91.3		
Alone	16	7.5	11	4.8		
Others	4	1.9	9	3.9		
Employment status					7.472	.006
Yes	132	62.3	171	74.0		
No	80	37.7	60	26.0		
Regular exercise					0.320	.572
Yes	74	34.9	87	37.7		
No	138	65.1	144	62.3		
Smoking status					1.307	.253
Yes	3	1.4	7	3.0		
No	209	98.6	224	97.0		
Alcohol consumption[a]						.003
Yes	1	0.5	12	5.2		
No	211	99.5	219	94.8		

Note. RDs = rheumatic disease.
[a]Fisher's exact test.

TABLE 2.
ANCOVA for Stress, Fatigue, Physical, and Mental Status Between Groups (N = 443)

Variable	RD Group		Comparison Group			
	Mean	*SD*	Mean	*SD*	*F*	*p*
Fatigue	37.70	13.85	33.06	12.46	12.05	.001
Stress	15.44	6.86	13.03	5.57	6.64	.010
Perceived physical health status	43.93	8.44	50.17	6.16	76.25	< .001
Physical functioning	69.34	29.97	86.68	22.40	45.44	< .001
Role physical	63.74	27.12	66.87	18.25	1.10	.296
Bodily pain	68.28	23.95	80.02	18.93	30.42	< .001
General health	32.88	22.81	47.34	26.31	41.41	< .001
Perceived mental health status	48.40	8.63	45.67	7.37	12.36	< .001
Vitality	53.89	22.56	61.46	21.13	11.27	.001
Social functioning	70.17	22.25	70.20	21.04	0.00	.969
Role emotional	71.70	23.55	66.21	17.08	8.25	.004
Mental health	68.51	18.55	66.05	16.81	2.12	.146

Note. ANCOVA = analysis of covariance; RD = rheumatic disease.

group and 13.03 (5.57) for the comparison group revealed a significant intergroup difference in stress ($p = .010$), with the RD group perceiving significantly greater stress.

Mean (*SD*) PCS scores were 43.93 (8.44) and 48.40 (8.63), respectively, for the RD and comparison groups, showing that perceived physical health status was poorer in the RD group. In addition, the scores for the four subscales of PCS were analyzed. The respective mean scores for physical function, bodily pain, and general health were 69.31, 68.28, and 32.88 in the RD group and 86.68, 80.02, and 47.34 in the comparison group, indicating a significant intergroup difference for each of the three subscales. No significant intergroup difference in role physical was found ($p = .296$). In summary, the RD group reported poorer physical functioning and general health and greater bodily pain than the comparison group. Moreover, mean (*SD*) MCS scores were 48.40 (8.63) and 45.67 (7.37), respectively, for the RD and comparison groups. The RD group reported significantly better perceived mental health status. Subsequent analysis of the scores of the four MCS subscales found the mean scores for vitality and role emotional to be 53.89 and 71.70 in the RD group and 61.46 and 66.21 in the comparison group, which identify a significant intergroup difference for these two subscales. No significant intergroup differences in social functioning ($p = .969$) or mental health ($p = .146$) were found. Thus, the RD group reported lower scores for vitality and higher scores for role emotional.

Discussion

RA was the most common disease reported in the RD group. This finding is similar to the findings reported in the population-based studies of Yu et al. (2013), which studied the general population in Taiwan, and Jokar and Jokar (2018), which studied a population of outpatients with RD in Mashhad, Iran. Moreover, Yu et al. found RA to be the most prevalent of the autoimmune RDs, with an incidence rate three times higher in women than men. The prevalence of RA in this study of 65.5% is higher than the 47.30% reported in Jokar and Jokar. A possible explanation for this is that the latter study included both men and women as subjects, whereas this study included women only. Participants in the RD group were significantly more likely to be unemployed than their comparison group peers. This finding partially echoes the results of a prior study (Wolfe & Michaud, 2009). Women with RDs frequently experience multiple disorders (e.g., pain extent, joint deformities, disrupted sleep) that lead to loss of function and an inability to continue working (Matcham, Rayner, Steer, & Hotopf, 2013; Westhoff, Dörner, & Zink, 2012). In this study, the participants in the RD group reported a lower mean consumption of alcohol than their healthy peers. Several researchers have identified a higher incidence of RDs among individuals with infrequent alcohol consumption than among individuals with baseline, low-to-moderate alcohol consumption (Bergström, Jacobsson, Nilsson, Wirfält, & Turesson, 2013; Jin, Xiang, Cai, Wei, &He, 2014). One possible explanation is the antinociceptive and anti-inflammatory effects of alcohol (Maxwell, Gowers, Moore, & Wilson, 2010).

In terms of stress, the findings of this study revealed higher levels of stress in the RD group than in the comparison group. Few prior studies have compared stress levels between individuals with RDs and individuals in the general, healthy population, with most focused on identifying RD-related stress (Davis et al., 2008; Jacobs et al., 2001). Curtis, Groarke, Coughlan, and Gsel (2005), who investigated 59 women with RA with a mean age of 60 years, found that women with higher perceived levels of stress had higher depression and that women with higher depression had lower adaptive coping. Furthermore, the results of Delgado (2007) found that patients with chronic illness who reported lower perceived levels of stress had a higher sense of coherence and spirituality.

Fatigue is an ambiguous symptom. Because of the lack of a single, widely accepted measurement instrument, the Fatigue Severity Scale and the vitality scale of SF-12 V2 were used in this study as a comprehensive measure of fatigue. This study found higher rates of severe fatigue and low vitality in the RD group. These results are similar to Godaert et al. (2002), who compared daily fatigue with repeated measures in women patients with SLE (n = 20) and with primary Sjögren's syndrome (n = 28) and in healthy women subjects (n = 30) and found significantly more severe levels of general and physical fatigue in patients with SLE and primary Sjögren's syndrome. In addition, the results of this study echo Overman et al. (2016), who used the RAND (SF)-36 Vitality scale to conduct an online measurement of fatigue in patients with RDs in several European countries and found significantly more severe fatigue in patients with FM than in those without. Chronic, widespread pain is a typical complaint among patients with FM, and related musculoskeletal conditions and mental disorders are known to confound related diagnoses (Häuser, Perrot, Sommer, Shir, & Fitzcharles, 2017). In this study, only one participant with RA reported concomitant FM. In clinical settings, chronic fatigue is a difficult condition to communicate to healthcare providers, and rheumatology nurses typically do not know how to manage fatigue in patients with RDs (Repping-Wuts, Sarah, Van Riel, & Van Achterberg, 2008). Thus, the findings of this study support the importance of obtaining an early diagnosis of fatigue to implement the self-management strategies necessary to cope with, ameliorate, and resolve fatigue.

Fatigue reflects bodily pain that limits physical functioning (Nijrolder, van der Windt, Twisk, & van der Horst, 2010). As expected, the RD group in this study reported significantly worse perceived physical health in terms of physical functioning, general health, and bodily pain. These findings reinforce the findings of Salaffi et al. (2009), who compared 380 patients with FM, 693 patients with RA, and 1,579 individuals from the general population in Italy using SF-36 scores and found that those with FM or RA reported more significantly impaired physical and mental health on all eight subscales than the general population. The partially different findings in Salaffi et al. may be because of that study's exclusion of patients with concomitant RDs and its nonexclusion of subjects with chronic illness comorbidities from the comparison groups. In contrast, this study excluded women with chronic disease comorbidities. The participants with RDs in this study reported greater role physical functioning difficulties than their healthy peers, although the intergroup difference did not reach significance. The role physical subscale is designed to measure the severity of role limitations caused by physical problems (Hoffman & Dukes, 2008; Ware et al., 1996). There are several possible explanations why the RD group in this study did not face role physical functioning limitations. First, more than 90% of the participants in the RD group were currently receiving medical treatment (i.e., prescribed oral drugs and biologic therapies). More than 98% of Taiwan's population is covered under universal National Health Insurance, which provides minimal-cost access to healthcare at nearly all healthcare facilities (Lee et al., 2010). Moreover, Pollard, Choy, Gonzalez, Khoshaba, and Scott (2006) revealed that biologic and disease-modifying antirheumatic drug therapies significantly improve joint activity, pain, and fatigue. Second, the RD group reported higher ratios of unemployment and being single (unmarried) than the comparison group. Third, the RD group reported better perceived mental health than the comparison group, particularly in the role emotional subscale. Matcham et al. (2014) associated longer RA disease duration with improved mental health. Disease duration may increase acceptance of a disease (Kiebles, Doerfler, & Keefer, 2010). In this study, mean disease duration in the RD group was 6.4 years. Thus, this relatively long duration of time may have positively influenced acceptance of chronic conditions.

A major limitation of this study is that all of the measures were based on self-reported data. In addition, the disease activity of RDs is known to manifest and abate unpredictably, which has been linked to poorer physical and psychological health. Cross-sectional studies gather subject data at one point in time and thus cannot elucidate the longitudinal effects of variations in disease activity on stress, fatigue, and perceived health status or support unidirectional effects. Moreover, data were collected from southern Taiwan only, which limits the generalizability of findings to populations in other areas. Finally, potential confounders such as past histories of trauma and abuse, which may have long-lasting effects on physical and mental health, were not investigated in this study.

Conclusions

The findings of this study indicate that RDs have a significant and negative impact on perceived stress and fatigue in women. The most significant impacts occurred in the following three domains of perceived physical health: physical functioning, bodily pain, and general health. In addition, with the exception of the vitality subscale, no adverse impact was found in the domains of perceived mental health. The underlying physical and psychological problems that induce RDs remain unclear. Future studies should focus on clarifying this issue to provide the evidence necessary to develop early interventions that will effectively improve the physical and psychological health of women with RDs. In conclusion, healthcare professionals should cooperate with clinical rheumatologists, psychologists, and physiotherapists to provide comprehensive care that includes long-term education to help patients with RD self-manage stress, restore vitality, relieve pain, and increase physical functioning.

Acknowledgments

This study was funded by a grant from the Ministry of Science and Technology (MOST 104-2314-B-127-001) in Taiwan. We are particularly indebted to the women who volunteered as participants.

Author Contributions

Study conception and design: HMH
Data collection: HMH, MFC
Data analysis and interpretation: HMH
Drafting of the article: HMH
Critical revision of the article: HMH, CHC

References

American College of Rheumatology. (2019). *What is rheumatic disease? Managing your rheumatic disease*. Retrieved from https://www.rheumatology.org/I-Am-A/Patient-Caregiver/Diseases-Conditions/Living-Well-with-Rheumatic-Disease/Managing-Your-Rheumatic-Disease

Bergström, U., Jacobsson, L. T. H., Nilsson, J. A., Wirfält, E., & Turesson, C. (2013). Smoking, low formal level of education, alcohol consumption, and the risk of rheumatoid arthritis. *Scandinavian Journal of Rheumatology, 42*(2), 123–130. https://doi.org/10.3109/03009742.2012.723744

Chen, S. Y., & Wang, H. H. (2007). The relationship between physical function, knowledge of disease, social support and self-care behavior in patients with rheumatoid arthritis. *The Journal of Nursing Research, 15*(3), 183–192.

Cohen, S., Kamarch, T., & Mermelstein, R. (1983). A global measure of perceived stress. *Journal of Health and Behavior, 24*, 385_396.

Crowson, C. S., Matteson, E. L., Myasoedova, E., Michet, C. J., Ernste, F. C., Warrington, K. J., ... Gabriel, S. E. (2011). The lifetime risk of adult-onset rheumatoid arthritis and other inflammatory autoimmune rheumatic diseases. *Arthritis and Rheumatism, 63*(3), 633–639. https://doi.org/10.1002/art.30155

Curtis, R., Groarke, A. M., Coughlan, R., & Gsel, A. (2005). Psychological stress as a predictor of psychological adjustment and health status in patients with rheumatoid arthritis. *Patient Education and Counseling, 59*(2), 192–198. https://doi.org/10.1016/j.pec.2004.10.015

Davis, M. C., Zautra, A. J., Younger, J., Motivala, S. J., Attrep, J., & Irwin, M. R. (2008). Chronic stress and regulation of cellular markers of inflammation in rheumatoid arthritis: Implications for fatigue. *Brain, Behavior, and Immunity, 22*(1), 24–32. https://doi.org/10.1016/j.bbi.2007.06.013

de Brouwer, S. J., van Middendorp, H., Kraaimaat, F. W., Radstake, T. R., Joosten, I., Donders, A. R., ... Evers, A. W. (2013). Immune responses to stress after stress management training in patients with rheumatoid arthritis. *Arthritis Research and Therapy, 15*(6), R200. https://doi.org/10.1186/ar4390

Delgado, C. (2007). Sense of coherence, spirituality, stress and quality of life in chronic illness. *Journal of Nursing Scholarship, 39*(3), 229–234.

Faul, F., Erdfelder, E., Lang, A. G., & Buchner, A. (2007). G*Power 3: A flexible statistical power analysis program for the social, behavioral, and biomedical sciences. *Behavior Research Methods, 39*(2), 175–191. https://doi.org/10.3758/BF03193146

Godaert, G. L., Hartkamp, A., Geenen, R., Garssen, A., Kruize, A. A., Bijlsma, J. W., & Derken, R. H. (2002). Fatigue in daily life in patients with primary Sjögren's syndrome and systemic lupus erythematosus. *Annals of the New York Academy of Sciences, 966*(1), 320–326. https://doi.org/10.1111/j.1749-6632.2002.tb04232.x

Goldblatt, F., & O'Neill, S. G. (2013). Clinical aspects of autoimmune rheumatic diseases. *The Lancet, 382*(9894), 797–808. https://doi.org/10.1016/S0140-6736(13)61499-3

Häuser, W., Perrot, S., Sommer, C., Shir, Y., & Fitzcharles, M. A. (2017). Diagnostic confounders of chronic widespread pain: Not always fibromyalgia. *Pain Reports, 2*(3), e598. https://doi.org/10.1097/PR9.0000000000000598

Hoffman, D. L., & Dukes, E. M. (2008). The health status burden of people with fibromyalgia: A review of studies that assessed health status with the SF-36 or the SF-12. *International Journal of Clinical Practice, 62*(1), 115–126. https://doi.org/10.1111/j.1742-1241.2007.01638.x

Jacobs, R., Pawlak, C. R., Mikeska, E., Meyer-Olson, D., Martin, M., Heijnen, C., ... Schmidt, R. E. (2001). Systemic lupus erythematosus and rheumatoid arthritis patients differ from healthy controls in their cytokine pattern after stress exposure. *Rheumatology, 40*(8), 868–875. https://doi.org/10.1093/rheumatology/40.8.868

Jin, Z., Xiang, C., Cai, Q., Wei, X., & He, J. (2014). Alcohol consumption as a preventive factor for developing rheumatoid arthritis: A dose–response meta-analysis of prospective studies. *Annals of the Rheumatic Diseases, 73*(11), 1962–1967. https://doi.org/10.1136/annrheumdis-2013-203323

Jokar, M., & Jokar, M. (2018). Prevalence of inflammatory rheumatic diseases in a clinic: Analysis of 12626 cases rheumatologic outpatient. *Rheumatology Research Journal, 3*(1), 21–27. https://doi.org/10.22631/RR.2017.69997.1037

Kiebles, J. K., Doerfler, B., & Keefer, L. (2010). Preliminary evidence supporting a framework of psychological adjustment to inflammatory bowel disease. *Inflammatory Bowel Diseases, 16*(10), 1685–1695. https://doi.org/10.1002/ibd.21215

Kongsved, S. M., Basnov, M., Holm-Christensen, K., & Hjollund, N. H. (2007). Response rate and completeness of questionnaires: A randomized study of internet versus paper-and-pencil versions. *Journal of Medical Internet Research, 9*(3), e25. https://doi.org/10.2196/jmir.9.3.e25

Krupp, L. B., LaRocca, N. G., Muir-Nash, J., & Steinberg, A. D. (1989). The fatigue severity scale: Application to patients with multiple sclerosis and systemic lupus erythematosus. *Archives of Neurology, 46*(10), 1121–1123. https://doi.org/10.1001/archneur.1989.00520460115022

Lange, L. J., & Piette, J. D. (2005). Perceived health status and perceived diabetes control: Psychological indicators and accuracy. *Journal of Psychosomatic Research, 58*(2), 129–137. https://doi.org/10.1016/j.jpsychores.2004.08.004

Lee, Y. C., Huang, Y. T., Tsai, W. N., Huang, S. M., Kuo, K. N., McKee, M., & Nolte, E. (2010). The impact of universal National Health Insurance on population health: The experience of

Taiwan. *BMC Health Services Research, 2010*(10), 225. https://doi.org/10.1186/1472-6963-10-225

Li, R., Sun, J., Ren, L. M., Wang, H. Y., Liu, W. H., Zang, X. W., ... Li, Z. G. (2012). Epidemiology of eight common rheumatic diseases in China: A large-scale cross-sectional survey in Beijing. *Rheumatology, 51*(4), 721–729. https://doi.org/10.1093/rheumatology/ker370

Matcham, F., Rayner, L., Steer, S., & Hotopf, M. (2013). The prevalence of depression in rheumatoid arthritis: A systematic review and meta-analysis. *Rheumatology, 52*(12), 2136–2148. https://doi.org/10.1093/rheumatology/ket169

Matcham, F., Scott, I. C., Rayner, L., Hotopf, M., Kingsley, G. H., Norton, S., ... Steer, S. (2014). The impact of rheumatoid arthritis on quality-of-life assessed using the SF-36: A systematic review and meta-analysis. *Seminars in Arthritis and Rheumatism, 44*(2), 123–130. https://doi.org/10.1016/j.semarthrit.2014.05.001

Maxwell, J. R., Gowers, I. R., Moore, D. J., & Wilson, A. G. (2010). Alcohol consumption is inversely associated with risk and severity of rheumatoid arthritis. *Rheumatology, 49*(11), 2140–2146. https://doi.org/10.1093/rheumatology/keq20

Nijrolder, I., van der Windt, D. A., Twisk, J. W., & van der Horst, H. E. (2010). Fatigue in primary care: Longitudinal associations with pain. *Pain, 150*(2), 351–357. https://doi.org/10.1016/j.pain.2010.05.030

Overman, C. L., Kool, M. B., Da Silva, J. A., & Geenen, R. (2016). The prevalence of severe fatigue in rheumatic diseases: An international study. *Clinical Rheumatology, 35*(2), 409–415. https://doi.org/10.1007/s10067-015-3035-6

Palagini, L., Mauri, M., Faraguna, U., Carli, L., Tani, C., Dell'Osso, L., ... Riemann, D. (2016). Insomnia symptoms, perceived stress and coping strategies in patients with systemic lupus erythematosus. *Lupus, 25*(9), 988–996. https://doi.org/10.1177/0961203316631630

Pollard, L. C., Choy, E. H., Gonzalez, J., Khoshaba, B., & Scott, D. L. (2006). Fatigue in rheumatoid arthritis reflects pain, not disease activity. *Rheumatology, 45*(7), 885–889. https://doi.org/10.1093/rheumatology/kel021

Repping-Wuts, H., Sarah, H., Van Riel, P., & Van Achterberg, T. (2008). Fatigue in patients with rheumatoid arthritis: British and Dutch nurses' knowledge, attitudes and management. *Journal of Advanced Nursing, 65*(4), 901–911. https://doi.org/10.1111/j.1365-2648.2008.04904.x

Rieger, K. L., Lobchuk, M. M., Duff, M. A., Chernomas, W. M., Campbell-Enns, H. J., Demczuk, L., ... West, C. H. (2018). Effectiveness of mindfulness-based arts interventions on psychological wellbeing and fatigue in adults with a physical illness: A systematic review protocol. *JBI Database of Systematic Reviews and Implementation Reports, 16*(7), 1476–1484. https://doi.org/10.11124/JBISRIR-2017-003446

Salaffi, F., Sarzi-Puttini, P., Girolimetti, R., Atzeni, F., Gasparini, S., & Grassi, W. (2009). Health-related quality of life in fibromyalgia patients: A comparison with rheumatoid arthritis patients and the general population using the SF-36 health survey. *Clinical and Experimental Rheumatology, 27*(56, Suppl.), S67–S74.

Sandıkç, S. C., & Özbalkan, Z. (2015). Fatigue in rheumatic diseases. *European Journal of Rheumatology, 2*(3), 109–113. https://doi.org/10.5152/eurjrheum.2015.0029

Sok, S. R., Ryu, J. S., Park, S. H., & Seong, M. H. (2019). Factors influencing self-care competence in Korean women with rheumatoid arthritis. *The Journal of Nursing Research, 27*(2), e16. https://doi.org/10.1097/jnr.0000000000000279

Taylor, A. H., & Dorn, L. (2006). Stress, fatigue, health, and risk of road traffic accidents among professional drivers: The contribution of physical inactivity. *Annual Review of Public Health, 27*, 371–391. https://doi.org/10.1146/annurev.publhealth.27.021405.102117

Ware, J. Jr., Kosinski, M., & Keller, S. D. (1996). A 12-item short-form health survey: Construction of scales and preliminary tests of reliability and validity. *Medical Care, 34*(3), 220–233.

Weinert, C., Cudney, S., & Spring, A. (2008). Evolution of a conceptual model for adaptation to chronic illness. *Journal of Nursing Scholarship, 40*(4), 364–372. https://doi.org/10.1111/j.1547-5069.2008.00241.x

Westhoff, G., Dörner, T., & Zink, A. (2012). Fatigue and depression predict physician visits and work disability in women with primary Sjögren's syndrome: Results from a cohort study. *Rheumatology, 51*(2), 262–269. https://doi.org/10.1093/rheumatology/ker208

Wolfe, F., & Michaud, K. (2009). Predicting depression in rheumatoid arthritis: The signal importance of pain extent and fatigue, and comorbidity. *Arthritis and Rheumatism, 61*(5), 667–673. https://doi.org/10.1002/art.24428

World Health Organization. (2018). *Chronic diseases and health promotion—Chronic rheumatic conditions*. Retrieved from http://www.who.int/chp/topics/rheumatic/en/

Yu, K. H., See, L. C., Kuo, C. F., Chou, I. J., & Chou, M. J. (2013). Prevalence and incidence in patients with autoimmune rheumatic diseases: A nationwide population-based study in Taiwan. *Arthritis Care and Research, 65*(2), 244–250. https://doi.org/10.1002/acr.21820

Zeng, Q. Y., Chen, R., Darmawan, J., Xiao, Z. Y., Chen, S. B., Wigley, R., ... Zhang, N. Z. (2008). Rheumatic diseases in China. *Arthritis Research & Therapy, 10*(1), R17. https://doi.org/10.1186/ar2368

17

Living With Diabetes: Perceived Barriers of Adolescents

Kübra Pınar GÜRKAN[1]* • Zuhal BAHAR[2]

ABSTRACT

Background: Type 1 diabetes mellitus is the most common endocrine disease during infancy and adolescence. Diabetes causes serious coping problems during adolescence because of the need for continuous observation and because of diabetes-related complications. Thus, adolescents must adapt to and effectively manage their diabetes.

Purpose: This study was designed to determine the perceived barriers to home care in adolescents with Type 1 diabetes using the Health Promotion Model.

Methods: Eighteen adolescents were selected from the qualified patients who applied to a diabetes polyclinic at a training and research hospital in western Turkey. Interview questions were created based on the Health Promotion Model. A phenomenological analysis of the data was conducted using the content analysis method.

Results: The barriers that participants identified as negatively impacting their ability to manage their disease effectively were categorized into the three themes of "negative feelings about having diabetes," "personal barriers," and "environmental barriers." The barriers identified included school, friends, family, fear of complications, lack of information, and personal characteristics, among others.

Conclusions/Implications for Practice: This qualitative study enables us to understand what patients feel because the participants explained their difficulties in managing their disease and in maintaining metabolic control. The findings provide an understanding of the subjective experiences of adolescent patients with diabetes. The findings of this study are intended to be helpful in restructuring training in clinics, raising diabetes awareness among teachers and students, socializing diabetic adolescents, and providing family-centered education.

KEY WORDS:
adolescent, Type 1 diabetes, home monitoring, health promotion, qualitative study.

Introduction

Type 1 diabetes mellitus (T1DM) is a chronic endocrine disease seen in childhood (Fortunato et al., 2016). A multidisciplinary team is required to set and achieve the goals of treatment, which are unique to each stage of childhood development. Pediatric diabetes nurses in the team are responsible for the education and care of children/adolescents with T1DM, which includes providing monitoring and consultancy services (American Diabetes Association, 2018). Research shows that nursing care is effective in increasing the ability of children with T1DM to self-manage their disease (Dobson et al., 2016; Samimi, Talakoub, & Ghazavi, 2018; Tiberg, Lindgren, Carlsson, & Hallström, 2016). Furthermore, a study performed in Portugal reported that most adolescents with Type 1 diabetes (87.4%) were happy with the consultancy services provided by their nurses (Pires, Aparício, & Duarte, 2016). Diabetes education plays a key role in managing this disease. According to the literature, Type 1 diabetes education provided by diabetes nurses, including psychological as well as behavioral strategies, is effective in altering the lifestyle of patients, which results in a reduction in hospitalizations and associated costs because of improved glycemic control (Cheraghi, Shamsaei, Mortazavi, & Moghimbeigi, 2015; O'Hara et al., 2017).

After diagnosing and treating T1DM, it is necessary to ensure that nursing care continues at home (Clapin et al., 2017; Tiberg et al., 2016). In the limited studies of T1DM home care, those who receive home care were found to incur 30% less in healthcare costs, to be satisfied with their healthcare, and to have more time for social activities (Tiberg et al., 2016).

Adolescence is a developmental crisis period, and the presence of a chronic disease in adolescence may undermine the sense of identity and independence and change the future plans of patients (Castensøe-Seidenfaden et al., 2017). These issues make it more difficult to manage this disease in the adolescent period. Thus, it is necessary to determine the cognitive and perceptual barriers faced by adolescents with T1DM to help them gain the skills necessary to manage their disease effectively. Pender's Health Promotion Model (HPM), used widely in public health nursing applications, is often used to determine these barriers. The HPM consists of individual features and concepts and specifically addresses behavior. Knowledge of behavior and attitudes toward a disease helps

[1]PhD, Lecturer, Faculty of Nursing, Department of Public Health Nursing, Dokuz Eylül University, Izmir, Turkey • [2]PhD, Professor, Faculty of Nursing, Department of Public Health Nursing, Okan University, Istanbul, Turkey.

determine the perceived barriers to and benefits of health promotion (Pender, Murgaugh, & Parsons, 2015). The results gained from this study should assist home care nurses to identify the barriers faced by adolescents with T1DM in managing their disease.

Qualitative studies have focused mainly on patients with Type 2 diabetes mellitus. Furthermore, the few qualitative studies that have been conducted with adolescent patients with T1DM were limited to investigating their school experiences and their mothers' experiences in having a child diagnosed with T1DM (Rostami, Parsa-Yekta, Najafi-Ghezeljeh, Vanaki, & Zarea, 2015; Schwartz, Denham, Heh, Wapner, & Shubrook, 2010). However, no study has used the HPM to investigate this issue holistically or to identify the difficulties that adolescents with T1DM face in managing their disease. Moreover, no qualitative study has been conducted on adolescents with T1DM in Turkey. Therefore, this study was designed to identify the barriers to sustaining the behaviors necessary for the effective management of T1DM.

Methods

Setting and Participants

A qualitative, phenomenological research approach was used in this study, which was conducted between June 1 and September 31, 2015, on 18 adolescents with T1DM who were registered in a training and research hospital in the western region of Turkey. Patients who came for a diabetes mellitus regular check were included in the study using a purposeful sampling method. The inclusion criteria were as follows: (a) being diagnosed with Type 1 diabetes for at least 1 year, (b) aged 11–17 years, (c) volunteering to participate in the study (adolescent and their parents), and (d) able to speak and understand Turkish. The exclusion criteria were as follows: (a) being diagnosed with Type 2 diabetes, (b) unable to complete the interviews, or (c) being diagnosed with mental retardation.

Data Collection

Interviews were conducted in a quiet, special interview room in the diabetes unit and were audio recorded. Data were collected through face-to-face interviews using semistructured interview questions. During the interview, probing questions were asked to obtain explanations and clarifications (Sandelowski, 2000). Interview durations ranged from 25 to 45 minutes (mean = 35 minutes). A semistructured interview guide was prepared (evaluation of the questions was performed by five experts and corrections were made in line with their recommendations) based on the qualitative research methods described in the HPM (Pender et al., 2015). The five interview questions were the following:

(1) Could you please describe your life with diabetes?
(2) What activities do you do to manage your diabetes (e.g., insulin injection, dosing, individual monitoring, exercise, and diabetes education)?
(3) How does having diabetes affect your life?
(4) What do you need to help you manage your diabetes?
(5) What difficulties do you face in managing your diabetes?/ What conditions affect your ability to manage your diabetes?

This method was chosen because it was applicable to adolescents; it could improve patients' health by determining individuals' self-competence, social support, and perceptions (perceptions of benefit and handicap); and it caused changes in their behavior. All of the interviews were conducted by the first researcher, who participated in relevant courses and workshops on qualitative research methods. Pre interviews were conducted with five patients, although the data obtained were not included in the statistical analysis.

Data Analysis

The data were analyzed using the content analysis method, which has been suggested for qualitative research (Creswell, Hanson, Clark Plano, & Morales, 2007; Olsen Roper et al., 2009; Yıldırım & Şimşek, 2011). The data were analyzed independently by two researchers using an inductive approach. First, audio recording transcription was performed. Second, the researchers analyzed each transcription line by line and coded the data. Third, the coded data were assigned to relevant subthemes, which the researchers determined by unanimous agreement. Finally, the main theme was created by integrating the subthemes. The main themes and subthemes were identified and compared with the patients' statements and their answers to the study questions. At the end of each participant's statement, the interview order, age, and gender of participants were recorded using abbreviations.

Study Trustworthiness

The researchers used Lincoln and Guba's (1985) four criteria of credibility, transferability, dependability, and confirmability to ensure the reliability of the data for use in qualitative studies. To ensure credibility, the interviews were conducted in a quiet and private place and the first researcher took notes during the recording. Two experienced researchers created categories and subcategories to describe the data and findings, with the first researcher and an independent researcher examining the data and the second researcher performing the content analysis. To ensure transferability, giving detailed information related to the stages of the research and the data collection method were clearly defined, the themes obtained were exemplified using direct quotations, and the interview data were transferred verbatim. The data for dependability were consistent, because most participants gave the same answers to a given question. An expert observed all phases of the study and verified that the interpretations and suggestions that were derived from the study reflected the data gathered. In addition, the data collection devices and the raw data were retained for confirmability.

Ethical Considerations

Ethical permission was received from the "Non-Invasive Clinical Studies Evaluation Commission" and from the hospital in which the study was conducted (Decision No. 2015/14-12; Protocol No. 2123-GOA). Informed consent was obtained from the participating adolescents and their parents.

Results

The mean age of the adolescent participants was 15.06 ± 1.7 years. Ten were male, the duration of T1DM diagnosis ranged from 1 to 14 years, and the mean HbA1c (glycated hemoglobin) level was 8.7 g/dl.

Barriers to diabetes management after discharge and home care needs for the participants were organized under three main themes: (a) negative feelings about having diabetes, (b) personal barriers, and (c) environmental barriers (Table 1).

Theme 1: Negative Feelings About Having Diabetes

This theme was further subdivided into two subthemes: denying being diabetic and caring about self-image.

Denying being diabetic

During in-depth interviews with the participants, it was found that their perceptions of their disease were negative.

> *...I am bored now. Why can't I just die? It was the question that I was thinking every minute. Why did I become a diabetic? I'm only 14 years old. Why me, while there are so many people out there?* (Fourth patient, aged 15 years, female)

> *Taking pills is not such a difficult thing. But the insulin represents a different dimension. It is a hard job to arrange it.* (First patient, aged 17 years, female)

Caring about self-image

Being an adolescent also affected participant attitudes toward managing their diabetes. They wanted to look good.

TABLE 1.
Theme and Subtheme

Theme	Subtheme
1. Negative feelings about having diabetes	Denying being diabetic Caring about self-image
2. Personal barriers	Lack of knowledge Fear of complications Personal traits
3. Environmental barriers	Family Friends School Provision of healthcare services

> *...Well, I do not like at all walking with a machine (glucometer) in my pocket.* (15th patient, aged 17 years, male)

Theme 2: Personal Barriers

This theme was composed of the three subthemes of lack of knowledge, fear of complications, and personal traits.

Lack of knowledge

Many patients said they had sufficient related knowledge. However, during the conversation, researchers noticed that adolescents lacked knowledge regarding diabetes management.

> *...Cigarette smoking is not harmful to diabetes. On the contrary, it is healthy. For example my blood sugar drops when I smoke. For example, I measure my blood sugar and it shows 300. Then I smoke a cigarette and I check my blood sugar ten minutes later and it shows 70....* (Seventh patient, aged 14 years, male)

Fear of complications

The participants stated that they feared macrovascular and microvascular complications, especially hypoglycemia. Because of hypoglycemia fears, adolescents did not want to go anywhere else.

> *...hyperglycaemia scares me. Nausea there is so scary, it is awful beyond belief. So, I eat too much.* (Fifth patient, aged 17 years, male)

> *...I feel very hungry. My hands and feet tremble. I feel so ill and I mostly want to go somewhere with my friends or family, but don't want to go anywhere alone.* (Seventh patient, aged 14 years, male)

In addition, some health professionals had warned the participants about diabetes complications. However, these warnings impacted their motivations negatively.

> *...Doctors sometimes say that you can go blind. This thought disturbs me.* (First patient, aged 17 years, female)

Personal traits

The personal traits of some of the participants negatively affected their ability to manage their disease. The participants reported difficulties in integrating exercise, blood glucose monitoring, and dietary requirements into their daily routine.

> *...I do not have any time for sports. Honestly, this is the biggest difficulty for me.* (18th patient, aged 15 years, female)

> *...It is a real torture for me to measure my blood sugar, to open it, to change the tip. It destroys my life for 5–10 minutes.* (Fifth patient, aged 17 years, male)

> *Measuring blood sugar is a problem also for me. I forget to measure it before meals.* (Fourth patient, aged 15 years, female)

> *...It (the glucometer) shows a high value all the time. In a word, I eat too much. I cannot prevent myself from eating a lot. When there is dessert at home, I eat it all.* (11th patient, aged 14 years, male)

Theme 3: Environmental Barriers

This theme was divided into the four subthemes of family, friends, school, and provision of healthcare services.

Family

Continuous warnings about diabetes management from their parents disturbed the participants and caused them to feel inadequate.

> *...my family still wants to measure my sugar. It's ridiculous, I'm fifteen years old.* (Second patient, aged 15 years, female)

Some of the participants reported experiencing family conflicts while performing diabetes self-care activities. As a result, they were angry with family members.

> *The family stops checking you after a while, and you get into the mode of "you do what you wanna do. They do not care."* (Fourth patient, aged 15 years, female)

> *...I am fed up with my parents', and particularly my mother's, constantly asking about my blood sugar values. I am fed up with their controlling my food all of the time. All I want is that they let me alone and trust me....* (Fifth patient, aged 17 years, male)

Friends

Participants noted that friend-related concerns encouraged them to violate their dietary restrictions.

> *...You have to keep up with your friends. If you fail this, then you feel excluded from them. For example, everyone eats ice cream, and if you do not eat, it becomes weird.* (Sixth patient, aged 16 years, female)

The participants noted that their friends continuously asked questions about their illness, which made them uncomfortable.

> *...I am sick of my friends' questions about diabetes. For example, my friends say "You have to take shots every day? I'd die if I had to do that."... It's so annoying.* (Fourth patient, aged 15 years, female)

School

The participants reported receiving negative attitudes and feedback from teachers, causing them to feel bad in class.

> *...One teacher does not believe me (that I have diabetes). They say "don't play games" (when I have a hypoglycaemia moment). None of them let me go out....* (First patient, aged 14 years, male)

The participants further noted difficulties in managing Type 1 diabetes at school.

> *...Foods at school are not appropriate for us.* (18th patient, aged 15 years, female)

Provision of healthcare services

Many of the participants stated that the length of the diabetes education that they received was inadequate.

> *...At first, I was scared and cried so much. I was scared so much to think how I would inject the insulin. What will I do if it drops or rises? They said, "You will know when it drops or rises, and you will do everything yourself." At that moment, there was so much information in front of me and the time was so inadequate. I was worried so much, saying how could I keep all this information in my mind.* (First patient, aged 17 years, female)

Discussion

In this study, all of the participants perceived multiple barriers that impeded their effective management of their Type 1 diabetes. Three main themes were identified in this context, including negative feelings about having diabetes, personal barriers, and environmental barriers.

Theme 1: Negative Feelings About Having Diabetes

The results of this study support that adolescents perceive diabetes as a disease that restricts their daily lives. In addition, the participants perceived themselves as different from their peers, an indication that they may not yet have accepted their diagnosis. Similar to the results described here, other studies have reported that children with diabetes feel different from their peers (Castensøe-Seidenfaden et al., 2017; Joensen, Filges, & Willaing, 2016; Kelo, Martikainen, & Eriksson, 2011). The "disease-related perceptions" of individuals with Type 1 diabetes are effective with regard to maintaining self-management behaviors. Moreover, it has been shown that the potential reactions of adolescents to a disease diagnosis include denial of the disease and refusal to accept treatment, particularly for diseases that are not visibly apparent (Castensøe-Seidenfaden et al., 2017). Individuals who held a positive point of view before, during, or after their behavior education or training are more likely to begin and maintain the desired behaviors. Similarly, adolescents with T1DM who hold negative attitudes toward their disease face relatively greater difficulties in adapting to their disease.

The participants in this study placed a high degree of importance on their appearance, which is attributable to their age and social conditioning. This factor was identified as a hindrance to effective disease management in this study as well as other studies in the literature (Boztepe, 2011; Marshall, Carter, Rose, & Brotherton, 2009). The biological properties of an individual are his or her age, gender, and puberty/menopause status. These individual factors must be considered, as they prevent adolescents from managing Type 1 diabetes effectively by affecting their cognitive processes, reactions, and health behaviors.

Theme 2: Personal Barriers

The results of this study support that lack of knowledge about the disease is a barrier in diabetes management. Studies in the literature highlight similar findings, indicating that low blood sugar, insulin injection, dietary restrictions, and lack of knowledge of these disease issues are among the most difficult issues for adolescents with T1DM (Kelo et al., 2011; Olsen Roper et al., 2009). A qualitative study conducted in Iran found that adolescents needed to have sufficient information regarding disease management to internalize their disease (Rostami et al., 2015). Lack of knowledge about diabetes management may constitute a barrier to self-care, leading to a loss of control over the body and, potentially, to negative effects on disease management self-efficacy. Successful diabetes management may be achieved by increasing the self-care information available to adolescents. One of the barriers to ensuring good glycemic control was found to be fear of disease management complications. Other studies have shown hypoglycemia to be the most common fear among families and children (Amiri, Vafa, & Gonder-Frederick, 2013; Barnard, Thomas, Royle, Noyes, & Waugh, 2010; Castensøe-Seidenfaden et al., 2017). The mood of the adolescent is affected by the disease. Studies have found that fear of hypoglycemia negatively affects the quality of life and increases the sensation of disease burden of adolescents and their families (Amiri et al., 2013). In addition, fear of hypoglycemia negatively affects glycemic control (Shepard, Vajda, Nyer, Clarke, & Gonder-Frederick, 2014). Fear of diabetes hypoglycemia results in a perceived increase in the difficulties associated with health self-management for adolescents with T1DM.

In addition, this study revealed that personal traits such as forgetfulness and laziness decreased diabetes management efficacy. In particular, the monitoring of blood sugar levels and following medical dietary recommendations were identified as the most difficult issues for the participants in this study, which is similar to findings previously described in the literature (Carroll & Marrero, 2006; Marshall et al., 2009). Other studies have shown that adolescents have identified disease management as a particularly difficult issue (Alderson, Sutcliffe, & Curtis, 2006; Herrman, 2006; Iannotti et al., 2006). Thus, it is important to identify approaches and strategies that effectively motivate individuals to manage their disease.

Theme 3: Environmental Barriers

This study identified parental support as a protective factor for diabetes management. Previous studies have indicated that conflicts experienced with parents cause adolescents to fail to manage their disease (Boztepe, 2011; Cameron et al., 2008; Lin, Mu, & Lee, 2008; Wang, Brown, & Horner, 2013). In this study, the participants stated that their family members concealed when they ate sweet and high-calorie foods out of sympathy, which negatively affected the participant's self-esteem. However, a similar finding has not been found in the literature. The findings of this article indicate that having a negative relationship with family members is considered by adolescents to be a barrier to effectively managing a disease.

The second subtheme was the problems that participants experienced related to their school environment. Other studies have similarly found that school-provided foods are not suitable for adolescents with T1DM, that these adolescents face difficulties in physical education classes, that they do not know how teachers will intervene in cases of hypoglycemia and hyperglycemia, and that they experience conflicts with teachers (Cameron et al., 2008; Kelo et al., 2011; Schwartz et al., 2010). The participants described the absences of an infirmary and a school nurse as barriers to managing their disease, although no other studies have been found to support this finding. The reason for this difference may be that there are no school nursing programs in Turkey. Furthermore, a lack of sufficient support from teachers and inadequate medical facilities at school may increase the perceived barriers to managing disease and may reduce perceived self-efficacy.

This study also revealed that friendship relationships among adolescents prevented the participants from implementing proper diabetes management. Children with T1DM tend to hide their disease because of concerns about being excluded from their friend groups (Wang et al., 2013; Yang, Lou, Lien, & Gau, 2018). During adolescence, when peer acceptance is extremely important, adolescents may not want to perform self-care behaviors to not appear different from peers and because of fears of rejection or feeling ashamed. School nurses may provide diabetes education to students and staff in both individual and group settings.

Among the barriers perceived by the participants toward the provision of adolescent health services, the issue of inadequate training was particularly highlighted, which echoes the findings of previous studies (Cheraghi et al., 2015; Jönsson, Hallström, & Lundqvist, 2012). This issue may be attributable to several reasons, including that diabetes nurses do not provide age-group-specific training, that training is not standardized, staffing shortages, and large numbers of patients. Receiving inadequate education on Type 1 diabetes reduces the self-efficacy of adolescents, which likely increases their perceived barriers to disease self-management.

Conclusions

The findings of this study show that adolescents with T1DM face multifaceted obstacles to self-management. Health professionals should work with parents, teachers, and peer groups to eliminate these obstacles. Moreover, policymakers should employ school nurses, who have important responsibilities in the school-based care of adolescents with T1DM. In addition, the psychosocial needs of adolescents should be taken into consideration when promoting diabetes self-management strategies. Providing diabetes education in schools may increase both the awareness of T1DM adolescents and the commitment of these adolescents to their schools. An experimental study has been planned by the authors to design nursing interventions to help adolescents with T1DM overcome their perceived barriers to disease self-management. Finally, focus group discussions are recommended for the parents of adolescents with Type 1 diabetes.

Limitations

One limitation of this study was that the sample group consisted of adolescents with T1DM from one hospital only. In addition, it is likely that the perspectives elicited in this study did not sufficiently reflect the full range of perspectives of adolescents with T1DM. Holding focus group interviews rather than individual interviews may have elicited significantly more diverse information based on interparticipant discussions and dialogue. Finally, despite the use of inductive questions in the interviews, some of the participants provided superficial answers, which is typical of people in this age group. This resulted in the short average duration of interviews.

Acknowledgment

The authors appreciate the patients who participated in this study.

Author Contributions

Study conception and design: KPG, ZB
Data collection: KPG
Data analysis and interpretation: KPG
Drafting of the article: KPG, ZB
Critical revision of the article: ZB

References

Alderson, P., Sutcliffe, K., & Curtis, K. (2006). Children as partners with adults in their medical care. *Archives of Disease in Childhood, 91*(4), 300–303. https://doi.org/10.1136/adc.2005.079442

American Diabetes Association. (2018). Standards of medical care in diabetes—2018. *Diabetes Care, 41*(1, Suppl.), S1–S2. https://doi.org/10.2337/dc18-Sint01

Amiri, F., Vafa, M., & Gonder-Frederick, L. (2013). Glycemic control, self-efficacy and fear of hypoglycemia among Iranian children with type 1 diabetes. *Journal of Diabetes & Metabolism, 4*(10), 2–5. https://doi.org/10.1016/j.jcjd.2014.12.011

Barnard, K., Thomas, S., Royle, P., Noyes, K., & Waugh, N. (2010). Fear of hypoglycaemia in parents of young children with type 1 diabetes: A systematic review. *BMC Pediatrics, 10*(1), 2–8. https://doi.org/10.1186/1471-2431-10-50

Boztepe, H. (2011). Problems experienced by adolescents with Type 1 diabetes with their parents and the solution suggestions. *Health and Society, 21*(3), 12–18. https://ssyv.org.tr/wp-admin/uploader/std2011-3/2.pdf (Original work published in Turkish)

Cameron, F. J., Skinner, T. C., De Beaufort, C. E., Hoey, H., Swift, P. G., Aanstoot, H., ... Danne, T. (2008). Are family factors universally related to metabolic outcomes in adolescents with Type 1 diabetes? *Diabetic Medicine, 25*(4), 463–468. https://doi.org/10.1111/j.1464-5491.2008.02399.x

Carroll, A. E., & Marrero, D. G. (2006). How do parents perceive their adolescent's diabetes: A qualitative study. *Diabetic Medicine, 23,* 1222–1224. https://doi.org/10.1111/j.1464-5491.2006.01961.x

Castensøe-Seidenfaden, P., Teilmann, G., Kensing, F., Hommel, E., Olsen, B. S., & Husted, G. R. (2017). Isolated thoughts and feelings and unsolved concerns: Adolescents' and parents' perspectives on living with type 1 diabetes—A qualitative study using visual storytelling. *Journal of Clinical Nursing, 26*(19–20), 3018–3030. https://doi.org/10.1111/jocn.13649

Cheraghi, F., Shamsaei, F., Mortazavi, S. Z., & Moghimbeigi, A. (2015). The effect of family-centered care on management of blood glucose levels in adolescents with diabetes. *International Journal of Community-Based Nursing and Midwifery, 3*(3), 177–180. https://www.ncbi.nlm.nih.gov/pmc/articles/PMC4495325/

Clapin, H., Hop, L., Ritchie, E., Jayabalan, R., Evans, M., Browne-Cooper, K., ... Davis, E. A. (2017). Home-based vs inpatient education for children newly diagnosed with type 1 diabetes. *Pediatric Diabetes, 18*(7), 579–587. https://doi.org/10.1111/pedi.12466

Creswell, J. W., Hanson, W. E., Clark Plano, V. L., & Morales, A. (2007). Qualitative research designs: Selection and implementation. *The Counseling Psychologist, 35*(2), 236–264. https://doi.org/10.1177/0011000006287390

Dobson, R., Whittaker, R., Jiang, Y., Shepherd, M., Maddison, R., Carter, K., ... Murphy, R. (2016). Text message-based diabetes self-management support (SMS4BG): Study protocol for a randomised controlled trial. *Trials, 17*(1), 179. https://doi.org/10.1186/s13063-016-1305-5

Fortunato, F., Cappelli, M. G., Vece, M. M., Caputi, G., Delvecchio, M., Prato, R., & Martinelli, D. (2016). Incidence of type 1 diabetes among children and adolescents in Italy between 2009 and 2013: The role of a regional childhood diabetes registry. *Journal of Diabetes Research, 2016,* 7239692. https://doi.org/10.1155/2016/7239692

Herrman, J. W. (2006). Children's and young adolescents' voices: Perceptions of the costs and rewards of diabetes and its treatment. *Journal of Pediatric Nursing, 21*(3), 211–221. https://doi.org/10.1016/j.pedn.2005.07.012

Iannotti, R. J., Schneider, S., Nansel, T. R., Haynie, D. L., Plotnick, L. P., Clark, L. M., & Simons-Morton, B. (2006). Self-efficacy, outcome expectations, and diabetes self-management in adolescents with type 1 diabetes. *Journal of Developmental and Behavioral Pediatrics, 27*(2), 98–105.

Joensen, L. E., Filges, T., & Willaing, I. (2016). Patient perspectives on peer support for adults with type 1 diabetes: A need for diabetes-specific social capital. *Patient Preference and Adherence, 10,* 1443–1451. https://doi.org/10.2147/PPA.S111696

Jönsson, L., Hallström, I., & Lundqvist, A. (2012). "The logic of care"—Parents' perceptions of the educational process when a child is newly diagnosed with type 1 diabetes. *BMC Pediatrics, 12*(1), 165. http://www.biomedcentral.com/1471-2431/12/165

Kelo, M., Martikainen, M., & Eriksson, E. (2011). Self-care of school-age children with diabetes: An integrative review. *Journal of Advanced Nursing, 67*(10), 2096–2108. https://doi.org/10.1111/j.1365-2648.2011.05682.x

Lin, H. P., Mu, P. F., & Lee, Y. J. (2008). Mothers' experience supporting life adjustment in children with T1DM. *Western Journal of Nursing Research, 30*(1), 96–110. https://doi.org/10.1177/0193945907302456

Lincoln, Y. S., & Guba, E. G. (1985). *Naturalistic inquiry* (1st ed.). Beverley Hills, CA: Sage.

Marshall, M., Carter, B., Rose, K., & Brotherton, A. (2009). Living with type 1 diabetes: Perceptions of children and their parents. *Journal of Clinical Nursing, 18,* 1703–1710. https://doi.org/10.1111/j.1365-2702.2008.02737.x

O'Hara, M. C., Hynes, L., O'Donnell, M., Nery, N., Byrne, M., Heller, S. R., ... Irish Type 1 Diabetes Young Adult Study Group. (2017). A systematic review of interventions to improve outcomes for young adults with Type 1 diabetes. *Diabetic Medicine, 34* (6), 753–769. https://doi.org/10.1111/dme.13276

Olsen Roper, S., Call, A., Leishman, J., Ratcliffe, G. C., Mandleco, B. L., Dyches, T. T., & Marshall, E. S. (2009). Type 1 diabetes: Children and adolescents' knowledge and questions. *Journal of Advanced Nursing, 65*(8), 1705–1714. https://doi.org/10.1111/j.1365-2648.2009.05033.x

Pender, N. J., Murdaugh, C. L., & Parsons, M. A. (2015). *Health promotion in nursing practice* (7th ed.). Upper Saddle River, NJ: Prentice Hall.

Pires, A., Aparício, G., & Duarte, J. (2016). PO22—Children's satisfaction with the diabetes nursing consultation. *Nursing Children and Young People, 28*(4), 101. https://doi.org/10.7748/ncyp.28.4.101.s100

Rostami, S., Parsa-Yekta, Z., Najafi-Ghezeljeh, T., Vanaki, Z., & Zarea, K. (2015). Self-perception in Iranian adolescents with diabetes: A qualitative study. *Journal of Diabetes & Metabolic Disorders, 14*(1), 2–9. https://doi.org/10.1186/s40200-015-0163-0

Samimi, Z., Talakoub, S., & Ghazavi, Z. (2018). Effect of telephone follow-up by nurses on self-care in children with diabetes. *Iranian Journal of Nursing and Midwifery Research, 23*(1), 26–28. https://doi.org/10.4103/1735-9066.220950

Sandelowski, M. (2000). Whatever happened to qualitative description? *Research in Nursing & Health, 23*(4), 334–340. https://doi.org/10.1002/1098-240X(200008)23:4<334::AID-NUR9>3.0.CO;2-G

Schwartz, F. L., Denham, S., Heh, V., Wapner, A., & Shubrook, J. (2010). Experiences of children and adolescents with type 1 diabetes in school: Survey of children, parents and schools. *Diabetes Spectrum, 23*(1), 47–55. https://doi.org/10.2337/diaspect.23.1.47

Shepard, J. A., Vajda, K., Nyer, M., Clarke, W., & Gonder-Frederick, L. (2014). Understanding the construct of fear of hypoglycemia in pediatric type 1 diabetes. *Journal of Pediatric Psychology, 39*(1), 1115–1125. https://doi.org/10.1093/jpepsy/jsu068

Tiberg, I., Lindgren, B., Carlsson, A., & Hallström, I. (2016). Cost-effectiveness and cost-utility analyses of hospital-based home care compared to hospital-based care for children diagnosed with type 1 diabetes; a randomised controlled trial; results after two years' follow-up. *BMC Pediatrics, 16*(1), 94. https://doi.org/10.1186/s12887-016-0632-8

Wang, Y. L., Brown, S. A., & Horner, S. D. (2013). The school-based lived experiences of adolescents with type 1 diabetes. *The Journal of Nursing Research, 21*(4), 235–243. https://doi.org/10.1097/jnr.0000000000000003

Yang, P. Y., Lou, M. F., Lien, A. S. Y., & Gau, B. S. (2018). Adolescent perceptions of peer responses to diabetes self-management: A qualitative study. *The Journal of Nursing Research, 26*(2), 104–111. https://doi.org/10.1097/jnr.0000000000000234

Yıldırım, A., & Şimşek, H. (2011). *Qualitative research methods in social sciences* (8th ed.). Ankara, Turkey: Tıpkı Press. (Original work published in Turkish).

18

Development of a Simple and Practical Delirium Screening Tool for Use in Surgical Wards

Keisuke KUBOTA[1*] • Akihiro SUZUKI[2] • Sachiko OHDE[3] • Ui YAMADA[4] • Ikumi FUJITANI[5] • Aya KOITABASHI[5]

ABSTRACT

Background: Delirium is an important and common medical condition, particularly in hospitalized patients, that is associated with adverse outcomes. The identification, prevention, and treatment of delirium are increasingly regarded as major public health priorities.

Purpose: The aim of this study was to create a simple-to-use screening tool for delirium in hospitalized patients using clinical manifestations of delirium regularly observed by nurses.

Methods: This study was conducted using data on 2,168 patients who had been admitted to the surgical ward between January 2011 and December 2014. Data were collected retrospectively from medical records. Univariate and multivariate analyses were performed, and a logistic regression model was constructed for the development of a predictive screening tool. After constructing a new screening tool for delirium, a receiver operating characteristic curve was drawn, the most appropriate cutoff value was decided, and the area under the curve was obtained. Bootstrapping was used for the internal model validation.

Results: A screening tool for delirium (Subjective Delirium Screening Scale by Nurse) with a total score of 5 points was constructed as follows: 2 points for disorientation and 1 point each for restlessness, somnolence, and hallucination. The area under the curve for the Subjective Delirium Screening Scale by Nurse was 81.9% (95% CI [77.9%, 85.8%]), and the most appropriate cutoff value was determined to be 2 (sensitivity of 61.0% and specificity of 96.7%). Bootstrapped validation beta coefficients of the predictive factors were similar to the original cohort beta coefficients.

Conclusions: We created a screening tool for delirium using factors that were regularly observed and recorded by nurses. This tool is simple and practical and has adequate diagnostic accuracy.

KEY WORDS:
delirium, screening tool, surgical ward.

Introduction

Delirium, characterized by an acute change in the level of consciousness, inattention, and disturbed cognitive function, is an important and common medical condition, particularly in hospitalized patients. Delirium is associated with adverse outcomes such as increased mortality, accidental falls, cognitive decline, functional dependence, and healthcare costs. The identification, prevention, and treatment of delirium are increasingly regarded as major public health priorities (Chaput & Bryson, 2012; Greer et al., 2011; Inouye, Westendorp, & Saczynski, 2014; O'Regan, Fitzgerald, Timmons, O'Connell, & Meagher, 2013).

In our hospital, we began addressing issues related to delirium beginning in 2011. These actions were as follows: early assessment of the risk of delirium after admission and repeated assessments thereafter, acquiring information on drugs with a risk for delirium (benzodiazepine, etc.), physical therapy (cognitive stimulation, promotion of good sleep, early mobilization, etc.), nutritional support (including avoidance of dehydration), family education, and early introduction of therapy using medications (quetiapine, risperidone, haloperidol, etc.; Inouye et al., 1999; Martinez, Tobar, & Hill, 2015; National Institute for Health and Care Excellence, 2010; Siddiqi et al., 2016; Zhang et al., 2013). Delirium was screened and diagnosed using the Delirium Screening Tool (DST) and the Confusion Assessment Method for the Intensive Care Unit (CAM-ICU). We have recently reported risk factors for delirium in patients hospitalized for more than 5 days in surgical wards (Kubota et al., 2018).

We then wanted to assess the incidence of delirium in our hospital before the implementation of the abovementioned actions (i.e., before 2011). However, DST and CAM-ICU were unavailable because we did not screen for delirium using these tools before 2011.

[1]PhD, MD, Professor, Department of Gastroenterological Surgery, St. Luke's International Hospital, Tokyo, Japan • [2]PhD, MD, Specialist, Department of Gastroenterological Surgery, St. Luke's International Hospital, Tokyo, Japan • [3]EdM, Professor, Center for Clinical Epidemiology, St. Luke's International University, Tokyo, Japan • [4]PhD, MD, Professor, Department of Psychosomatic Medicine, St. Luke's International Hospital, Tokyo, Japan • [5]RN, Advanced Practice Nurse, Nursing Department of Gastroenterological Surgery, St. Luke's International Hospital, Tokyo, Japan.

Therefore, the aim of this study was to devise a convenient screening tool for delirium in patients hospitalized for more than 5 days in surgical wards, using clinical observations that are typically recorded by nurses subjectively in clinical records. This new screening tool would allow us to obtain information on whether or not a patient had delirium by checking past records retrospectively.

Methods

This study was approved by the local ethical committee of St. Luke's International Hospital (#16-09). Written informed consent had been provided by all of the patients at admission for use of their data for publication.

The study was conducted using data collected retrospectively from hospital medical records on 2,168 patients who had been admitted to the surgical ward of St. Luke's International Hospital for 5 days or more between January 2011 and December 2014 (Kubota et al., 2018). The most frequent surgeries in our hospital are appendectomy, cholecystectomy, and herniorrhaphy. Their clinical paths for hospitalization range between 3 and 4 days. We rarely encounter delirium in short-term hospitalization patients. In one study of postoperative delirium, entry criteria included the expectation of a hospital stay of more than 48 hours after surgery (DeCrane et al., 2011). General hospitals in Japan typically hospitalize patients for 1–2 days before surgery (Kubota et al., 2018). Therefore, we considered 5 days or more as a sufficiently long period of hospitalization for the purposes of this study.

Clinical variables obtained from the medical records included age, gender, underlying disease, results of DST and CAM-ICU, observational factors recorded by nurses, length of hospital stay, and mortality. Factors observed and recorded by nurses subjectively included hypomotivation, somnolence, hallucinations, visual hallucinations, auditory hallucinations, disorientation, disturbance, insomnia, depression, and restlessness. A list of over 50 signs and symptoms were observed and recorded by nurses in an electronic medical chart. The nurses routinely observed the patients and recorded "yes or no" for each sign or symptom in the usual clinical settings. In this study, we selected 10 psychological problems among the list of items and analyzed the data electronically.

In this study, the definition of delirium onset was made when the score for either the DST or CAM-ICU was positive for delirium. Univariate analysis was performed to investigate the relationship between each factor observed and recorded by nurses subjectively and delirium as determined by either the DST or CAM-ICU. To select the final predictive factors and develop a scoring formula, a multivariate analysis was performed using all of the candidate observed factors in the univariate analysis. Scores for each corresponding factor were obtained based on the beta value from the final prediction model.

On the basis of these results, a screening tool for delirium (Subjective Delirium Screening Scale by Nurse: SDS-N) was constructed. We calculated the total SDS-N score for each patient and the sensitivities and specificities for each cutoff value of the SDS-N score. A receiver operating characteristic curve was then drawn, and the area under the curve (AUC) was obtained.

For internal validation, a bootstrapping technique with 1,000 iterations was used to simulate unbiased expected future performance. The internal validity of a predictive logistic regression model may best be estimated using bootstrapping analysis, which provides stable estimates with low bias (Ohde et al., 2010; Steyerberg et al., 2001). All analyses were performed using SPSS Version 22.0 (IBM, Inc., Armonk, NY, USA).

Results

Table 1 shows the background characteristics of the patients included in this study. Delirium was identified in 205 of the 2,168 patients (9.5%).

Table 2 shows the results of the univariate analysis of the relationship between delirium and factors observed subjectively and recorded by nurses. According to the results of the univariate analysis, logistic regression analysis was constructed, with all of the identified factors determined to be candidate predictors by the univariate analysis (Table 3). Disorientation, restlessness, somnolence, and hallucination were identified as statistically independent factors of delirium in the multivariate analysis. Disorientation was identified as the factor with the greatest effect, with an odds ratio of 9.632.

On the basis of these results, a simple and practical screening tool for delirium (SDS-N) with a total score of 5 points

TABLE 1.
Characteristics of Study Patients (N = 2,168)

Characteristic	*n*	%
Age (years; *M* and *SD*)	65	15.4
Range	16–100	
Gender		
Male	1,255	57.9
Female	913	42.1
Underlying disease		
Gastrointestinal cancer	860	39.7
Other malignancy	33	1.5
Gastrointestinal disorder	1,018	47.0
Hernia	154	7.1
Others	103	4.7
Surgery		
Yes	1,531	70.6
No	637	29.4
Length of stay (*M* and *SD*)	15.7	19.2
Range	5–412	
Outcome		
Improved	2,076	95.8
Died	92	4.2

TABLE 2.

Results of Univariate Analysis of the Relationship Between Delirium and Nurse-Observed Factors (N = 2,168)

	Delirium				
	No (*n* = 1,963)		Yes (*n* = 205)		
Factor	*n*	%	*n*	%	*p*
Hypomotivation					
No	1,958	99.7	202	98.5	
Yes	5	0.3	3	1.5	.007
Somnolence					
No	1,949	99.3	193	94.1	
Yes	14	0.7	12	5.9	<.001
Hallucination					
No	1,941	98.9	131	63.9	
Yes	22	1.1	74	36.1	<.001
Visual hallucination					
No	1,962	99.9	199	97.1	
Yes	1	0.1	6	2.9	<.001
Auditory hallucination					
No	1,963	100.0	194	94.6	
Yes	0	0	11	5.4	<.001
Disorientation					
No	1,900	96.8	83	40.5	
Yes	63	3.2	122	59.5	<.001
Disturbance					
No	1,958	99.7	204	99.5	
Yes	5	0.3	1	0.5	.546
Insomnia					
No	1,936	98.6	189	92.2	
Yes	27	1.4	16	7.8	<.001
Depression					
No	1,959	99.8	204	99.5	
Yes	4	0.2	1	0.5	.420
Restlessness					
No	1,897	96.6	91	44.4	
Yes	66	3.4	114	55.6	<.001

TABLE 3.

Results of Logistic Regression Analysis of the Predictors of Delirium

Factor	Adjusted Odds Ratio	95% CI	Score Point	*p*
Disorientation	9.632	[5.403, 17.171]	2	<.001
Restlessness	4.336	[2.386, 7.878]	1	<.001
Somnolence	3.605	[1.130, 11.498]	1	.030
Hallucination	2.916	[1.498, 5.678]	1	.002

TABLE 4.

Sensitivities and Specificities for Each SDS-N Score

SDS-N Score	Sensitivity (%)	Specificity (%)
1	67.3	94.9
2	61.0	96.7
3	52.2	97.8
4	35.1	99.1
5	1.0	99.9

Note. SDS-N = Subjective Delirium Screening Scale by Nurse.

was constructed as follows: 2 points for disorientation and 1 point each for restlessness, somnolence, and hallucination, as shown below:

$$[\text{SDS–N}] = [\text{Disorientation}]*2 + [\text{Restlessness}] + [\text{Somnolence}] + [\text{Hallucination}].$$

We calculated the total SDS-N score for each patient and drew a receiver operating characteristic curve. Table 4 shows the sensitivities and specificities for each cutoff value of the SDS-N score when the cutoff values were changed from 1 to 5. The AUC of this novel screening tool was 81.9% (95% CI [77.9%, 85.8%]; Figure 1). On the basis of these results, the

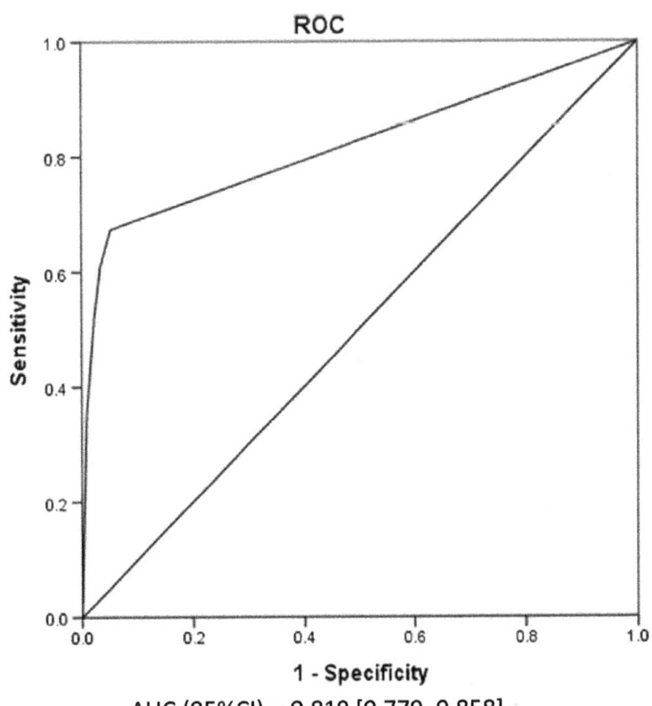

Figure 1. Receiver operating characteristic (ROC) curve for the Subjective Delirium Screening Scale by Nurse.
AUC = area under the curve.

TABLE 5.
Bootstrap Validation of the Model and Comparison With the Original Model

Factor	Logistic Regression Beta Coefficient	Bootstrapped Beta Coefficient	95% CI
Disorientation	2.265	2.278	[1.575, 2.997]
Restlessness	1.467	1.468	[0.687, 2.130]
Somnolence	1.282	1.280	[−0.086, 2.399]
Hallucination	1.070	1.093	[0.322, 1.875]

most appropriate cutoff value was determined as 2 (sensitivity: 61.0%; specificity: 96.7%).

We then conducted bootstrap cross-validation with 1,000 iterations for the SDS-N. Table 5 shows the originally observed beta coefficient and the bootstrapped validation beta coefficient. Scores assigned to each predictive factor were identical in both the original and bootstrapped results, which supports that this model is relatively robust.

Discussion

We conducted this study to construct a chart-based DST to be administered to patients hospitalized for more than 5 days in surgical wards using clinical observations that are typically recorded by nurses subjectively. In the study group, delirium was screened and diagnosed using the CAM-ICU and DST. We then searched for key factors associated with delirium to create a chart-based tool: SDS-N. The SDS-N included four predictive factors for delirium screening: disorientation, restlessness, somnolence, and hallucination. The AUC showed good accuracy (AUC = 0.819, 95% CI [0.779, 0.858]). Delirium was diagnosed with a sensitivity of 61.0% and a specificity of 96.7% in comparisons with the DST and CAM-ICU. However, caution is still advised in applying the AUC, as subjective observational diagnoses often miss or fail to recognize the onset of delirium (Inouye, Foreman, Mion, Katz, & Cooney, 2001).

Some reviews have reported currently available assessment tools for delirium (Grover & Kate, 2012; van Meenen, van Meenen, de Rooij, & ter Riet, 2014). Our colleagues, Kobayashi et al., introduced the Chi-Square Automatic Interaction Detector Decision Tree Analysis Model, which is an easy-to-implement model for detecting the development of delirium in patients in medical wards (Kobayashi, Takahashi, Arioka, Koga, & Fukui, 2013). In addition, the NEECHAM Confusion Scale (Neelon, Champagne, Carlson, & Funk, 1996) and the Nursing Delirium Screening Scale (Gaudreau, Gagnon, Harel, Tremblay, & Roy, 2005) are based on nursing assessments similar to the SDS-N, with 80%–90% sensitivity and specificity. As these scales include specifically determined items and the recording of each item uses a scale, they are not suitable for use in research such as that conducted in this study. The Chart-based Delirium Identification Instrument was developed to identify delirium retrospectively from information that is typically included on medical charts (Inouye et al., 2005). However, this scale is overly complicated and difficult to apply in daily clinical settings, and although potentially helpful for determining delirium in individual patients, it may not be suited for screening large numbers of patients. The SDS-N developed in this study has an advantage over existing screening tools in that it is simple and practical because it includes only factors that are regularly observed subjectively and recorded by nurses. Furthermore, the SDS-N has shown adequate diagnostic accuracy.

Various interventions, including Multicomponent Interventions and Hospital Elder Life Program, have been proposed as strategies to prevent delirium in hospitalized patients (Inouye et al., 1999; Martinez et al., 2015). Several practice guidelines, for example, the National Institute for Health and Care Excellence guidelines, have encouraged the establishment of multicomponent interventions programs to prevent the incidence of delirium (National Institutes for Health and Care Excellence, 2010), which have subsequently been shown to be effective in reducing the incidence, duration, and severity of delirium and in decreasing healthcare costs.

A major limitation of this study is our exclusive focus on cognitive disturbances such as disorientation, restlessness, somnolence, and hallucination and exclusion of important symptoms such as acute onset and fluctuation in the new SDS-N tool. We are now conducting a prospective cohort study of delirium focused on dementia and cerebrovascular disease. In addition, diagnostic accuracy in this study was evaluated in comparison with the DST and CAM-ICU, which are also screening tools. Our newly developed tool should be evaluated in comparison with a standard diagnostic tool such as the *Diagnostic and Statistical Manual of Mental Disorders, Fifth Edition*. Another limitation of this study was its retrospective design. Replication of the results is needed using a study with a prospective design and external validation.

In conclusion, the SDS-N, a novel screening tool for delirium in patients hospitalized for more than 5 days in surgical wards, was created in this study using factors that are typically recorded by nurses subjectively in clinical settings. The developed tool is simple and practical and has adequate diagnostic accuracy.

Acknowledgments

We thank the colleagues of the Gastroenterological Surgery Department, including Takuto Yoshida, Aoi Fujikawa, Takayuki Watanabe, Takashi Taketa, Taketo Matsubara, Hiroki Sunagawa, Seiji Ohigashi, and Shintaro Sakurai, for their daily clinical practice and data collection efforts. We further thank Chika Horikawa and Aya Ohizumi of the Center for Information Systems for their special assistance in collecting data.

Author Contributions

Study conception and design: KK, AS
Data collection: IF, AK
Data analysis and interpretation: SO

Drafting of the article: KK
Critical revision of the article: UY

References

Chaput, A. J., & Bryson, G. L. (2012). Postoperative delirium: Risk factors and management: Continuing professional development. *Canadian Journal of Anesthesia, 59*(3), 304–320. https://doi.org/10.1007/s12630-011-9658-4

DeCrane, S. K., Sands, L., Ashland, M., Lim, E., Tsai, T. L., Paul, S., ... Leung, J. M. (2011). Factors associated with recovery from early postoperative delirium. *Journal of PeriAnesthesia, 26*(4), 231–241. https://doi.org/10.1016/j.jopan.2011.03.001

Gaudreau, J. D., Gagnon, P., Harel, F., Tremblay, A., & Roy, M. A. (2005). Fast, systematic, and continuous delirium assessment in hospitalized patients: The nursing delirium screening scale. *Journal of Pain and Symptom Management, 29*(4), 368–375. https://doi.org/10.1016/j.jpainsymman.2004.07.009

Greer, N., Rossom, R., Anderson, P., MacDonald, R., Tacklind, J., Rutks, I., ... Wilt, T. J. (2011). *Delirium: Screening, prevention, and diagnosis—A systematic review of the evidence* [Internet]. Washington, DC: U.S. Department of Veterans Affairs.

Grover, S., & Kate, N. (2012). Assessment scales for delirium: A review. *World Journal of Psychiatry, 2*(4), 58–70. https://doi.org/10.5498/wjp.v2.i4.58

Inouye, S. K., Bogardus, S. T. Jr., Charpentier, P. A., Leo-Summers, L., Acampora, D., Holford, T. R., ... Cooney, L. M. Jr. (1999). A multicomponent intervention to prevent delirium in hospitalized older patients. *New England Journal of Medicine, 340*(9), 669–676. https://doi.org/10.1056/NEJM199903043400901

Inouye, S. K., Foreman, M. D., Mion, L. C., Katz, K. H., & Cooney, L. M. Jr. (2001). Nurses' recognition of delirium and its symptoms: Comparison of nurse and researcher ratings. *Archives of Internal Medicine, 161*(20), 2467–2473. https://doi.org/10.1001/archinte.161.20.2467

Inouye, S. K., Leo-Summers, L., Zhang, Y., Bogardus, S. T. Jr., Leslie, D. L., & Agostini, J. V. (2005). A chart-based method for identification of delirium: Validation compared with interviewer ratings using the confusion assessment method. *Journal of the American Geriatrics Society, 53*(2), 312–318. https://doi.org/10.1111/j.1532-5415.2005.53120.x

Inouye, S. K., Westendorp, R. G., & Saczynski, J. S. (2014). Delirium in elderly people. *Lancet, 383*(9920), 911–922. https://doi.org/10.1016/S0140-6736(13)60688-1

Kobayashi, D., Takahashi, O., Arioka, H., Koga, S., & Fukui, T. (2013). A prediction rule for the development of delirium among patients in medical wards: Chi-Square Automatic Interaction Detector (CHAID) decision tree analysis model. *American Journal of Geriatric Psychiatry, 21*(10), 957–962. https://doi.org/10.1016/j.jagp.2012.08.009

Kubota, K., Suzuki, A., Ohde, S., Yamada, U., Hosaka, T., Okuno, F., ... Kishida, A. (2018). Age is the most significantly associated risk factor with the development of delirium in patients hospitalized for more than five days in surgical wards: Retrospective cohort study. *Annals of Surgery, 267*(5), 874–877. https://doi.org/10.1097/SLA.0000000000002347

Martinez, F., Tobar, C., & Hill, N. (2015). Preventing delirium: Should non-pharmacological, multicomponent interventions be used? A systematic review and meta-analysis of the literature. *Age and Ageing, 44*(2), 196–204. https://doi.org/10.1093/ageing/afu173

National Institute for Health and Care Excellence. (2010). *Delirium: Diagnosis, prevention and management—Clinical guideline [CG103]*. London, England: Author.

Neelon, V. J., Champagne, M. T., Carlson, J. R., & Funk, S. G. (1996). The NEECHAM Confusion Scale: Construction, validation, and clinical testing. *Nursing Research, 45*(6), 324–330.

Ohde, S., Hayashi, A., Takahasi, O., Yamakawa, S., Nakamura, M., Osawa, A., ... Fukui, T. (2010). A 2-week prognostic prediction model for terminal cancer patients in a palliative care unit at a Japanese general hospital. *Palliative Medicine, 25*(2), 170–176. https://doi.org/10.1177/0269216310383741

O'Regan, N. A., Fitzgerald, J., Timmons, S., O'Connell, H., & Meagher, D. (2013). Delirium: A key challenge for perioperative care. *International Journal of Surgery, 11*(2), 136–144. https://doi.org/10.1016/j.ijsu.2012.12.015

Siddiqi, N., Harrison, J. K., Clegg, A., Teale, E. A., Young, J., Taylor, J., ... Simpkins, S. A. (2016). Interventions for preventing delirium in hospitalised non-ICU patients. *Cochrane Database of Systematic Reviews*, 3, CD005563. https://doi.org/10.1002/14651858.CD005563.pub3

Steyerberg, E. W., Harrell, F. E. Jr., Borsboom, G. J., Eijkemans, M. J., Vergouwe, Y., & Habbema, J. D. (2001). Internal validation of predictive models: Efficiency of some procedures for logistic regression analysis. *Journal of Clinical Epidemiology, 54*(8), 774–781. https://doi.org/10.1016/S0895-4356(01)00341-9

van Meenen, L. C., van Meenen, D. M., de Rooij, S. E., & ter Riet, G. (2014). Risk prediction models for postoperative delirium: A systematic review and meta-analysis. *Journal of the American Geriatrics Society, 62*(12), 2383–2390. https://doi.org/10.1111/jgs.13138

Zhang, H., Lu, Y., Liu, M., Zou, Z., Wang, L., Xu, F. Y., ... Shi, X. Y. (2013). Strategies for prevention of postoperative delirium: A systematic review and meta-analysis of randomized trials. *Critical Care, 17*(2), R47. https://doi.org/10.1186/cc12566

19

The Effects of Shared Decision Making on Different Renal Replacement Therapy Decisions in Patients With Chronic Kidney Disease

Ya-Fang HO[1] • Yu-Chi CHEN[2] • Chiu-Chin HUANG[3] • Wen-Yu HU[4] • Kuan-Chia LIN[5] • I-Chuan LI[6*]

ABSTRACT

Background: The prevalence and incidence of end-stage renal disease (ESRD) in Taiwan are the highest of any country in the world. The different renal replacement therapies that are adopted by patients with ESRD significantly affect their social roles and daily life. However, because of the complexities of different renal replacement therapies, patients may be unsure of which to choose.

Purpose: The aim of this study was to explore the effectiveness of a shared decision-making (SDM) program regarding different renal replacement therapies for patients with chronic kidney disease.

Methods: A quasi-experimental design was conducted at two similar regional hospitals in Miaoli County, Taiwan. One hospital hosted the intervention group, and the other hospital hosted the control group. The 31 participants in the intervention group took part in a SDM program. The 36 control group participants took part in the pre-ESRD care program. Data collection included demographic and disease characteristics, decisional conflict scale, and decision self-efficacy scale. Results were analyzed using independent *t* test, Fisher's exact test, generalized estimating equation, and paired *t* tests.

Results: The study results revealed that the intervention group experienced a significant increase in decision self-efficacy and a significant decrease in decisional conflict at 1 month after receiving the SDM intervention in comparison to before and immediately after receiving the intervention. Moreover, the intervention group had higher decision self-efficacy and lower decisional conflict than the control group.

Conclusions/Implications for Practice: The SDM program may be an effective intervention for complex decision-making processes, such as the process involved in making renal replacement treatment decisions. The SDM program group intervention improved decisional conflict and decision self-efficacy. Thus, to improve patients' decision-making processes, the application of an SDM program focused on the personal values and opinions of patients with ESRD will be necessary. Physicians and case managers of patients with ESRD should act in complementary and cooperative roles in SDM programs.

KEY WORDS:
chronic kidney disease, renal replacement therapy, shared decision-making, decision self-efficacy, decisional conflict.

Introduction

End-stage renal disease (ESRD) is the most serious stage of kidney disease. In 2010, the number of patients with ESRD worldwide receiving renal replacement therapies was 2.62 million, and the need for dialysis was projected to double by 2030 (Liyanage et al., 2015). For many years, the incidence and prevalence of ESRD in Taiwan has been the highest in the world (U.S. Renal Data System, 2018). Currently, aside from renal transplantation, most patients with ESRD primarily receive either hemodialysis or peritoneal dialysis treatments (National Health Research Institutes, Taiwan, ROC, 2015). For patients with ESRD, renal replacement therapies are critical to survival. In addition, different renal replacement therapies have an impact on patients physically, socially, and financially in ways that often increase emotional distress (Chiaranai, 2016). For both renal replacement treatment therapies, patients must be willing to continue receiving treatment for the rest of their lives, which is why it is important for patients to choose the treatment that is personally the most acceptable and suitable. Therefore, the government of Taiwan has implemented a "pre-ESRD care program" since 2007 to delay the progression of this disease in patients with chronic kidney disease (CKD) and to prepare patients with ESRD in advance for

[1]*PhD, RN, Assistant Professor, School of Nursing & Graduate Institute of Nursing, China Medical University, Taiwan, ROC* • [2]*PhD, RN, Associate Professor, Institute of Clinical Nursing, School of Nursing, National Yang-Ming University, Taiwan, ROC* • [3]*MD, Chair Professor, China Medical University Hospital, Taiwan, ROC* • [4]*PhD, RN, Professor, School and Graduate Institute of Nursing, College of Medicine, National Taiwan University, and Director, Nursing Department, National Taiwan University Hospital, Taiwan, ROC* • [5]*PhD, Professor, Institute of Hospital and Health Care Administration, Community Medicine Research Center, Preventive Medicine Research Center, National Yang-Ming University, Taiwan, ROC* • [6]*PhD, RN, Professor, Institute of Community Health Care, National Yang-Ming University, Taiwan, ROC.*

future choices regarding renal replacement therapy (Ministry of Health and Welfare, Taiwan, ROC, 2018).

About 64% of patients with CKD who were enrolled in the pre-ESRD care program had used temporary catheters during dialysis treatment (Lai et al., 2018). Moreover, approximately 52.7% of patients with ESRD who entered dialysis treatment had completed emplacement of an arteriovenous fistula beforehand (Taiwan Society of Nephrology, Taiwan, ROC, 2018). On the basis of these data, the pre-ESRD care program has had limited use in the predialysis preparation of patients with ESRD. A possible reason for this is the use of one-way education rather than preference-based counseling by kidney disease case managers regarding renal replacement therapy decisions. The quality of preference-based decisions depends on the patient having the knowledge necessary to select the treatment that is most consistent with personal preferences (Causarano et al., 2015). However, in Taiwan, the preferences, values, needs, and concerns of patients are not often heard by physicians. In addition, CKD is a disease that affects predominantly older adults, who often have a level of education that is lower than the general population. These patients may be afraid to express their opinions and preferences and, instead, choose to rely on physicians to make decisions regarding renal replacement therapy. This reliance leaves many patients insufficiently prepared to understand information about the treatments or the different outcomes of treatment choices.

Patients are in the best position to accommodate their own interests as to how to fit disease-related changes into daily life. Thus, patients need to be encouraged and assisted to choose the most appropriate renal replacement therapy proactively rather than relying passively on physician decisions. A balanced decision between patients and/or their families and physicians is preferred. Thus, in Western countries, the concept of shared decision making (SDM) has been adopted to emphasize patient autonomy and empowerment in making treatment decisions (Obeidat et al., 2013). Through the SDM process, healthcare providers communicate evidence and information regarding different therapies, whereas the patient develops their opinions and preferences. This exchange of information helps ensure that patients understand the relevant information as well as possible, thereby reducing decision conflicts (Charles et al., 1997; Gionfriddo et al., 2014).

SDM programs are still in the development stage in Taiwan. The relevant evidence on Taiwan SDM programs is still rare, and there is no standardized description of either the content or form of related interventions. The lack of related evidence for different renal replacement therapy decisions in patients with CKD means that the most effective and comprehensive formats have yet to be established. Given that improved knowledge and patient preferences are cornerstones of decision making, it is crucial that SDM be explored in the context of renal replacement therapy decisions.

Although several hospitals have applied SDM concepts in renal replacement therapy programs, robust evidence is still needed to support the effects by comparing program results with pre-ESRD care programs. Thus, the purpose of this study was to compare the effects of decision self-efficacy and decisional conflict between patients receiving the pre-ESRD care program and patients receiving the SDM program.

Intervention Framework

Charles et al. (1997) proposed four operational definitions of SDM: (a) healthcare providers and the patient must both be involved, (b) both parties must share information, (c) both parties must take steps to build consensus on the preferred treatment options, and (d) agreement must be reached on the treatment to be implemented. The SDM process includes the following three stages: exchange of information, deliberations regarding different treatment options, and reaching agreement on a final decision; healthcare providers and patients must be involved in all three phases (Charles et al., 1997, 1999). Charles et al. reported that SDM should be regarded as a process of patient empowerment. Related studies have pointed out that empowerment may be used to effectively improve confidence and ability in renal transplant patients with regard to self-care behaviors, which promotes patient willingness to proactively make decisions to change (Hsiao et al., 2016). Therefore, healthcare providers may share complete information through the SDM empowerment process to enhance patient knowledge and ability to make decisions and introduce a spirit of respect for autonomy in the decision-making process (Charles et al., 1997). The concept of empowerment has a patient-centered emphasis. Therefore, building a partnership based on trust and encouraging participation are the necessary starting points for SDM. After providers create an atmosphere of trust, patients will be more willing to share their preferences and opinions.

Thus, the fundamental principles of SDM are that providers and patients participate together, that both parties establish a relationship of trust and share information, that providers share complete information and patients share preferences, and that patients' final choices be respected by providers. The three processes and four elements of this study were developed in accordance with the ideas of SDM outlined in Charles et al. (1997). These three processes are exchange of information, deliberation on different treatment options, and reaching agreement on a final decision.

Methods

Research Design

This research was designed as a quasi-experimental study that used two groups of repeated measurements. The intervention group was the SDM group, who received the SDM program proposed in this study. The control group was the pre-ESRD group, who received the current pre-ESRD program, which is provided as the standard under Taiwan's National Health Insurance system. Data were collected using structured questionnaires from August 2017 to January 2018.

Sample and Setting

This study used purposive sampling to recruit participants from two nephrology clinics of the regional hospital in Miaoli County, Taiwan. To prevent contamination, one of the two regional hospitals hosted the intervention group, and the other hosted the control group. The study population consisted of patients diagnosed with CKD who had participated in the pre-ESRD care program. The inclusion criteria were an estimated glomerular filtration rate of $\leq$ 30 ml/min/1.73 m^2, at least 20 years of age, intact cognition, and the ability to communicate in Mandarin or Taiwanese. Otherwise, qualified patients with dementia, intellectual disabilities, or cancer were excluded as well as those with absolute contraindications for hemodialysis or peritoneal dialysis.

G*Power Version 3.1.9.2 (Heinrich Heine Universitat, Dusseldorf, Germany) was used to calculate the required sample size to set an effect size of 0.3, which is suggested by Ottawa Hospital and Health Research Institute (OHHRI) if the outcome variable used is "decisional conflict" of SDM effect (OHHRI, 2015). The statistical method of analysis of variance (the repeated measures between factors) was used to estimate the sample size. On the basis of Cohen, a power size of 0.8 or more was considered relatively appropriate (Cohen, 1992). Therefore, based on power = 0.8, alpha level = .05, effect size = 0.3, number of groups = 2, number of measurements = 3, and correlation among repeated measures = .5, the appropriate sample size for the analysis was 31 participants in each group. Furthermore, in consideration of a potential loss rate up to 20% (Schulz & Grimes, 2008), a total of 72 participants (36 in each group) were recruited.

Study Intervention

Intervention group

The components of the SDM program in this study included physician training, decision support tool development, telephone interviews, and clinical consultations with a renal disease case manager.

Before conducting interventions with the participants, four physicians who agreed to participate attended the SDM education training designed and provided by the first author. This 30-minute educational training course included an introduction to the intervention process and the concept of SDM as well as instructions on how to inform and encourage patients to participate in SDM. To minimize bias, physicians followed a standard structure to ensure that patients were informed and encouraged in a consistent manner. Then, the first author led a role-play session to confirm that physicians' instructions to patients were consistent with one another.

Three clinical consultation sessions were performed for each participant by the renal disease case manager. If family members accompanied the participant, they also participated in the clinical consultation. The focus of the first clinical consultation was on establishing an equal partnership of mutual trust, making participants aware of their disease condition, and encouraging acceptance of the possibility that they might need to be on dialysis in the future, to motivate active participation in decision making. The focus of the second clinical consultation was on providing information on use of the decision support tool to select one of the renal replacement therapies, as well as on the advantages, disadvantages, and complications associated with the therapy options. The decision support tool was a simple, paper-based tool designed for easy use by both the researcher and the participants. It was evidence-based and included information regarding the symptoms of ESRD and treatment options as well as the benefits and risks of different renal replacement therapies. In addition, this tool assisted in clarifying values and confirming related knowledge for each participant, encouraged by the renal disease case manager. The third clinical consultation involved deliberations about different treatment options until agreement was reached on a final decision. The values and preferences of the participants were summarized based on the results of the second consultation and used to consider the feasibility of different renal replacement therapies. Finally, a consensus was reached, and participant choices were treated with respect.

Three telephone interviews were conducted by the renal disease case manager with each participant for continuity of care and to assist in resolving any problems encountered during each consultation.

Control group

The participants in the control group received standard care provided under the pre-ESRD program, which included education from the renal disease case manager using a leaflet to introduce renal replacement therapies and the advantages and disadvantages of each treatment option.

Measurements

A structured questionnaire was used to obtain information and included a demographic and disease characteristics datasheet, the decisional conflict scale (DCS), and the decision self-efficacy scale (DSES).

Demographic and Disease Characteristics Datasheet

The demographic information collected included age, gender, education, employment, marital status, living condition, and number of children. The disease characteristics information collected included the glomerular filtration rate, CKD stage, and number of chronic diseases.

Decisional Conflict Scale

The DCS was developed by the OHHRI to measure personal perceptions of uncertainty in making choices among different treatments. This scale has five subscales, including the informed, values clarity, supported, uncertainty, and effective decision subscales. It is a 16-item, five-response instrument. The scores are first summed, then divided by 16, and then multiplied by 25 to produce a total score ranging from 0 to 100, with higher scores indicating more conflict (OHHRI, 2015). The total scale has been validated with internal consistency coefficient scores of .78–.92, respectively, when tested on individuals considering whether to receive flu vaccinations and considering breast cancer screening options (O'Connor, 1995). These scores are similar to the internal consistency coefficient score in this study of .90 for the entire DCS. In O'Connor's study, the internal consistency coefficient of each subscale ranged from .58 to .92, which is similar to the range in this study of .65–.89 for each subscale.

Decision Self-Efficacy Scale

The DSES assesses the respondent's self-confidence or belief in their abilities with respect to decision making. The DSES, also developed by the OHHRI, is an 11-item, five-response instrument. The scores are first summed, then divided by 11, and then multiplied by 25 to produce a total score ranging from 0 to 100, with 100 representing complete self-efficacy and 0 representing a complete lack of self-efficacy (OHHRI, 2014). In testing, the DSES internal consistency coefficients ranged from .78 to .84 (Bunn & O'Connor, 1996). The internal consistency coefficient of the DSES in this study was .93.

Research Procedures

This study was conducted in one nephrology health education room at each of the two regional hospitals. One hospital provided the intervention group participants, and the other provided the control group participants. The study was carried out between August 2017 and January 2018. A list of patients currently using nursing case management services was obtained through the pre-ESRD care program regularly provided at the two hospitals. The renal disease case managers of the two hospitals identified prospective participants from a list of patients. Patients who agreed to participate completed the baseline questionnaire either on their own or with the help of the renal disease case manager. Before conducting the intervention, the first author and the renal disease case manager of the control group took part in an interview training session, with both discussing the questionnaire to be used until consensus was reached.

All data were collected by the renal disease case manager. The participants completed the baseline questionnaires, which included the demographic and disease characteristics datasheet, the DCS, and the DSES. After completing the baseline questionnaire before a regular appointment, the participants in the control group received the standard pre-ESRD care program, whereas the participants in the intervention group received a structured explanation of their condition from the physician and were then encouraged to participate in SDM. After completing their regular appointments, the intervention group participants returned to the nephrology health education room for their first clinical consultation. One month later, when these participants returned to the clinic for their regular appointment, the renal disease case manager conducted the second clinical consultation. The third clinical consultation occurred 1 month after the second clinical consultation. The renal disease case manager conducted three telephone interviews, respectively, 1 week and 3 weeks after the first clinical consultation and 2 weeks after the second clinical consultation. Immediately after the intervention, the participants in both groups completed the first posttest (T1) questionnaire, which included the DCS and the DSES. One month after the completion of the intervention, all of the participants completed the second posttest (T2) questionnaire (Figure 1).

Ethical Considerations

The study purpose was explained to potential participants who met the selection criteria, and written informed consent was obtained from all of the participants. The study protocol was approved by the research ethics committee of a medical university hospital in central Taiwan (CRREC-106-058).

Data Analysis

All of the statistical analyses were carried out using IBM SPSS Statistics Version 22.0 (IBM, Armonk, NY, USA). A *t* test and chi-squared test (Fisher's exact test was performed if an expected value was < 5) were performed to compare the basic information of the intervention and control groups. We carried out at a two tailed significant level of less than .05. To confirm the effectiveness of the intervention, the intragroup differences between the pre- and postintervention questionnaires were analyzed using a paired *t* test, whereas intergroup differences before and after the intervention for each questionnaire were analyzed using generalized estimating equations. To minimize the probability of Type I error, Bonferroni correction was used to correct the *p* value in the intervention effectiveness. For the paired *t* test, a two-tailed significance level of .017 was conducted. A significance level of .025 was used in the generalized estimating equations.

Results

Of the 72 eligible patients who were initially recruited as participants, 67 completed the three questionnaire measurements (response rate: 93%). The five participants who were lost to follow-up were all in the intervention group. One was lost due to hospitalization, three refused to continue, and one did not return to the clinic. The response rate was 86% in the intervention group and 100% in the control group.

Demographic and Clinical Characteristics and Baseline Decision Measure Outcomes

Table 1 shows the baseline demographic and clinical characteristics of the intervention and control groups. According to the results of the *t* test and chi-square test, except for number of chronic diseases ($t = 3.297$, $p = .002$), there were no statistically significant differences between the two groups in terms of demographic or clinical characteristics.

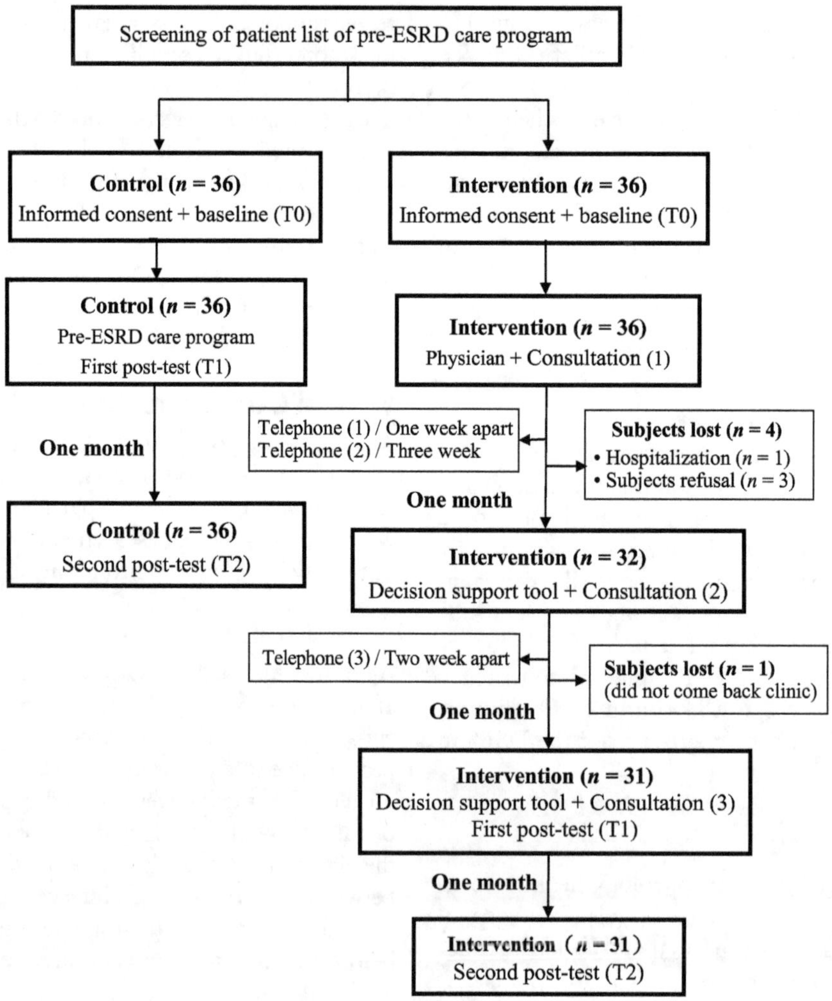

Figure 1. Intervention procedure. ESRD = end-stage renal disease.

The groups were similar in terms of their baseline DSES scores but differed in terms of their DCS scores. For the DCS, the groups had similar scores for the informed, values clarity, and supported subscales, but significantly different scores for the uncertainty and effective decision subscales. Using an unpaired t test (p = .014), the intervention group experienced significantly more conflict than the control group. Thus, the uncertainty and effective decision conflicts of the intervention group were significantly greater than those of the control group (p < .001 and p = .01, respectively; Table 2).

Between- and Within-Subject Effects

Table 3 shows the scores for decisional conflict and decision self-efficacy at baseline (T0), immediately following the intervention (T1), and at 1 month after the intervention (T2) as well as the changes in scores among these three time points. A paired t test was used to compare the differences between the intervention group DSES scores at T0 and T1; participants' DSES scores improved after the intervention, and the difference was statistically significant (t = 11.609, p < .001). Furthermore, the DSES scores for the intervention group decreased slightly but not significantly between T1 and T2 (t = −1.520, p = .139) and, at T2, remained significantly higher than at T0 (mean difference = 26.25, SD = 20.1; t = 7.287, p < .001). These results confirm that the effects of the intervention used in this study persisted for at least 1 month after the end of the intervention. Conversely, no statistically significant difference in DSES scores were observed for the control group across the three time points, indicating that the pre-ESRD care program does not significantly affect decision self-efficacy.

A comparison of the intervention group showed that DCS scores decreased significantly between T0 and T1 (t = −17.665, p < .001), and although DCS scores subsequently increased significantly between T1 and T2 (t = 2.540, p < .05), the difference between T0 and T2 was statistically significant (t = −14.337, p < .001). These results show not only that the intervention group experienced a reduction in decisional conflict but also that the effects of the intervention persisted for at least 1 month. The DCS scores of the control group also decreased from T0 to T1 as well as from T0 to T2, but only the difference in scores between T0 and T1 was statistically significant (t = −3.475, p < .001), indicating that, although the pre-ESRD care program

TABLE 1.
Demographic and Clinical Characteristics of Participants

Variable	Total (n = 67) n (%)	Intervention (n = 31) n (%)	Control (n = 36) n (%)	t/χ^2	p
Age in years, M (SD)	65.4 (11.9)	63.5 (13.8)	67.1 (9.89)	−1.250	.216
Gender				1.032	.310
Male	39 (58.2)	16 (51.6)	23 (63.9)		
Female	28 (41.8)	15 (48.4)	13 (36.1)		
Education				2.953[a]	.251
Elementary school or below	35 (52.3)	13 (41.9)	22 (61.1)		
Junior high school	9 (13.4)	6 (19.4)	3 (8.30)		
High school or above	23 (34.3)	12 (38.7)	11 (30.6)		
Employment status				0.305	.580
Unemployed	52 (77.6)	25 (80.6)	27 (75.0)		
Employed	15 (22.4)	6 (19.4)	9 (25.0)		
Marital status				0.183	.668
Married	45 (67.2)	20 (64.5)	25 (69.4)		
Single	22 (32.8)	11 (35.5)	11 (30.6)		
Living condition				2.854[a]	.434
Living alone	10 (14.9)	5 (16.1)	5 (13.9)		
Living with spouse	14 (20.9)	5 (16.1)	9 (25.0)		
Living with children	17 (25.4)	6 (19.4)	11 (30.6)		
Living with spouse and children	26 (38.8)	15 (48.4)	11 (30.6)		
No. of children, M (SD)	2.64 (1.60)	2.65 (1.68)	2.64 (1.53)	0.016	.987
GFR, M (SD)	14.9 (7.64)	15.4 (8.03)	14.4 (7.37)	0.517	.607
Stage				0.0002	.988
Stage 4	26 (38.8)	12 (38.7)	14 (38.9)		
Stage 5	41 (61.2)	19 (61.3)	22 (61.1)		
No. of chronic diseases, M (SD)	2.67 (1.05)	3.10 (1.04)	2.31 (0.92)	3.297	.002

Note. GFR = glomerular filtration rate.
[a]Fisher's exact test.

reduced decisional conflicts immediately after the program, this effect was not sustained.

Table 4 shows the differences in DSES and DCS scores between the two groups before and after the intervention. To reduce the interference factor, "number of chronic diseases" was included in the model analysis. The results show that the DSES degrees of score change between T0 and T1, and T0 and T2, respectively, in the intervention group were significantly greater; the differences were statistically significant in both cases ($B = 27.6$, $SE = 3.8$, $p < .001$; $B = 25.8$, $SE = 4.8$,

TABLE 2.
Baseline DSES and DCS Comparison, Intergroup

Variable	Total (n = 67) M	SD	Intervention (n = 31) M	SD	Control (n = 36) M	SD	t	p
DSES	55.05	17.7	51.83	18.5	57.83	16.8	−1.390	.169
DCS	64.11	12.2	67.89	8.1	60.85	14.1	2.541	.014
Informed	61.82	19.0	66.67	16.5	57.64	20.3	1.978	.052
Values clarity	67.29	16.7	70.97	15.6	64.12	17.2	1.692	.095
Supported	56.72	15.9	56.18	11.6	57.18	19.0	−0.262	.794
Uncertainty	73.13	13.1	79.30	12.3	67.82	11.5	3.944	< .001
Effective	62.22	13.4	66.73	11.1	58.33	14.2	2.668	.010

Note. DSES = decision self-efficacy scale; DCS = decision conflict scale.

TABLE 3.
Differences in DSES and DCS, Intragroup at Different Time Points

Variable	Intervention (*n* = 31)					Control (*n* = 36)				
	M	*SD*	95% CI	Paired-*t*	*p*	*M*	*SD*	95% CI	Paired *t*	*p*
DSES										
T0	51.83	18.5				57.83	16.8			
T1	82.11	11.6				60.50	8.6			
T2	78.08	13.8				58.25	8.6			
T1–T0	30.28	14.5	[24.9, 35.6]	11.609	< .001	2.67	17.4	[−3.2, 8.6]	0.920	.364
T2–T0	26.25	20.1	[18.9, 33.6]	7.287	< .001	0.42	19.6	[−6.2, 7.1]	0.129	.898
T2–T1	−4.03	14.8	[−1.4, 9.5]	−1.520	.139	−2.25	8.9	[−5.3, 0.8]	−1.515	.139
DCS										
T0	67.89	8.1				60.85	14.1			
T1	20.82	10.8				50.17	11.4			
T2	26.56	12.5				55.67	8.8			
T1–T0	−47.08	14.8	[−41.6, −52.5]	−17.665	< .001	−10.68	18.4	[−16.9, −4.4]	−3.475	< .001
T2–T0	−41.33	16.1	[−35.4, −47.2]	−14.337	< .001	−5.18	17.2	[−10.9, 0.6]	−1.810	.079
T2–T1	5.75	12.6	[1.1, 10.4]	2.540	.016	5.50	8.1	[2.8, 8.2]	4.091	< .001

Note. Two-tailed significance level = .017. DSES = decision self-efficacy scale; DCS = decision conflict scale; T0 = baseline; T1 = first posttest; T2 = second posttest.

$p < .001$). Meanwhile, the degree of change in the DCS scores of the intervention group was 36.4 points lower, whereas the T0 to T2 score change range was 36.1 points lower than that of the control group; the differences were statistically significant in both cases ($B = -36.4$, $SE = 4.0$, $p < .001$; $B = -36.1$, $SE = 4.0$, $p < .001$). These results confirm that the proposed intervention was more effective than the pre-ERSD care program in reducing decisional conflict and that the effect of the proposed intervention lasted for at least 1 month.

Discussion

The results of this study indicate that the SDM process increases decision self-efficacy significantly more than the standard pre-ESRD care program for patients with CKD and that its effects persist for at least 1 month. This finding is consistent with previous studies that evaluated changes in decision self-efficacy of patients with Type 2 diabetes following their use of patient decision aids and of patients with breast cancer following their use of decision supports (Bailey et al., 2016; Causarano et al., 2015).

Kane et al. (2014) conducted a systematic review and found that physicians who invited their patients to participate in SDM helped patients understand their right to choose their treatments and obtain greater support. Because of cultural factors, a high percentage of patients in Taiwan are predisposed not to challenge the authority of medical professionals. Therefore, without the support of a physician, even when patients

TABLE 4.
Intergroup Differences in Intervention Effectiveness of DSES and DCS

Variable	DSES				DCS			
	B	*SE*	95% CI	*p*	*B*	*SE*	95% CI	*p*
Intercept	64.1	4.1	[56.1, 72.1]	< .001	58.9	3.1	[52.8, 65.1]	< .001
Group								
Intervention vs. Control	−3.8	4.4	[−12.4, 4.7]	.382	6.4	2.8	[0.8,−11.9]	.024
Time								
T1 vs. T0	2.7	2.9	[−2.9, 8.3]	.351	−10.7	3.0	[−16.6, −4.7]	< .001
T2 vs. T0	0.4	3.2	[−5.9, 6.7]	.896	−5.2	2.8	[−10.7, 0.4]	.066
No. of chronic diseases	−2.7	1.2	[−5.2, −0.3]	.027	0.8	0.9	[−0.9, 2.6]	.347
Group × Time								
Intervention × T1 and Control × T1	27.6	3.8	[20.1, 35.1]	< .001	−36.4	4.0	[−44.2, −28.5]	< .001
Intervention × T2 and Control × T2	25.8	4.8	[16.4, 35.2]	< .001	−36.1	4.0	[−43.9, −28.3]	< .001

Note. Significance level = .025. DSES = decision self-efficacy scale; DCS = decision conflict scale; T0 = baseline; T1 = first posttest; T2 = second posttest.

are informed about their treatment options, they do not feel entitled to participate in the decision-making process. In this study, "medical staff clearly inform and encourage patients to participate" was used in the intervention group to increase the confidence and willingness of patients to participate in decision making. The intensity of self-efficacy may be influenced by the speech of significant figures in an individual's life (Bandura, 1977). This may explain the effectiveness of the intervention in our study to some extent. With clear information and encouragement from physicians, the participants in the intervention group were able to effectively and significantly increase their confidence to make treatment decisions.

According to Bandura (1977), self-efficacy is also enhanced by emotional arousal when a patient obtains support from others. In this study, the roles of the physician and the renal disease case manager in SDM were complementary and cooperative. The physician was the initiator, and the case manager was the guide who assisted each patient through the SDM process. In addition, the case manager continued to use encouragement and appreciation in the intervention process to make patients feel that they had the ability to understand the information related to different renal replacement therapies. The verbal praise of medical staff contributed to the improvement of patient self-efficacy, and the more patients trust healthcare providers, the greater the effect of verbal praise (Y. Y. Lee & Lin, 2008). Thus, the case manager played an important role in supporting and guiding the participants through the SDM process. Establishing a trusting relationship further strengthens the verbal persuasion effect of case managers, who aim to provide encouragement and show appreciation, thereby indirectly improving patient decision-making self-efficacy.

The DCS is used to assess the conflict and uncertainty that individuals perceive regarding which course of action to take when facing a choice that involves risk, regret, or personal values. The intervention group participants reported a more significant reduction in decisional conflict than their peers who received standard pre-ESRD care program education. This finding is consistent with the results of Causarano et al. (2015) and Bailey et al. (2016). Uncertainty is the most significant factor of influence on decisional conflict, with subfactors including lack of knowledge about treatment options, unclear personal values, and insufficient support (Légaré et al., 2012). In this study, in addition to providing knowledge, the sharing of values and opinions among patients and case managers based on relationships of mutual trust was an important component of the consultation process. Berrios-Rivera et al. (2006) found that the establishment of a trusting relationship encourages patients to share their concerns, which may then be solved with assistance, further strengthening patient trust in providers (Y. Y. Lee & Lin, 2008). Therefore, the consultation and discussion process proposed in this study creates a positive reinforcement cycle. When patients are willing to share their values and opinions, their decisional conflict may be effectively reduced. Many scholars have advocated the positive role of decision aids in improving patient knowledge, assisting patients to explore their personal values, and structurally guiding patients to discuss important issues with providers to define personal values more clearly and reduce decisional conflict (S. C. Lee, 2016; Stacey et al., 2014). Patient knowledge may be improved through the process of information exchange. When patients are better able to participate in decision making and present their values and opinions, conflicts will be reduced. Moreover, decision aids play an important role in improving patient knowledge and reducing decisional conflict.

In this study, telephone consultations were used to provide additional knowledge to help reduce psychological pressures related to the decision-making process. Sun and Hsu (2017) pointed out that giving patients emotional support during the decision-making process through activities such as regular telephone interviews allows patients to express fears and uneasiness and effectively reduces decisional conflict. Therefore, the effectiveness of the intervention in this study was better than that of the standard pre-ESRD program.

The standard pre-ESRD care program that is currently provided in the Taiwan healthcare system was developed with the goal of limiting the workforce and time burdens on medical institutions. Under this program, each patient receives the same educational content, and thus, it is easy to neglect the personal values and opinions of individual patients. Moreover, this program pays little attention to the nurse–patient relationship and the relationship of trust between patients and case managers. Lacking this relationship of trust, patients are unlikely to discuss expectations and opinions or to participate in medical decisions. This may be the reason why the control group did not experience sustained improvement in decision self-efficacy or in decisional conflict despite immediate postprogram gains for both.

No previous study has examined the effectiveness of SDM in different renal replacement therapies for patients with CKD. This study provides preliminary evidence that the proposed program improves decisional conflict and decision self-efficacy significantly better than the standard pre-ESRD program. These results may provide a reference for applying SDM in the standard pre-ESRD program. To improve patient decision making, care services should focus on the personal values and opinions of each patient. It is recommended that physicians and renal disease case managers should also work in complementary and cooperative ways in SDM programs. The case manager should provide not only adaptive education but also clinical consultation appointments. Because SDM is phased, the case manager and the patient must meet several times for discussions.

Limitations

This study is affected by several limitations. First, because of human resource limitations, physicians did not participate in the third (final) clinical consultation. Because the final clinical consultation involves the patient making decisions, having physicians participate may further strengthen the decision-making self-efficacy of patients and reduce decisional conflicts. Second, the sample used in this study comprised selected patients with CKD at two regional teaching hospitals in Miaoli County, Taiwan. Therefore, the generalization of study results is limited. Third, because of the relatively long (6-month) recruitment period, it was impossible to control for interference factors such as changes in renal function or CKD stage, which may have affected the inferences of the results. Finally, family involvement in SDM may have affected the results of the study. Furthermore, variance in the ability of family members to accompany patients during clinical consultations inevitably affected the patients and the effect of the interventions.

Conclusions

The SDM program may be an effective intervention to help patients navigate the complex process of making patient-centered decisions regarding renal replacement treatment. The intervention significantly improved the decision self-efficacy of patients with CKD and reduced their decisional conflicts with regard to different renal replacement therapies.

Acknowledgments

The authors would like to thank all of the patients who agreed to participate. The assistance of the renal disease case managers and physicians in the study process is gratefully acknowledged.

Author Contributions

Study conception and design: YFH, ICL, CCH, WYH
Data collection: YFH
Data analysis and interpretation: YFH, ICL, KCL
Drafting of the article: YFH, ICL
Critical revision of the article: ICL, YCC

References

Bailey, R. A., Pfeifer, M., Shillington, A. C., Harshaw, Q., Funnell, M. M., VanWingen, J., & Col, N. (2016). Effect of a patient decision aid (PDA) for type 2 diabetes on knowledge, decisional self-efficacy, and decisional conflict. *BMC Health Services Research, 16*, 10. https://doi.org/10.1186/s12913-016-1262-4

Bandura, A. (1977). Self-efficacy: Toward a unifying theory of behavioral change. *Psychological Review, 84*(2), 191–215. https://doi.org/10.1037//0033-295X.84.2.191

Berrios-Rivera, J. P., Street, R. L. Jr., Garcia Popa-lisseanu, M. G., Kallen, M. A., Richardson, M. N., Janssen, N. M., ... Suarez-Almazor, M. E. (2006). Trust in physicians and elements of the medical interaction in patients with rheumatoid arthritis and systemic lupus erythematosus. *Arthritis and Rheumatism, 55*(3), 385–393. https://doi.org/10.1002/art.21988

Bunn, H., & O'Connor, A. (1996). Validation of client decision-making instruments in the context of psychiatry. *Canadian Journal of Nursing Research, 28*(3), 13–27.

Causarano, N., Platt, J., Baxter, N. N., Bagher, S., Jones, J. M., Metcalfe, K. A., ... Zhong, T. (2015). Pre-consultation educational group intervention to improve shared decision-making for postmastectomy breast reconstruction: A pilot randomized controlled trial. *Support Care Cancer, 23*(5), 1365–1375. https://doi.org/10.1007/s00520-014-2479-6

Charles, C., Gafni, A., & Whelan, T. (1997). Shared decision-making in the medical encounter: What does it mean? (or it takes at least two to tango). *Social Science & Medicine, 44*(5), 681–692. https://doi.org/10.1016/S0277-9536(96)00221-3

Charles, C., Gafni, A., & Whelan, T. (1999). Decision-making in the physician-patient encounter: Revisiting the shared treatment decision-making model. *Social Science & Medicine, 49*(5), 651–661.

Chiaranai, C. (2016). The lived experience of patients receiving hemodialysis treatment for end-stage renal disease: A qualitative study. *The Journal of Nursing Research, 24*(2), 101–108. https://doi.org/10.1097/jnr.0000000000000100

Cohen, J. (1992). A power primer. *Psychological Bulletin, 112*(1), 155–159.

Gionfriddo, M. R., Leppin, A. L., Brito, J. P., Leblanc, A., Boehmer, K. R., Morris, M. A., ... Montori, V. M. (2014). A systematic review of shared decision making interventions in chronic conditions: A review protocol. *Systematic Reviews, 3*, 38. https://doi.org/10.1186/2046-4053-3-38

Hsiao, C. Y., Lin, L. W., Su, Y. W., Yeh, S. H., Lee, L. N., & Tsai, F. M. (2016). The effects of an empowerment intervention on renal transplant recipients: A randomized controlled trial. *The Journal of Nursing Research, 24*(3), 201–210. https://doi.org/10.1097/jnr.0000000000000115

Kane, H. L., Halpern, M. T., Squiers, L. B., Treiman, K. A., & McCormack, L. A. (2014). Implementing and evaluating shared decision making in oncology practice. *CA: A Cancer Journal for Clinicians, 64*(6), 377–388. https://doi.org/10.3322/caac.21245

Lai, M. J., Chou, C. Y., & Lu, S. H. (2018). Factors associated with starting dialysis using a temporary catheter among patients with chronic kidney disease. *VGH Nursing, 35*(3), 278–288. https://doi.org/10.6142/VGHN.201809_35(3).0007 (Original work published in Chinese)

Lee, S. C. (2016). Treatment decision making process of cancer patients. *The Journal of Nursing, 63*(5), 12–18. https://doi.org/10.6224/JN.63.5.12 (Original work published in Chinese)

Lee, Y. Y., & Lin, J. L. (2008). Patient-physician trust, outcome expectations and self-efficacy in diabetic patients' self-care. *Taipei City Medical Journal, 5*(3), 304–319. https://doi.org/10.6200/TCMJ.2008.5.3.02 (Original work published in Chinese)

Légaré, F., Leblanc, A., Robitaille, H., & Turcotte, S. (2012). The decisional conflict scale: Moving from the individual to the dyad level. *The Journal of Evidence and Quality in Health Care, 106*(4), 247–252. https://doi.org/10.1016/j.zefq.2012.02.021 (Original work published in German)

Liyanage, T., Ninomiya, T., Jha, V., Neal, B., Patrice, H. M., Okpechi, I., ... Perkovic, V. (2015). Worldwide access to treatment for end-stage kidney disease: A systematic review. *The Lancet, 385*(9981), 1975–1982. https://doi.org/10.1016/S0140-6736(14)61601-9

Ministry of Health and Welfare, Taiwan, ROC. (2018). *Nationwide multidisciplinary pre-end stage renal disease (pre-ESRD) care program.* Retrieved from https://www.nhi.gov.tw/Content_List.aspx?n=D5CC89AE36D48E5E&topn=CA428784F9ED78C9 (Original work published in Chinese)

National Health Research Institutes, Taiwan, ROC. (2015). *Timing, preparation and selection of patients with chronic kidney disease receiving renal replacement therapy. 2015 Taiwan chronic kidney disease clinical guidelines.* Retrieved from http://w3.nhri.org.tw/nhri_org/rl/lib/NewWeb/nhri/html/B-5/B-5_son_05.htm#I (Original work published in Chinese)

Obeidat, R. F., Homish, G. G., & Lally, R. M. (2013). Shared decision making among individuals with cancer in non-Western cultures: A literature review. *Oncology Nursing Forum, 40*(5), 454–463. https://doi.org/10.1188/13.ONF.454-463

O'Connor, A. M. (1995). Validation of a decisional conflict scale. *Medical Decision Making, 15*(1), 25–30. https://doi.org/10.1177/0272989X9501500105

Ottawa Hospital and Health Research Institute. (2014). *Sample tool: Decision self-efficacy.* Retrieved from https://decisionaid.ohri.ca/eval_self.html

Ottawa Hospital and Health Research Institute. (2015). *Traditional decisional conflict scale (DCS)—Statement format: 16 Item 5 response categories.* Retrieved from https://decisionaid.ohri.ca/eval_dcs.html

Schulz, K. F., & Grimes, D. A. (2008). Sample size slippages in randomized trials: Exclusions and the lost and wayward (J. H. Lin, Trans.). In H. D. Chen (Ed.), *The Lancet handbook of essential concepts in clinical research* (pp. 171–172). Taipei City, Taiwan, ROC: Elsevier Taiwan. (Original work published 2006)

Stacey, D., Légaré, F., Col, N. F., Bennett, C. L., Barry, M. J., Eden, K. B., . . . Wu, J. H. (2014). Decision aids for people facing health treatment or screening decisions. *The Cochrane Database of Systematic Reviews, 4,* CD001431. https://doi.org/10.1002/14651858.CD001431.pub4

Sun, W. N., & Hsu, H. T. (2017). Discourse of decision conflict. *The Kaohsiung Journal of Nursing, 34*(1), 25–35. https://doi.org/10.6692/KJN-2017-34-1-3 (Original work published in Chinese)

Taiwan Society of Nephrology, Taiwan, ROC. (2018). *2018 Annual report on kidney disease in Taiwan.* Retrieved from https://www.tsn.org.tw/UI/L/L002.aspx (Original work published in Chinese)

U.S. Renal Data System. (2018). *2018 ADR chapters: End-stage renal disease (ESRD) in the United States—International comparisons.* https://www.usrds.org/2018/view/Default.aspx

20

A Systematic Review of Behavioral Outcomes for Leadership Interventions Among Health Professionals

Michelle CLEARY[1]* • Rachel KORNHABER[2] • Deependra Kaji THAPA[3] • Sancia WEST[4] • Denis VISENTIN[5]

ABSTRACT

Background: Healthcare requires effective leadership to improve patient outcomes, manage change, and achieve organizational goals.

Purpose: The purpose of this study was to evaluate interventions aimed at improving leadership behavior in health professionals.

Methods: A systematic literature review of key databases (PubMed, CINAHL, Embase, and Scopus) was performed in September 2018. Data were extracted and synthesized.

Results: Thirty-three articles from 31 studies met the inclusion criteria. Self-reported leadership behavior showed a significant postprogram improvement. Objective observations were more likely to show improved leadership behavior than subjective observations. Face-to-face delivery of leadership development was more effective than online delivery. Interventions incorporating the elements of personal development planning, self-directed learning, workplace-based learning, and reflection were more likely to develop leadership behavior.

Conclusions/Implications for Practice: Leadership interventions had a beneficial effect on the leadership behaviors of participants based on both subjective and objective changes in behavior. In addition to focusing on individual skill development, interventions that aim to develop leadership should consider the organizational, social, cultural, and political contexts in which behavioral change is expected. Workplace-based learning should be included in program development.

KEY WORDS:
health professionals, leadership, leadership interventions, program development, systematic review.

Introduction

Quality healthcare is dependent on effective organizational factors, including interdisciplinary teamwork, a supportive culture, and good leadership (Barr & Dowding, 2019; Marchionni & Ritchie, 2008; McAlearney, 2008). As the healthcare system has evolved to align business and medical imperatives (Murdock & Brammer, 2011), the tendency to separate leadership and administration from clinical care has given way to leadership development becoming a core approach in physician, nurse, and allied health training (Ackerman et al., 2019).

The development of leadership skills among healthcare professionals aims to improve performance, allow for succession planning, facilitate organizational change, and achieve organizational goals (Collins & Holton, 2004; Turner, 2019). Effective leadership grows an accountable culture that is aligned with these goals (Peters, 2019), which improves patient outcomes (Suhonen et al., 2019).

Research has shown the importance of developing leadership in health professionals, including specific clinical leadership skills (Cleary et al., 2005; Cutcliffe & Cleary, 2015; Daly et al., 2014). However, discussions of skills and capabilities in the literature often emphasize what should happen instead of evaluating successful strategies. Studying the comparative degrees of success of different leadership development programs allows future endeavors to benefit from previous experiences to better target strategies. For example, one study highlighted the importance of the context of the proposed change for successful leadership in complex healthcare environments (Kwamie et al., 2014). This study found that leadership change was not sufficiently institutionalized, directing future studies to consider context to enable a more reflexive organizational culture. Another study found that the development of leadership in physicians focused on individual skills rather than enhancing collaborative capacity (Frich et al., 2015).

Strategies to enhance leadership behavior have important effects on both public health workplaces and healthcare (Dellve et al., 2007; Jiménez et al., 2017). This systematic review seeks to evaluate the evidence of interventions aimed at improving leadership behavior in health professionals.

[1]*PhD, RN, Professor, School of Nursing, College of Health and Medicine, University of Tasmania, Sydney, NSW, Australia* • [2]*PhD, RN, Associate Professor, School of Nursing, College of Health and Medicine, University of Tasmania, Sydney, NSW, Australia* • [3]*MPH, MSc, Research Assistant, School of Nursing, College of Health and Medicine, University of Tasmania, Sydney, NSW, Australia* • [4]*PhD, RN, Research Assistant, School of Nursing, College of Health and Medicine, University of Tasmania, Sydney, NSW, Australia* • [5]*PhD, Senior Lecturer, School of Health Sciences, College of Health and Medicine, University of Tasmania, Sydney, NSW, Australia.*

Methods

Study Design and Search Methods

The Preferred Reporting Items for Systematic Reviews and Meta-Analyses guidelines (Liberati et al., 2009) were used in this study to systematically review studies concerning the effectiveness of leadership development/intervention programs in improving leadership behavior in health professionals. A literature search was conducted in September 2018 of several databases, including PubMed, CINAHL, Embase, and Scopus. No time restriction was applied to these database searches. Boolean connectors combined Medical Subject Headings and the following search terms: leadership*, health personnel, allied health personnel, nursing, physicians, program development, intervention*, and program evaluation.

For example, the search strategy for CINAHL was ([MH nurses OR TI nursing OR AB nursing OR MH Allied Health Personnel OR MH Occupational Therapists OR MH Social Workers OR MH Physical Therapists OR TI physiotherapist OR AB physiotherapist OR MH Physicians] AND [MH Leadership OR TI "transformational leadership" OR AB "transformational leadership"] AND [MH Program Development OR TI intervention* OR AB intervention* OR MH Program Evaluation]) NOT student* NOT undergraduate NOT baccalaureate NOT supervision NOT mentor*. Across the four databases, the search was modified for variations in syntax and Medical Subject Headings terms.

Eligibility Criteria

The eligibility for inclusion encompassed qualitative or quantitative peer-reviewed articles published in English evaluating leadership development programs/interventions on leadership behavior among health professionals across health sectors. All prospective interventions that were designed to develop or enhance leadership were included. Kirkpatrick's evaluation model (Kirkpatrick & Kirkpatrick, 2009), which describes four evaluation levels of reaction (Level 1), knowledge (Level 2), behavioral change (Level 3), and system results (Level 4), was used to classify the outcome of leadership interventions. This review only included studies reporting behavior change (Level 3). Studies without interventions; studies not primarily addressing health professionals; studies on students, supervision, or mentorship; theoretical articles; commentaries; editorials; and review articles were excluded.

Search Outcomes

The search identified 660 articles, with an additional 34 articles identified in the reference lists of the identified studies and through hand searching. After the removal of 214 duplicates, the titles and abstracts of 480 articles were screened, resulting in the removal of an additional 361 articles. The remaining 119 articles were subject to full text review, resulting in the removal of an additional 39 articles. After removing one article (Blaney, 2012) because of the lack of reported findings, the

Figure 1
Flow Diagram of Studies Identified, Screened, Assessed for Eligibility, and Included

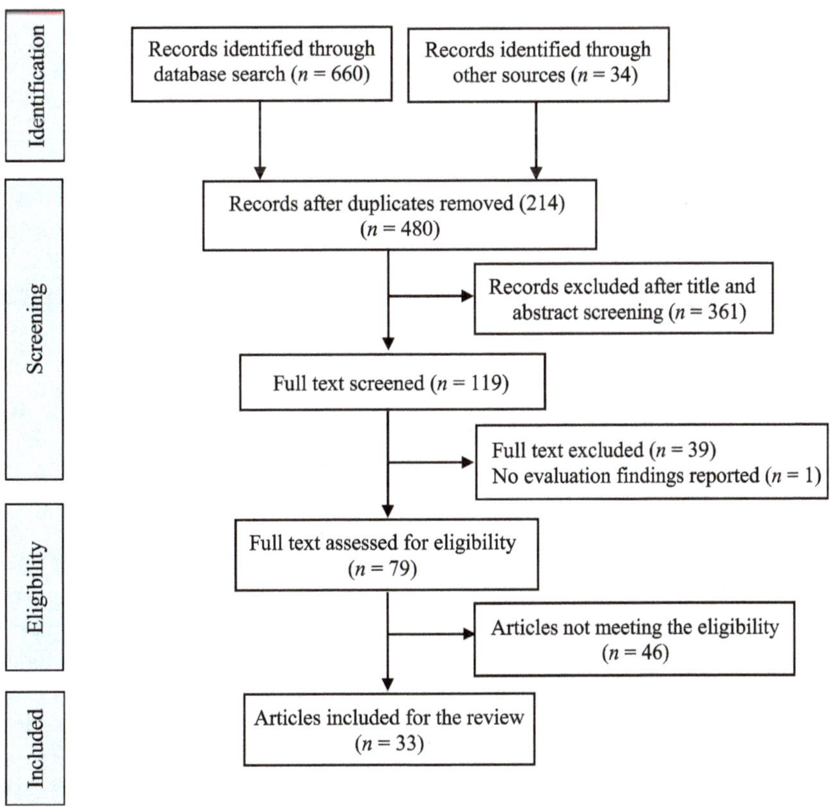

remaining 79 articles were assessed for eligibility, of which 33 (from 31 studies) met the inclusion criteria (see Figure 1).

Data Extraction and Synthesis

A data extraction sheet was developed in consensus with all of the authors and finalized using an iterative process. Two of the authors extracted the information from the included articles in five domains: (a) study characteristics, namely, author, publication year, country, objective(s), and study design; (b) study settings and participants; (c) intervention characteristics, namely, duration, content, and training methods; (d) behavioral outcome and assessment, namely, assessment measures and follow-up; and (e) significant findings (see Table 1). The other authors assessed the data, with discrepancies resolved by consensus. In line with the previous reviews of leadership interventions (Collins & Holton, 2004; Frich et al., 2015), the reported behavioral outcomes were differentiated into subjective and objective assessments of the behaviors. The results of this review are presented in narrative form.

Results

Characteristics of the Studies

The characteristics of the included studies are presented in Table 1. Of the 31 included studies, 19 used quantitative methods, five used qualitative methods, and seven used mixed methods to measure the intervention outcomes. Seventeen of the studies used a pretest–posttest design, and the remaining 14 used only a posttest (with or without follow-up) design. Only five of the included studies used a control group(s) for comparison. Ten of the studies were conducted in the United States; seven, in Canada; six, in the United Kingdom; two each, in Australia and Ireland; and three, in other European countries. One study was conducted in both the United States and Canada. The included studies were published between 2002 and 2016.

Study Settings and Participants

Most of the included studies evaluated different types of leadership development programs in clinical settings. Study participants included nurses in 12 studies, physicians in six studies, healthcare educators in three studies, and mixed-group participants (including physicians, nurses, clinical managers, ward managers, allied health professionals, and administrators) in 10 studies. The number of trainees who participated in the interventions ranged from eight to 48 in qualitative and seven to 550 in quantitative and mixed-methods studies. Female participants outnumbered male participants in many of the studies. Some studies did not exclusively report the number of participants who provided the evaluation data used in analyses.

In addition to the participants, key stakeholder informants were used in nine studies to provide information using observer evaluations of leadership behavior (objective behavior) of the participants (Study nos. 3, 4, 7, 10, 18, 23, 26, 30, 33). These informants included participants' immediate supervisors, peers and colleagues, dyad partners, and patients.

Intervention Characteristics

The interventions differed in terms of duration, content, and mode of delivery. The duration of the interventions ranged from a half-day workshop (Gilfoyle et al., 2007) to a 4-year program that was integrated into standard clinical training (Agius et al., 2015). Eleven studies reported on interventions lasting for 12 months or longer, whereas five studies had intervention lasting for less than 1 week. Five studies (Study nos. 5, 10, 17, 19, 32) did not specify the duration of the intervention. The intervention dose also varied across the studies, and the time devoted to the intervention was difficult to ascertain in many studies.

Despite the diversity across interventions in terms of training content, most interventions addressed leadership, group dynamics, teamwork, communication, personal development, change management, conflict resolution, time management, and supervision skills. Some studies also included clinical skills such as perioperative issues in geriatric care (delirium, functional assessment, polypharmacy, and discharge planning; Levine et al., 2008) and pediatric resuscitation (resuscitation skills and avoidance of fixation errors; Gilfoyle et al., 2007).

All of the included studies used face-to-face training, with the exception of Brown et al. (2003), which used an online leadership course. Maddalena and Fleet (2015) employed both face-to-face and online modules. The interventions used different types of teaching/learning methods, among which group-based workshops were the most common, with many studies using more than one type of training method. Other methods included lectures, coaching, 360° feedback, mentorship, learning reflection, group discussion, team activities, plenary sessions, role play, presentation, and simulation exercises. Some of the studies also included work-based action learning in which participants developed their own action plan and implemented this plan over the intervention period. Five studies (Study nos. 4, 9, 10, 19, 32) did not clearly specify the mode of training delivery.

Outcome Measures

This review only included studies reporting the behavioral outcomes of the leadership interventions. Most of the included studies ($n = 21$) reported only subjective behavioral outcomes, consisting of intervention-related, self-reported alterations in behavior. Gilfoyle et al. (2007) reported objective behavior in which participants were asked to participate in a mock leadership scenario. The remaining nine studies reported on both subjective and objective behaviors. Nine studies used standard scales to measure leadership behavior, of which four used the Leadership Practices Inventory (LPI; Table 2).

Eight studies (Study nos. 3, 5, 10, 11, 13, 14, 22, 28) used only one measurement during the postintervention

Table 1
Study Characteristics, Leadership Intervention, and Behavioral Outcomes

No.	Author (Year) / Country	Objective	Study Setting and Participant	Study Design	Intervention Duration
1.	Agius et al. (2015) / United Kingdom	To determine the impact of Medical Leadership Programme (MLP) at an individual and service level for the delivery of patient care.	Eight physicians participated in MLP	Qualitative, pre, mid, and post program	Four-year program integrated into the clinical training.
2.	Bergman et al. (2009) / Sweden	To assess the impact of two different leadership programs (long-term and 1-week) on healthcare managers' attitudes toward and the views on leadership.	53 (45 female) managers, mostly nurses (34 in long-term support group and 19 in 1-week) 39 responded both before and after questionnaires and 30 participated in focus group interviews	Mixed methods, before and 6 months after program	Long-term (3-hour sessions conducted 9 times in a year, for an average of 17 months) versus 1 week.
3.	Boomer & McCormack (2010) / Northern Ireland	To evaluate a 3-year practice development program for clinical nurse leaders.	48 clinical leaders from 16 units Data collected from key stakeholders, which included patients, facilitators, nursing and service managers, and nursing staff	Qualitative, postprogram	3 years
4.	Boyle & Kochinda (2004)/ United States	To test an intervention to enhance collaborative communication among nurse and physician leaders in two intensive care units (ICUs).	10 (eight female) clinical leaders (seven nurses and three physicians) Mean age: 39.8 years Average years in their respective leadership positions: 4.7 Participants also included the unit staff of the trainees	Quantitative, single-arm pre–post and 6 months of follow-up	8 months (six modules of 23.5 hours in total).

Intervention Content	Teaching Method	Behavioral Outcome and Assessment	Significant Finding
Leadership, health and public policy, organizational development, governance, future challenges of health, and public leadership	Integrated training model comprising academic and vocational components	Subjective Semistructured qualitative interviews and reviews of achievement	The participants reported evidence on showing personal qualities, working with others, managing services, improving services, and setting direction.
Group dynamics, teamwork, communication, leadership, conflict management	1-week course, reflection, and long-term support group	Subjective Questionnaire and focus groups	Both leadership programs strengthened the managers in their leadership roles. The long-term support groups helped the managers to structure and cope with everyday leadership situations in their occupational environment. The 1-week course was good for inexperienced managers and the long-term support groups for more experienced managers.
Leadership development	Work-based action learning, workshops The team met monthly to solve problems, plan activities, and analyze and synthesize data	Subjective and objective Qualitative interview, observations	Process outcomes showing growth as leaders contributing to cultural shifts (becoming more reflexive; becoming proactive; valuing teamwork and becoming more accessible, reachable, and approachable; and becoming a facilitator). Stakeholders showed practice change including teamwork among staff, friendliness and professionalism, better communication with staff and patients, efficient management of waiting lists, learning culture, good working relationships, reflective practice, role modeling behaviors, managing performance, and challenging poor practice.
Collaborative communication, leadership, coordination, problem solving, conflict management, team culture	Not clear	Subjective and objective Investigator-developed Collaboration Skills Simulation Vignette test and a modified ICU Nurse–Physician Questionnaire	Postintervention mean score on the Collaborative Communication Simulation Vignette (possible score range: 0–100) increased from 56.7 in pretest to 75.3 in posttest ($p = .021$). During follow-up, participants reported a significant improvement in self-perception of leadership characteristics exhibited, and satisfaction with leadership, and communication skills ($p < .05$). The unit staff reported improved collaborative communication, problem solving, and nursing leadership.

(continues)

Table 1
Study Characteristics, Leadership Intervention, and Behavioral Outcomes, Continued

No.	Author (Year) / Country	Objective	Study Setting and Participant	Study Design	Intervention Duration
5.	Brown et al. (2003)/ United States	To describe the results of an evaluative research project that examined outcomes of a web-based nursing leadership course.	33 registered nurse students	Quantitative, single-arm postprogram	Not clear
6.	Castillo & James (2013)/ United Kingdom	No specific objective(s) stated.	120 participants (therapists, ward managers, senior nurses, midwives, school nurses, and other managers) participated in improving the Frontline Leaders program (eight cohorts). Not clear how many were involved in the program evaluation	Quantitative, posttest and 1-year follow-up	Around 6 days of contact spread over 8 months.
7. 8.	Cunningham & Kitson (2000a) Cunningham & Kitson (2000b)/ United Kingdom	To test whether the Clinical Nurse Leadership program improved the clinical leadership capability of participants.	28 (22 female) participants (four senior nurses and 24 ward sisters) in four acute hospital trusts Questionnaires were also completed by the colleagues on the wards of the participants	Quantitative, single-arm, pre–post design	18 months

Intervention Content	Teaching Method	Behavioral Outcome and Assessment	Significant Finding
Not clear	Online nursing leadership course	Subjective Researcher-developed questionnaire	More than 71% participants reported the course caused them to reevaluate their communication patterns, develop lifelong learning skills, and improve their critical thinking. More than 65% indicated the course led them to reevaluate personal leadership style and improve ability to offer concrete reasons for opinions. Participants reported confidently applying change strategies, conflict resolution, case management, ethical decision management, and different leadership and management styles.
Leadership styles, coaching and feedback skills, delivering and sustaining change	Lecture, practice-based project, coaching, 360° feedback	Subjective 360° feedback tool	After program, 360° feedback revealed improvements in behavior of the participants especially in acting in feedback, asking people's points of view, and effectively providing positive feedback. 70% of the participants reported impact of the training on their leadership behavior such as encouraging nurses to solve problems and involving colleagues during difficult situations. Nursing managers reported using their new skills to role model and encourage critical thinking.
Personal development, 360° feedback, undertaking observations of care and patient narratives	Personal development plan, action learning, workshop, storytelling, mentorship	Subjective and objective Multifactor Leadership Questionnaire (MLQ)	Participants self-assessed significant changes for the inspiration ($p = .024$), active management by exception ($p < .001$), effectiveness ($p = .033$), and satisfaction ($p < .001$) dimensions of MLQ. Participants' colleague assessed significant improvements for the attributed charisma ($p = .043$), inspiration ($p = .049$), idealized contribution ($p = .039$), extra effort ($p = .002$), and effectiveness ($p = .042$) dimensions of MLQ.

(continues)

Table 1
Study Characteristics, Leadership Intervention, and Behavioral Outcomes, Continued

No.	Author (Year) / Country	Objective	Study Setting and Participant	Study Design	Intervention Duration
9.	Dannels et al. (2008)/ United States and Canada	To determine whether the participants of Executive Leadership in Academic Medicine (ELAM) program aspire leadership, show mastery of leadership competencies, and attain leadership position.	78 female (professor and assistant professor) of the ELAM program compared with 468 matched controls from the Association of American Medical Colleges (AAMC) Faculty Roster and 26 women who had applied to the program but had not been accepted	Quantitative, pre and 4–5 years of follow-up, two control groups	1 year
10.	Debono et al. (2016)/ Australia	To examine the effects of "Take the Lead" program on job performance, nursing leadership, and patient experience.	30 (27 female) nursing unit managers (NUMs) and 30 (26 female) supervisors of the participants	Mixed method, postprogram	Not specified
11.	Duffield (2005)/ Australia	To describe a master class for NUMs.	18 NUMs from four hospitals, 14 evaluated	Quantitative, 6 months after program	Monthly classes for 1 year.
12.	Fennimore & Wolf (2011)/ United States	To describe an innovative approach to the development of successful nursing leaders across an integrated healthcare system.	25 nurse managers participated in the Leadership Development pilot program for Nursing Middle Managers program, 21 completed follow-ups	Mixed method, pre and 6 months of follow-up	Five 8-hour sessions conducted every alternative week for 2 months.

Intervention Content	Teaching Method	Behavioral Outcome and Assessment	Significant Finding
Executive leadership	Not clear	Subjective Researcher-developed questionnaire	Program participants reported significant improvements on 12 of 16 leadership indicators (seven leadership competencies, three administrative leadership attainments, and two leadership aspirations) compared with control groups. During follow-up, a significantly higher number of ELAM participants reported attaining higher administrative positions (63.5%) compared with the AAMC (22.5%) and nonparticipant (37%) groups. No difference in results related to academic level.
Communication, lean thinking, financial management, rostering, and leadership	Not specified	Subjective and objective Semistructured telephone interviews, researcher-developed questionnaire	Program participants exhibited improvements in job performance and leadership skills. 70% of participants and 83% of supervisors reported positive changes in job performance since their participation in the program. Most participants and supervisors reported a positive impact on leadership skills and behaviors.
Motivating staff, time management, enhancing staff performance, changing unit culture, coping with change, team building, applying leadership in practice, communication	Coaching, experiential learning, "trust walk," sharing narrations	Subjective A 26-item Likert scale evaluation	All the participants "strongly agreed" (on a 5-point Likert scale) that the program had allowed them to express opinions, stretched their mind, and encouraged networking and learning from each other. Participants reported changes in leadership behavior.
Understanding the leader within, art of nursing management, financial management, human resource issues	Assigned leadership readings, lecture, discussion, self-assessment tools, homework assignments	Subjective Modified Nurse Manager Inventory Tool and qualitative feedback	Participants reported an average raw score improvement of 0.68 for 15 different competency areas 6 months after the intervention, with an average increase of 26.7% in the domain of "the science of managing people," 20.9% in "the art of leading people," and 27.0% in "creating the leader within." Qualitative data depicted improvement in behavioral competencies in use of a reflection as a leadership behavior, foundational thinking, human resource management, and shared decision making.

(continues)

Table 1

Study Characteristics, Leadership Intervention, and Behavioral Outcomes, Continued

No.	Author (Year) / Country	Objective	Study Setting and Participant	Study Design	Intervention Duration
13.	Ford et al. (2008)/ Ireland	To describe the benefits of the Clinical Leadership program for participants, commissioners, and service users.	16 Directors of Nursing had an equivalent level of responsibility	Qualitative, postprogram	10 months
14.	Gagliano et al. (2010)/ United States	The development, implementation, and experience of the Physician Leadership Development Program.	52 midcareer physicians having leadership responsibilities in clinical practices from 12 departments at an academic medical center	Mixed method, postprogram each session and at the end of the program	2-year program, monthly 4-hour sessions, and three full-day intensive sessions.
15.	Gifford et al. (2011)/ Canada	To describe the planning and evaluation of a leadership intervention to facilitate nurses' use of guideline recommendations for diabetic foot ulcers in home healthcare.	13 nurse managers and clinical leaders	Mixed method, posttest and 3 months of follow-up	3 months: one workshop (6 hours) and three follow-up teleconferences.
16.	Gilfoyle et al. (2007)/ Canada	To evaluate learning outcomes of a leadership intervention to determine whether residents acquire and retain team leadership skills in pediatric advanced resuscitation.	15 pediatric residents	Quantitative, posttest and 6 months of follow-up with wait-list control	Half-day workshop.
17.	Graham & Jack (2008)/ United Kingdom	To evaluate how an executive nursing team developed their leadership characteristics using a professional development program.	Seven senior nurses in an acute hospital trust	Quantitative, pre and post	Not specified

Intervention Content	Teaching Method	Behavioral Outcome and Assessment	Significant Finding
Personal development, service improvement	Workshop, coaching, storytelling, mentorship, action learning, learning reflection	Subjective Qualitative feedback	Participants perceived increased self-belief resulting in improved ability to hold team members to account for their actions, lead improvement initiatives, and foster greater collaborative relationships through increased rapport.
Organizational leadership, financial management, management strategy, applied skills and tools	Lectures, case-based discussion	Subjective Researcher-developed questionnaire and group discussion	79% participants reported that they had altered their approach to specific projects or problems. Participants also reported taking larger challenges in their departments.
Leadership and planned change theory, barriers and facilitators to guideline utilization, chart audit, findings of nursing care	Identification of clinical indicators and development of action plan, reflection on leadership, discussion on leadership strategies	Subjective Researcher-developed questionnaire and interviews	During postprogram (3 months of follow-up), participants felt that leadership behaviors were influenced by the intervention. Participants reported changed leadership performance including increased engagement with staff and more, clear implementation goals. All perceived the intervention to have influenced them as leaders of guideline implementation.
Teamwork, communication, technical skills on resuscitation, avoidance of fixation errors	Group discussion, plenary session, simulation, workshop	Objective Researcher-developed questionnaire	Scores on mock leadership scenario for assigning roles, limitations of team, communication, and team atmosphere among participants were significantly higher compared with baseline and control groups.
Future perspectives of healthcare and nursing, leadership, personal development	Workshops: presentation of seminar papers and an action learning group format	Subjective Researcher-developed questionnaire	Quantitative results showed no significant change (pre–post) in behavioral aspects of leadership. Participants cited developing leadership skills during postintervention, including enabling others to make decisions, reviewing staff potential, risk taking, inspiring others, and enhancing creative thinking. Participants described better able to be action focused, democratic, and participative.

(continues)

Table 1
Study Characteristics, Leadership Intervention, and Behavioral Outcomes, Continued

No.	Author (Year) / Country	Objective	Study Setting and Participant	Study Design	Intervention Duration
18.	Krugman & Smith (2003)/ United States	To describe the development and evaluation of a permanent charge nurse role and report outcomes of this leadership model over 4 years.	104 permanent charge nurses	Quantitative, single-arm pre, post, and yearly follow-up for 4 years	2-day training workshop and follow-up at Year 2 and Year 3 based on the gaps identified.
19.	Lee et al. (2010)/ Canada	To examine the effects of a Leadership Development Initiative on the emotional health and well-being of healthcare managers.	86 (72 female) completed both presurvey and postsurvey. 13 senior leaders/directors, 20 managers, 23 operational leaders, 16 in collaborative roles, and 14 junior supervisors	Mixed method, pre and post	Not specified
20.	Leeson & Millar (2013)/ United Kingdom	To describe a short leadership program for nurse and allied health professional leaders.	Number of trainees not specified; 17/66 returned the evaluation questionnaire	Quantitative, postprogram and follow-up	2-day training workshop and follow-up at 6 weeks.
21.	Levine et al. (2008)/ United States	To describe a 2 day educational intervention for chief residents from multiple disciplines combining training in leadership and teaching in geriatric care.	47 trainees (44 chief residents) participated in three cohorts over 3 years	Mixed method, pre and post with two follow-ups at 6 and 12 months	2 days
22.	Macphee et al. (2012)/ Canada	To describe nurse leaders' perspectives of the outcomes of a formal leadership development program.	27 front-line and midlevel nurse leaders participating in the Nursing Leadership Institute program	Qualitative, postprogram	1 year

Intervention Content	Teaching Method	Behavioral Outcome and Assessment	Significant Finding
Role of the charge nurse, leadership theory, communication, delegation, conflict resolution, stress management	Workshop	Subjective and objective Leadership Practices Inventory (LPI)	Significant increase in three of the five leadership practices: challenging the process; inspiring a shared vision; and modeling the way. Observers reported a significant decrease in modeling the way, enabling others to act, and encouraging the heart. Participants rated themselves higher than observers on most of the five subscales.
Not specified	Not specified	Subjective LPI Qualitative postprogram: three focus groups and 13 individual interviews	Aspects of self-assessed leadership did not show a significant improvement except in the "inspiring a shared vision" dimension of LPI ($p < .01$). Participants expressed reluctance in changing leadership behavior when faced with continual barriers.
7 Habits for Healthcare program aims to enable participants to take initiative and responsibility, focus on priorities, practice continuous improvement, and decrease stress.	Facilitated workshop, reflection, discussion, group activities	Subjective Researcher-developed questionnaire	Delegate improvements included prioritizing, planning, and assertiveness; taking responsibility for actions; professional workplace relationships; and teamwork.
Management of perioperative issues including delirium, functional assessment, polypharmacy, and discharge planning	Fictional case discussion, mini lectures, interactive seminars, and one-to-one mentoring	Subjective Researcher-developed questionnaire, group and individual interviews	During follow-up, participants reported improved care of older patients, better leadership and conflict resolution skills, better teaching, and more interdisciplinary collaboration. Participants believed that the training would inform their future work as physicians.
Leadership development, evidence-based empowerment	A 4-day workshop, mentoring, organizational supports to implement leadership projects and virtual networking	Subjective Telephone interviews	Nurse leaders reported increased self-confidence with respect to carrying out their roles and responsibilities, positive changes in their leadership styles, and perceptions of staff recognition of positive stylistic changes.

(continues)

Table 1
Study Characteristics, Leadership Intervention, and Behavioral Outcomes, Continued

No.	Author (Year) / Country	Objective	Study Setting and Participant	Study Design	Intervention Duration
23.	Maddalena & Fleet (2015)/ Canada	To document the process used to develop an innovative Physician Management and Leadership Program.	37 participants (35 physicians) and stakeholders	Quantitative, pre, post, and 6 months of follow-up	Seven modules each of 4–7 hours in classroom and three online modules Intervention duration not specified.
24.	Malling et al. (2009)/ Denmark	To evaluate the effect of a leadership course after a Multisource Feedback (MSF) procedure compared with MSF alone regarding the development of leadership skills over time.	87 consultants responsible for postgraduate education at clinical departments 42 intervention (20 analyzed) and 45 control (nine analyzed)	Quantitative, pre–post, controlled	6 months, a 7-day course (2- to 3-day residential modules and a follow-up day).
25.	Margolis et al. (2013)/ United States	To evaluate the effects of the Interdisciplinary Leadership Development Program (ILDP) on Maternal and Child Health (MCH) trainees.	208 MCH trainees divided into ILDP participants and controls	Quantitative, postprogram survey and interviews 1–8 years	A 3-day leadership intensive workshop.
26.	Martin et al. (2012)/ Switzerland	To evaluate the impact of the adapted Royal College of Nursing Clinical Leadership Programme on the development of leadership competencies of nurse leaders.	14 (nine female) nurse leaders from a university hospital Data were also collected from 403 supervisors and colleagues of the participants	Quantitative results reported from a mixed methods study Pre–post and 6 months of follow-up	147 contact hours in 18 days over a 12-month period, with a follow-up day 6 months later.

Intervention Content	Teaching Method	Behavioral Outcome and Assessment	Significant Finding
Leadership approach, strategic planning, managing competing priorities, change management, communications, patient safety, performance development	Team and individual problem-solving activities, role playing, online exercises	Subjective and objective The follow-up evaluation consisted data from stakeholders and peers/staff regarding impact of the program on participants' leadership skills and performance	During follow-up, participants reported planned changes in the workplace because of program participation, with > 95% feeling better prepared for their leadership responsibilities. Participants self-reported more effective communication, enhancement of teamwork, development of new policies and procedures, effective conflict resolution, altered approaches to various workplace issues, and increased awareness of potentially valuable partnerships. Stakeholders/observers also reported participants applying skills learned from the program in the workplace such as conflict resolution, problem solving, and quality care initiatives.
Pedagogical knowledge, supervision skills, personal development, leadership, research	Residential workshop, team assignments, reflection	Subjective MSF instrument	No significant improvement in pre–post MSF score or between intervention and control groups.
Conflict resolution, cultural competence, minority health, and family–professional collaboration	Workshop	Subjective Researcher-developed questionnaire	Program participants reported more frequent use of interdisciplinary practices compared with nonparticipants. Participants reported using the skills to improve a specific program, organization structure/functioning, partnership, and influenced policy.
Not specified	Lectures, one-to-one coaching, action learning sets, 360° feedback, and workshops	Subjective and objective LPI	Both the participants and observer assessments showed a significant postprogram improvement in two of the five subscales: "inspiring a shared vision" and "challenging the process," which was sustained over 6 months of follow-up.

(continues)

Table 1
Study Characteristics, Leadership Intervention, and Behavioral Outcomes, Continued

No.	Author (Year) / Country	Objective	Study Setting and Participant	Study Design	Intervention Duration
27.	McAlearney et al. (2005) United States	To describe the background, development, and evaluation of a leadership program.	52 physicians (two cohorts) from an academic hospital	Quantitative, pre–post, and 1-year follow-up	20 months (hourly sessions monthly and half-day sessions twice yearly).
28.	Singer et al. (2011)/ United States	To describe a safety-oriented leadership training program for hospital managers and to assess behavior change.	108 (100, 61 female, analyzed). 12 multidisciplinary management groups comprising physicians, nurses, clinicians, and administrators	Qualitative, postprogram per session	15 months, four full-day sessions with one 2-hour follow-up.
29.	Steinert et al. (2003)/ Canada	To describe a 2-day workshop on executive skills for medical faculty and the results of an evaluation conducted 1 year later.	20 (16 analyzed) medical faculty from the Department of Family Medicine	Quantitative, postprogram and 1 year of follow-up	2 days
30. 31.	Tourangeau et al. (2003), Tourangeau (2003)/ Canada	To determine effect of Nursing Leadership Institute leadership training on self- and observer-reported leadership behavior.	67 (66 female) nurses (30 established leaders and 37 aspiring leaders) from 28 healthcare organizations Mean age: 44 years 56 dyad partners, 227 peers, and 31 supervisors	Quantitative, pre–post	5-day residency program and a follow-up booster weekend at 3 months.

Intervention Content	Teaching Method	Behavioral Outcome and Assessment	Significant Finding
Teamwork, leadership, transformational change, collaborative decision making, strategic planning, conflict resolution	Interactive discussions, presentations, teamwork, seminars	Subjective Researcher-developed questionnaire	At 1-year follow-up, participants were more effective in their current leadership roles (mean = 4.2) and working in teams (mean = 4.0), were better able to lead teams (mean = 4.3), and experienced new and expanded leadership roles (mean = 4.0). Physicians improved leadership behavior in decision making, conflict resolution, business planning, and managing people.
Appreciative inquiry, team-based leadership, communication, project management	Simulation exercise, group work, project management exercise, interviews	Subjective Analysis of transcripts from group sessions	The training increased awareness and use of leadership behaviors among managers leading to new routines and coordinated effort. Improvements included caring for patients, encouraging their staff to speak up, facilitating teamwork and communication, mobilizing resources, and seeking input. Participants rated (on a scale of 0–10) an average training impact of 8.4 at postprogram and 6.9 at 15 months of follow-up across targeted behaviors.
Time management, determining goals and priorities, leadership styles, conducting effective meetings	Workshop	Subjective Researcher-developed questionnaire	At 1 year, many participants determined their priorities more clearly, altered their time management strategies, and planned more effective meetings. Less change was noted in leadership styles and skills.
Nursing practice, business of healthcare, leadership practices, and use of self	Didactic sessions, self-reflection, small group discussion and problem-solving, coaching, and networking opportunities	Subjective and objective LPI	No significant increase in self-scores of leadership practices postprogram. Established leaders reported using more leadership behaviors than aspiring leaders in three leadership areas (challenging the process, inspiring a shared vision, and encouraging the heart). Peers reported significant increases for all five leadership practices. Supervisors and dyad partners reported significant increases for challenging the process and inspiring a shared vision.

(continues)

Table 1
Study Characteristics, Leadership Intervention, and Behavioral Outcomes, Continued

No.	Author (Year) / Country	Objective	Study Setting and Participant	Study Design	Intervention Duration
32.	Werrett et al. (2002)/ United Kingdom	To evaluate the first phase of the Leading an Empowered Organization leadership program.	550 (502 female) nurses and midwives 181 participants completed the posttest.	Quantitative, before and 3 months after program	Not specified
33.	Weston et al. (2008)/ United States	To evaluate the impact of Arizona Nurse Leadership Model on leadership knowledge and skills in novice first-line nurse supervisors.	Entry-level nursing and healthcare supervisors and managers and their immediate supervisors Sample size not reported	Quantitative, before and 2 months after program	4-day educational program spread over 2 months.

period. Nine studies (Study nos. 1, 2, 7, 17, 19, 24, 30, 32, 33) used two assessments during the preintervention and postintervention periods, and seven studies collected follow-up data (Study nos. 4, 12, 18, 21, 23, 26, 27). Dannels et al. (2008) used baseline assessments and a 4- to 5-year follow-up period. The remaining six studies (Study nos. 6, 15, 16, 20, 25, 29) used measurements during the postintervention and follow-up periods. Follow-up periods ranged from 6 weeks (Leeson & Millar, 2013) to 8 years (Margolis et al., 2013).

Effectiveness of the Interventions

Key findings related to the effects of the interventions on subjective and objective leadership behaviors are summarized in Table 2.

Subjective behavior

Subjective behavior outcomes included participants' self-reported change in behavior as a result of the leadership intervention. Of the nine studies that used standard scales to measure these outcomes, six reported a significant postprogram improvement. Among the four studies that used the LPI, three showed significant improvements on different subscales of the LPI. Significant improvements in "inspiring a shared vision" (Krugman & Smith, 2003; Lee et al., 2010; Martin et al., 2012), "challenging the process" (Krugman & Smith, 2003; Martin et al., 2012), and "modeling the way" (Krugman & Smith, 2003) were observed. In the case of Tourangeau (2003), the increase in LPI scores was not significant.

Cunningham and Kitson (2000b), using the Multifactor Leadership Questionnaire, reported significant changes in the dimensions of inspiration, active management by exception, effectiveness, and satisfaction among the nurses participating in the Clinical Nurse Leadership program. Werrett et al. (2002) found significant pre–post improvements in the Importance–Performance Scale, particularly in aspects of team and management issues, staff development, and assertiveness. Boyle and Kochinda (2004) found a significant increase in postintervention scores (56.7 in pretest to 75.3 in posttest, $p = .021$) on the Collaborative Communication Simulation Vignette (maximum score = 100). Moreover, the follow-up results showed significant improvements in self-perceived leadership and leadership and communication skills satisfaction (measured using an ICU Nurse–Physician Questionnaire) among participants. Fennimore and Wolf (2011), using a modified Nurse Manager Inventory Tool, reported an average improvement of 0.68 in scores across 15 different competency areas among nurses who participated in the Leadership Development for Nursing Middle Managers program. Competency showed major improvements, particularly in the areas of "the science of managing people," "the art of leading people," and "creating the leader within." In Malling et al. (2009), the improvement in pre–post Multisource Feedback (MSF) was not significant for the intervention group (who received both the leadership intervention

Intervention Content	Teaching Method	Behavioral Outcome and Assessment	Significant Finding
Content not specified	Not specified	Subjective Importance–Performance Scale	Significant improvement for performance in aspects of practice related to team issues, management issues, staff support and development, and creative management and assertiveness. Self-development improved but was not significant. Participants highlighted team building and personal development outcomes.
Leadership, performance measures, team building, negotiations and conflict management, communications, time management	Group assignment, case study, presentation	Subjective and objective Researcher-developed questionnaire	Both participants and supervisors rated increased competence in all areas with largest improvements in negotiating, managing conflict, and dealing with difficult people. Participants identified applying conflict management, time management, and communication skills in their workplace.

and MSF) and between the intervention and control groups, the latter of which received MSF only.

Maddalena and Fleet (2015) found that more than 95% of the participants were better prepared for leadership responsibilities, with participants reporting planned changes in the workplace because of program participation. Weston et al. (2008) reported that participants applied learned skills such as conflict, time management and communication skills. Chief residents who participated in a 2-day leadership intervention reported better leadership and conflict resolution skills, more collaboration between disciplines (Levine et al., 2008) as well as the belief that the training would affect their future work as physicians. Physicians who participated in a 20-month leadership program reported increased effectiveness in their leadership role (mean = 4.2 on a 5-point scale), teamwork abilities (mean = 4.0), ability to lead teams (mean = 4.3), and experience of new and expanded leadership roles (mean = 4.0; McAlearney et al., 2005).

Three of the four studies with control groups showed increased leadership competencies and changed behavior among the intervention groups compared with controls. Dannels et al. (2008) found significant improvements on 12 of the 16 leadership indicators for participants in the intervention group. Follow-up results also showed a significantly higher number of participants reporting attainment of a higher administrative position. Bergman et al. (2009) compared long-term support groups with a 1-week leadership intervention for healthcare managers and found that both interventions strengthened leadership roles. The 1-week course was better for inexperienced managers, whereas the long-term group benefited experienced managers. Interdisciplinary Leadership Development Program participants improved their interdisciplinary practices more than nonparticipants (Margolis et al., 2013). Malling et al. (2009) did not find significant differences in pre–post MSF between intervention and control groups.

Castillo and James (2013) found that 70% of the training participants reported improved leadership behavior because of training, including being a role model, encouraging problem solving, and critical thinking. Moreover, Debono et al. (2016) found that 70% of participants reported improvements in job performance after the leadership program. In Gagliano et al. (2010), 79% of the physicians participating in the Leadership Development Program reported a change in their approach to specific projects and greater positivity in addressing problems. In addition, more than 65% of the nurses who participated in a web-based leadership course reported improved confidence in applying skills such as change management, conflict resolution, and ethical decision making (Brown et al., 2003).

Other qualitative studies also had similar results, with participants reporting changed leadership behavior and performance because of the intervention (Boomer & McCormack, 2010; Ford et al., 2008; Gifford et al., 2011; Macphee et al., 2012). Participants reported consciously seeking positive

Table 2
Subjective and Objective Behavior Findings for Intervention Effectiveness

Scale	Key Finding
Subjective Behavior	
Leadership Practices Inventory	Significant improvements in "inspiring a shared vision" (Krugman & Smith, 2003; Lee et al., 2010; Martin et al., 2012), "challenging the process" (Krugman & Smith, 2003; Martin et al., 2012), and "modeling the way" (Krugman & Smith, 2003). Tourangeau et al. (2003) showed no significant improvements.
Multifactor Leadership Questionnaire	Significant improvements in dimensions of inspiration, active management by exception, effectiveness, and satisfaction (Cunningham & Kitson, 2000b).
Importance–Performance Scale	Significant improvements—especially in team and management issues, staff development, and assertiveness (Werrett et al., 2002).
Collaborative Communication Simulation Vignette	Significantly higher postintervention scores (Boyle & Kochinda, 2004).
ICU Nurse–Physician Questionnaire	Significant improvement at follow-up in self-perceived leadership as well as leadership and communication skills satisfaction (Boyle & Kochinda, 2004).
Modified Nurse Manager Inventory Tool	Significant improvements, particularly in the dimensions "the science of managing people," "the art of leading people," and "creating the leader within" (Fennimore & Wolf, 2011).
Multisource Feedback	No significant improvement in the intervention group and no difference compared with the control group (Malling et al., 2009).
Other assessments	Better prepared for leadership responsibilities and workplace reform (Maddalena & Fleet, 2015).
	Applying conflict and time management as well as communication skills (Weston et al., 2008).
	Better leadership and conflict resolution skills; improved collaboration. Training would affect their future work (Levine et al., 2008).
	Increased leadership effectiveness, teamwork, and ability to lead and develop new and expanded leadership roles (McAlearney et al., 2005).
	Participants became more proactive, better at prioritizing and planning, and took responsibility for actions (Leeson & Millar, 2013).
	Improved leadership behavior, including being a role model, encouraging problem solving, and critical thinking (Castillo & James, 2013).
	Improvements in job performance (Debono et al., 2016).
	Modified approach to projects and addressing problems positively (Gagliano et al., 2010).
	Reevaluation of leadership skills and confidence in applying skills such as change management, conflict resolution, and ethical decision making (Brown et al., 2003).
	Improved action-focused, democratic, and participative approaches (Graham & Jack, 2008).
	At 1-year follow-up, participants were less satisfied with the changes they could make in leadership style and skills (Steinert et al., 2003).
Objective Behavior	
Leadership Practices Inventory completed by observers	Observers reported significant subscale improvements in "inspiring a shared vision" and "challenging the process" (Martin et al., 2012).
	Supervisors and dyad partners both reported significant improvements in "challenging the process" and "inspiring a shared vision," and peers reported significant improvements across all five subscales (Tourangeau et al., 2003).
	Observers reported significant decreases in the subscales "modeling the way," "enabling others to act," and "encouraging the heart" (Krugman & Smith, 2003).
Multifactor Leadership Questionnaire completed by observers	Observers reported significant improvements in the charisma, inspiration, idealized contribution, extra effort, and effectiveness dimensions (Cunningham & Kitson, 2000a, 2000b).
Modified ICU Nurse–Physician Questionnaire completed by unit staff	Significant improvements in collaborative communication, problem solving, and leadership (Boyle & Kochinda, 2004).

(continues)

Table 2
Subjective and Objective Behavior Findings for Intervention Effectiveness, Continued

Scale	Key Finding
Other assessments	Positive impact on leadership skills and improvement in job performance (Debono et al., 2016). Improvements in leadership behaviors of conflict management (Maddalena & Fleet, 2015; Weston et al., 2008), problem solving (Maddalena & Fleet, 2015), dealing with difficult people (Weston et al., 2008), and better teamwork and communication (Boomer & McCormack, 2010). Significantly improved performance in a mock leadership scenario at 6 months of follow-up compared with baseline and control groups (Gilfoyle et al., 2007).

behavioral change such as having a positive attitude, encouraging others to speak up, facilitating communication, and seeking input from colleagues (Singer et al., 2011). Other behavioral changes reported included becoming more reflexive (Boomer & McCormack, 2010; Fennimore & Wolf, 2011), facilitating teamwork (Study nos. 3, 6, 20, 23, 28, 32), effective conflict resolution (Brown et al., 2003; Levine et al., 2008; Maddalena & Fleet, 2015; Weston et al., 2008), and time management (Steinert et al., 2003; Weston et al., 2008).

Graham and Jack (2008) found no significant pre–post change in the quantitative results related to leadership behavior among leadership program participants. However, participants in qualitative interviews described being better able to be action focused, democratic, and participative. Steinert et al. (2003), at 1-year follow-up, found the participants in their study less satisfied with the changes they could make in leadership style and skills.

Interventions that incorporated the elements of personal development planning, self-directed learning, and reflection achieved relatively better results. Developing a leadership action plan and a practice-based action learning project (Study nos. 3, 6, 7, 13, 15, 17, 21, 26) was particularly effective in supporting the participants to operationalize leadership strategies and become more engaged with unit staff.

Objective behavior

Nine of the included studies reported objective behavior outcomes, including behavioral change exhibited by the participants as observed and rated by supervisors, colleagues, peers, and/or staff from the working unit of the participants (Table 2). Gilfoyle et al. (2007) used a mock leadership scenario to assess the effect of a leadership intervention, and hence it was considered an objective outcome in this review.

Three studies administered the LPI to the observers of the training participants. Martin et al. (2012) found that observers reported significant improvements in the "inspiring a shared vision" and "challenging the process" subscales of the LPI. Tourangeau et al. (2003) distinguished the observers into supervisors, dyad partners, and peers, with supervisors and dyad partners both reporting significant improvements in "challenging the process" and "inspiring a shared vision" and peers reporting significant improvements in all of the five subscales of the LPI. Conversely, in Krugman and Smith (2003), observers reported a significant decrease in the "modeling the way," "enabling others to act," and "encouraging the heart" subscales of the LPI. Observers, including colleagues of the participants, reported significant improvements in the dimensions of charisma, inspiration, idealized contribution, extra effort, and effectiveness on the Multifactor Leadership Questionnaire (Cunningham & Kitson, 2000a, 2000b). The unit staff in Boyle and Kochinda (2004) reported significant improvements in collaborative communication, problem solving, and nursing leadership, as measured using a modified ICU Nurse–Physician Questionnaire at 6 months of follow-up.

The supervisors of nurses participating in the leadership program reported a positive impact on the leadership skills (79%) and job performance (83%) of the nurses who participated in the program (Debono et al., 2016). In other studies, the observers rated postintervention improvements in leadership behaviors such as conflict management (Maddalena & Fleet, 2015; Weston et al., 2008), problem solving (Maddalena & Fleet, 2015), dealing with difficult people (Weston et al., 2008), and better teamwork and communication (Boomer & McCormack, 2010). Gilfoyle et al. (2007) found significantly improved performance during a 6-month follow-up of the mock leadership scenario among trainees who participated in a half-day workshop compared with both baseline and the control group.

Discussion

The primary aim of this study was to review the behavioral outcomes of leadership interventions that were conducted on health professionals. This review shows the beneficial effects on the leadership behavior of participants across a range of leadership interventions. Specific behavioral improvements as perceived by participants as well as observers were observed postprogram for most courses. The participants were found to implement more efficient processes and to engage more frequently with staff (Debono et al., 2016). Six of the nine studies that used standard leadership behavior scales (Study nos. 4, 7, 18, 19, 26, 32) showed significant postprogram improvement. Castillo and James (2013) identified change in organizational culture, with constructive use of feedback and improved communication. Both participants and observers reported the effective use of learned skills such as conflict resolution, communication, time management, teamwork, problem solving, critical thinking, and being reflective.

This review identified that the methods and processes used to implement leadership interventions are important in improving leadership behavior among participants. In this review, programs that targeted personal development, self-direction, and reflection were more likely to produce behavioral outcomes. Moreover, activities that were designed to assist participants to operationalize leadership strategies were particularly effective. Leadership action plans and practice-based action projects assisted participants to implement practical leadership strategies and promote staff engagement. Moreover, these action plans provided a tangible framework for showing leadership behavior and tracking the progress of leadership development (Gifford et al., 2011).

Among the included studies that used observer (e.g., supervisor, peer, or unit staff) ratings, most found that observers rated the participants' leadership behavior higher than participant self-ratings (Martin et al., 2012; Tourangeau, 2003; Tourangeau et al., 2003; Weston et al., 2008). Thus, objective observations are more likely to show the benefits of the leadership interventions. In general, objective behavior, as reported by the observers, improved from preintervention to postintervention. Unit staff perceived changes in participant behavior as the participants became more approachable, encouraging, and supporting (Maddalena & Fleet, 2015).

There is evidence across the studies showing improved leadership development where interventions use face-to-face delivery and showing that participants valued the opportunities provided by this mode of delivery. Participants from the included studies that used online course also preferred face-to-face delivery and reported that the absence of nonverbal cues and body language impeded their learning progress (Brown et al., 2003). Furthermore, participants in the included studies that used face-to-face courses valued the networking opportunities (Debono et al., 2016; Levine et al., 2008) and feedback from peers (Gagliano et al., 2010). Participants perceived these events as an opportunity to collaborate with other like-minded professionals (Lee et al., 2010).

This review identified the difficulties of and barriers to translating learned knowledge and skills into action. Steinert et al. (2003) argued that one of the reasons for failing to implement behavioral changes was the absence of dedicated workshop time during the sessions to apply their newly learned skills. In addition, leadership behavioral change may require time and experience. Other training areas such as resilience have shown context and experience as important to effective training outcomes (Cleary et al., 2018). Boomer and McCormack (2010) identified that lack of support from organization leaders adversely affected the articulation of learned skills into practice. Lee et al. (2010) further observed that, although leadership development programs often promote and encourage leadership practice, recurrent organizational barriers make participants reluctant to initiate and continue efforts to change. The increasing incongruities between workplace reality and leadership idealism promoted in training programs may result in a sense of isolation, skepticism, and frustration among program participants (Spiers et al., 2010). Furthermore, participants who are involved in a leadership development intervention may hold the preconception that senior executives are not in favor of change and that organizational culture inhibits change (Lee et al., 2010). Iles and Preece (2006) posited that "leadership development" differs from "the development of leaders." Interventions aiming to develop leadership, in addition to focusing on individual skill development, should consider the social, cultural, and political contexts of the organization in which behavioral change is expected. Leadership should not be considered as an individual activity but rather as a collective cultural activity with collective identity, interdependence, and collaborative accountability.

Program Implications

Efforts to improve leadership behavior among health professionals should involve the active collaboration and support of senior executives. As leadership is a team process, the entire organization should facilitate sustainable change in leadership. Face-to-face courses are recommended, as they support collegial feedback and provide networking opportunities to positively impact learning, behavioral change, and professional development. Training should incorporate elements of work-based and experiential learning. Interventions in which participants determine behavioral change needs, develop action plans, and have opportunities to apply these in real scenarios are more likely to succeed. Assessments performed with participants before training help identify the appropriate content and focuses for training interventions (Collins & Holton, 2004). Changing leadership behavior is a long-term process that requires continuous and sustained interventions and long-term follow-up.

Research Implications

Few studies have assessed the leadership behavior of health professionals using a robust evaluation design. Studies evaluating leadership interventions with a focus on leadership behavior should use specific leadership behavioral outcome measures, a strong evaluation design, and multiple outcome assessments. Studies should consider confounders that may have significantly affect leadership behavior. In evaluating leadership interventions, Saleh et al. (2004) recommended considering factors such as the support of senior executives, organizational culture (openness to change), organizational resources, and the opportunity to apply learning. Randomized control designs with wait-list controls and studies with an adequate sample size and follow-up periods are required to identify the long-term effects of the interventions.

Limitations

The considerable heterogeneity among the studies precluded a quantitative synthesis of the results. In addition, this review found that most interventions focus on individuals and thus ignore teamwork and collaboration. Most of the included studies on the behavioral impact of leadership interventions adopted a narrow set of outcome measures that primarily addressed self-reported behavioral change. Furthermore, as only a few of the included studies used control groups and none used a randomized control trial design, it is possible that other, unaccounted-for factors may have contributed to the outcomes. This review may also experience publication bias, as negative and nonsignificant findings may not have been published. The use of small sample sizes and self-selected convenience sampling in most of the included studies is another limitation that may affect the outcomes of this review. Finally, in many of the included studies, the researchers were also responsible for implementing the change in training programs and/or developing the training resources.

Conclusions

The culture of healthcare is defined by constant development, where effective leadership is central to addressing and managing change. Leadership development programs produce positive results, including implementation of efficient processes, staff engagement, and improved satisfaction for patients and staffs. This review identified many supporting factors for successful leadership development programs. Interventions that are designed to promote leadership development require preplanning, leadership needs assessments, considerations of organizational context, strong focuses on self-awareness and collaboration, experiential work-based learning to apply skills within the desired context, and proper evaluation and incentivization. The successful development of leadership in healthcare professionals promotes evidence-based best practice, positive organizational culture, and improved patient outcomes and keeps healthcare responsive to its ever-changing environment.

Acknowledgments

This work was supported by University of Tasmania funding awarded under the UTAS Research Theme: Better Health Research Development Grant Scheme, supported by the Office of the Deputy Vice-Chancellor and the Faculty of Health (C0025653).

Author Contributions

Study conception and design: MC, DV, RK, DKT
Data collection: MC, DV, RK, DKT
Data analysis and interpretation: All authors
Drafting of the article: All authors
Critical revision of the article: All authors

References

Ackerman, M., Malloch, K., Wade, D., Porter-O'Grady, T., Weberg, D., Zurmehly, J., & Raderstorf, T. (2019). The master in healthcare innovation: A new paradigm in healthcare leadership development. *Nurse Leader, 17*(1), 49–53. https://doi.org/10.1016/j.mnl.2018.09.010

Agius, S. J., Brockbank, A., Baron, R., Farook, S., & Hayden, J. (2015). The impact of an integrated medical leadership programme. *Journal of Health Organization and Management, 29*(1), 39–54. https://doi.org/10.1108/JHOM-09-2013-0188

Barr, J., & Dowding, L. (2019). *Leadership in health care* (4th ed.). Sage Publications Limited.

Bergman, D., Fransson-Sellgren, S., Wahlström, R., & Sandahl, C. (2009). Healthcare leadership: Impact of short-term intensive and long-term less intensive training programmes. *Leadership in Health Services, 22*(2), 161–175. https://doi.org/10.1108/17511870910953805

Blaney, P. (2012). Senior nursing leadership—Capacity building at the global level. *International Nursing Review, 59*(1), 40–47. https://doi.org/10.1111/j.1466-7657.2011.00953.x

Boomer, C. A., & McCormack, B. (2010). Creating the conditions for growth: A collaborative practice development programme for clinical nurse leaders. *Journal of Nursing Management, 18*(6), 633–644. https://doi.org/10.1111/j.1365-2834.2010.01143.x

Boyle, D. K., & Kochinda, C. (2004). Enhancing collaborative communication of nurse and physician leadership in two intensive care units. *Journal of Nursing Administration, 34*(2), 60–70. https://doi.org/10.1097/00005110-200402000-00003

Brown, S. T., Kirkpatrick, M. K., & Wrisley, C. D. (2003). Evaluative parameters of a web-based nursing leadership course from the learners' perspectives. *Journal of Nursing Education, 42*(3), 134–137.

Castillo, C., & James, S. (2013). How to turn ward managers into leaders. *Nursing Times, 109*(9), 18–19.

Cleary, M., Freeman, A., & Sharrock, L. (2005). The development, implementation, and evaluation of a clinical leadership program for mental health nurses. *Issues in Mental Health Nursing, 26*(8), 827–842. https://doi.org/10.1080/01612840500184277

Cleary, M., Kornhaber, R., Thapa, D. K., West, S., & Visentin, D. (2018). The effectiveness of interventions to improve resilience among health professionals: A systematic review. *Nurse Education Today, 71*, 247–263. https://doi.org/10.1016/j.nedt.2018.10.002

Collins, D. B., & Holton, E. F. (2004). The effectiveness of managerial leadership development programs: A meta-analysis of studies from 1982 to 2001. *Human Resource Development Quarterly, 15*(2), 217–248. https://doi.org/10.1002/hrdq.1099

Cunningham, G., & Kitson, A. (2000a). An evaluation of the RCN clinical leadership development programme: Part 1. *Nursing Standard, 15*(12), 34–37. https://doi.org/10.7748/ns2000.12.15.12.34.c2953

Cunningham, G., & Kitson, A. (2000b). An evaluation of the RCN clinical leadership development programme: Part 2. *Nursing Standard, 15*(13–15), 34–40. https://doi.org/10.7748/ns2000.12.15.13.34.c2956

Cutcliffe, J., & Cleary, M. (2015). Nursing leadership, missing questions, and the elephant (s) in the room: Problematizing the discourse on nursing leadership. *Issues in Mental Health Nursing, 36*(10), 817–825. https://doi.org/10.3109/01612840.2015.1042176

Daly, J., Jackson, D., Mannix, J., Davidson, P. M., & Hutchinson, M. (2014). The importance of clinical leadership in the hospital setting. *Journal of Healthcare Leadership, 6*, 75–83. https://doi.org/10.2147/JHL.S46161

Dannels, S. A., Yamagata, H., McDade, S. A., Chuang, Y.-C., Gleason, K. A., McLaughlin, J. M., Richman, R. C., & Morahan, P. S. (2008). Evaluating a leadership program: A comparative, longitudinal study to assess the impact of the Executive Leadership in Academic Medicine (ELAM) program for women. *Academic Medicine, 83*(5), 488–495. https://doi.org/10.1097/ACM.0b013e31816be551

Debono, D., Travaglia, J. F., Dunn, A. G., Thoms, D., Hinchcliff, R., Plumb, J., Milne, J., Erez-Rein, N., Wiley, J., & Braithwaite, J. (2016). Strengthening the capacity of nursing leaders through multifaceted professional development initiatives: A mixed method evaluation of the 'Take the Lead' program. *Collegian, 23*(1), 19–28. https://doi.org/10.1016/j.colegn.2014.09.005

Dellve, L., Skagert, K., & Vilhelmsson, R. (2007). Leadership in workplace health promotion projects: 1- and 2-year effects on long-term work attendance. *European Journal of Public Health, 17*(5), 471–476. https://doi.org/10.1093/eurpub/ckm004

Duffield, C. (2005). A master class for nursing unit managers: An Australian example. *Journal of Nursing Management, 13*(1), 68–73. https://doi.org/10.1111/j.1365-2834.2004.00489.x

Fennimore, L., & Wolf, G. (2011). Nurse manager leadership development: Leveraging the evidence and system-level support. *Journal of Nursing Administration, 41*(5), 204–210. https://doi.org/10.1097/NNA.0b013e3182171aff

Ford, P., Wynne, M., Rice, M., & Grogan, C. (2008). A partnership approach to leadership development for directors of nursing in older people's services in Ireland—Articulating the impact. *Journal of Nursing Management, 16*(2), 159–166. https://doi.org/10.1111/j.1365-2834.2007.00840.x

Frich, J. C., Brewster, A. L., Cherlin, E. J., & Bradley, E. H. (2015). Leadership development programs for physicians: A systematic review. *Journal of General Internal Medicine, 30*(5), 656–674. https://doi.org/10.1007/s11606-014-3141-1

Gagliano, N. J., Ferris, T., Colton, D., Dubitzky, A., Hefferman, J., & Torchiana, D. (2010). A physician leadership development program at an academic medical center. *Quality Management in Healthcare, 19*(3), 231–238. https://doi.org/10.1097/QMH.0b013e3181eb13ab

Gifford, W., Davies, B., Tourangeau, A., & Lefebre, N. (2011). Developing team leadership to facilitate guideline utilization: Planning and evaluating a 3-month intervention strategy. *Journal of Nursing Management, 19*(1), 121–132. https://doi.org/10.1111/j.1365-2834.2010.01140.x

Gilfoyle, E., Gottesman, R., & Razack, S. (2007). Development of a leadership skills workshop in paediatric advanced resuscitation. *Medical Teacher, 29*(9), e276–e283. https://doi.org/10.1080/01421590701663287

Graham, I. W., & Jack, E. (2008). Promoting leadership: The development of a nurse executive team in an acute hospital trust. *Journal of Nursing Management, 16*(8), 955–963. https://doi.org/10.1111/j.1365-2834.2008.00915.x

Iles, P., & Preece, D. (2006). Developing leaders or developing leadership? The academy of chief executives' programmes in the north east of England. *Leadership, 2*(3), 317–340. https://doi.org/10.1177/1742715006066024

Jiménez, P., Bregenzer, A., Kallus, K. W., Fruhwirth, B., & Wagner-Hartl, V. (2017). Enhancing resources at the workplace with health-promoting leadership. *International Journal of Environmental Research and Public Health, 14*(10), 1264. https://doi.org/10.3390/ijerph14101264

Kirkpatrick, D. L., & Kirkpatrick, J. D. (2009). *Implementing the four levels: A practical guide for effective evaluation of training programs* (2nd ed.). Berrett-Koehler.

Krugman, M., & Smith, V. (2003). Charge nurse leadership development and evaluation. *Journal of Nursing Administration, 33*(5), 284–292. https://doi.org/10.1097/00005110-200305000-00004

Kwamie, A., van Dijk, H., & Agyepong, I. A. (2014). Advancing the application of systems thinking in health: Realist evaluation of the leadership development programme for district manager decision-making in Ghana. *Health Research Policy and Systems, 12*, 29. https://doi.org/10.1186/1478-4505-12-29

Lee, H., Spiers, J. A., Yurtseven, O., Cummings, G. G., Sharlow, J., Bhatti, A., & Germann, P. (2010). Impact of leadership development on emotional health in healthcare managers. *Journal of Nursing Management, 18*(8), 1027–1039. https://doi.org/10.1111/j.1365-2834.2010.01178.x

Leeson, D., & Millar, M. (2013). Using the 7 habits programme to develop effective leadership. *Nursing Management, 20*(6), 31–37. https://doi.org/10.7748/nm2013.10.20.6.31.e1123

Levine, S. A., Chao, S. H., Brett, B., Jackson, A. H., Burrows, A. B., Goldman, L. N., & Caruso, L. B. (2008). Chief resident immersion training in the care of older adults: An innovative interspecialty education and leadership intervention. *Journal of the American Geriatrics Society, 56*(6), 1140–1145. https://doi.org/10.1111/j.1532-5415.2008.01710.x

Liberati, A., Altman, D. G., Tetzlaff, J., Mulrow, C., Gøtzsche, P. C., Ioannidis, J. P. A., Clarke, M., Devereaux, P. J., Kleijnen, J., & Moher, D. (2009). The PRISMA statement for reporting systematic reviews and meta-analyses of studies that evaluate health care interventions: Explanation and elaboration. *PLOS MEDICINE, 6*(7), e1000100. https://doi.org/10.1371/journal.pmed.1000100

Macphee, M., Skelton-Green, J., Bouthillette, F., & Suryaprakash, N. (2012). An empowerment framework for nursing leadership development: Supporting evidence. *Journal of Advanced Nursing, 68*(1), 159–169. https://doi.org/10.1111/j.1365-2648.2011.05746.x

Maddalena, V., & Fleet, L. (2015). Developing a Physician Management & Leadership Program (PMLP) in Newfoundland and Labrador. *Leadership in Health Services, 28*(1), 35–42. https://doi.org/10.1108/LHS-02-2014-0012

Malling, B., Mortensen, L., Bonderup, T., Scherpbier, A., & Ringsted, C. (2009). Combining a leadership course and multi-source feedback has no effect on leadership skills of leaders in postgraduate medical education. An intervention study with a control group. *BMC Medical Education, 9*(1), 72. https://doi.org/10.1186/1472-6920-9-72

Marchionni, C., & Ritchie, J. (2008). Organizational factors that support the implementation of a nursing best practice guideline. *Journal of Nursing Management, 16*(3), 266–274. https://doi.org/10.1111/j.1365-2834.2007.00775.x

Margolis, L. H., Rosenberg, A., Umble, K., & Chewning, L. (2013). Effects of interdisciplinary training on MCH professionals, organizations and systems. *Maternal and Child Health Journal, 17*(5), 949–958. https://doi.org/10.1007/s10995-012-1078-8

Martin, J. S., Mccormack, B., Fitzsimons, D., & Spirig, R. (2012). Evaluation of a clinical leadership programme for nurse leaders. *Journal of Nursing Management, 20*(1), 72–80. https://doi.org/10.1111/j.1365-2834.2011.01271.x

McAlearney, A. S. (2008). Using leadership development programs to improve quality and efficiency in healthcare. *Journal of Healthcare Management, 53*(5), 319–331.

McAlearney, A. S., Fisher, D., Heiser, K., Robbins, D., & Kelleher, K. (2005). Developing effective physician leaders: Changing cultures and transforming organizations. *Hospital Topics, 83*(2), 11–18.

Murdock, J., & Brammer, C. (2011). A successful model of leadership development for community practice physicians. *Physician Executive, 37*(2), 52–54.

Peters, L. (2019). Leading culture change: Moving from here to there. In L. Peters (Ed.), *The simple truths about leadership* (pp. 73–96). Palgrave Macmillan. https://doi.org/10.1007/978-3-030-03958-5_7

Saleh, S. S., Williams, D., & Balougan, M. (2004). Evaluating the effectiveness of public health leadership training: The NEPHLI experience. *American Journal of Public Health, 94*(7), 1245–1249. https://doi.org/10.2105/AJPH.94.7.1245

Singer, S. J., Hayes, J., Cooper, J. B., Vogt, J. W., Sales, M., Aristidou, A., Gray, G. C., Kiang, M. V., & Meyer, G. S. (2011). A case for safety leadership team training of hospital managers. *Health Care Management Review, 36*(2), 188–200. https://doi.org/10.1097/HMR.0b013e318208cd1d

Spiers, J. A., Cummings, G. G., Langenhoff, P., Sharlow, J., & Bhatti, A. (2010). "But we can't go back": The effect of raising expectations through organizational leadership development and consequences of failure to follow through. *Journal of Leadership Studies, 4*(1), 6–19. https://doi.org/10.1002/jls.20151

Steinert, Y., Nasmith, L., & Daigle, N. (2003). Executive skills for medical faculty: A workshop description and evaluation. *Medical Teacher, 25*(6), 666–668. https://doi.org/10.1080/0142159032000150485

Suhonen, R., Stolt, M., & Charalambous, A. (2019). Supporting individualised nursing care by leadership. In R. Suhonen, M. Stolt, & E. Papastavrou (Eds.), *Individualized care: Theory, measurement and practice* (1st ed., pp. 195–205). Springer International Publishing.

Tourangeau, A. E. (2003). Building nurse leader capacity. *Journal of Nursing Administration, 33*(12), 624–626.

Tourangeau, A. E., Lemonde, M., Luba, M., Dakers, D., & Alksnis, C. (2003). Evaluation of a leadership development intervention. *Nursing Leadership, 16*(3), 91–104.

Turner, P. (2019). Assessing health professionals for succession and leadership roles. In P. Turner (Ed.), *Leadership in healthcare: Delivering organisational transformation and operational excellence* (pp. 263–293). Palgrave Macmillan.

Werrett, J., Griffiths, M., & Clifford, C. (2002). A regional evaluation of the impact of the leading an empowered organisation leadership programme. *NT Research, 7*(6), 459–470. https://doi.org/10.1177/136140960200700607

Weston, M. J., Falter, B., Lamb, G. S., Mahon, G., Malloch, K., Provan, K. G., Roe, S., & Werbylo, L. (2008). Health care leadership academy: A statewide collaboration to enhance nursing leadership competencies. *The Journal of Continuing Education in Nursing, 39*(10), 468–472. https://doi.org/10.3928/00220124-20081001-09

21

Properties of the Early Symptom Measurement of Post-Stroke Depression: Concurrent Criterion Validity and Cutoff Scores

Jufang LI[1,6] • Linda Denise OAKLEY[2,6] • Roger L. BROWN[3] • Yun LI[4] • Yong LUO[5]*

ABSTRACT

Background: Early-stage post-stroke depression (PSD) increases the risk of stroke-related disability and mortality in the first year of recovery. Presently available screening measures were developed to assess major depression, and none used a PSD screening criterion that was systematically developed and tested in populations of patients with acute stroke.

Purpose: The purpose of this study was to evaluate the concurrent criterion validity and cutoff scoring of the Early Symptom Measurement of Post-Stroke Depression (ESM-PSD) instrument in hospitalized patients with acute stroke.

Methods: Purposive recruitment of newly admitted patients yielded a qualified sample of 139 nonaphasic participants who were 7–30 days post mild-to-moderate stroke confirmed by computed tomography and magnetic resonance images. Participants responded to the ESM-PSD and Hamilton Rating Scale for Depression-24 (HAMD-24).

Results: The mean number of post-stroke days was 11.99 (*SD* = 7.68). Cronbach's alpha estimates of internal consistency were ESM-PSD = .90 and HAMD-24 = .76. ESM-PSD measurement sensitivity and specificity were superior. The following three ESM-PSD cutoff scores, determined by the receiver operating characteristic curve, were used to assess clinically relevant early-symptom levels: no PSD < 14.5, low PSD = 14.5–25.5, moderate PSD = 25.5–45.5, high PSD ≥ 45.5.

Conclusion/Implications for Practice: ESM-PSD cutoff scores show the expected correspondence with mild–moderate–severe HAMD-24 symptoms, which was evidenced by the high area under the receiver operating characteristic curve. Planned follow-up research will assess the efficacy of using ESM-PSD scores to detect increased risk of major depression onset in patients with acute stroke.

Key Words:
post-stroke depression (PSD), concurrent criterion validity, patients with acute stroke, cutoff scores.

Introduction

Early-stage post-stroke depression (PSD) refers to PSD occurring within the first 30 days post-stroke, which is the time period of peak symptom onset (Gao, 2015; Zhang, Zeng, & Liu, 2015). Research has shown that more than one third of hospitalized patients with stroke are likely to develop symptoms of early-stage PSD (Towfighi et al., 2017). With incidence rates ranging from 25% to 79%, PSD following mild-to-moderate stroke is both common and one of the most severe complications in patients with acute stroke (Mitchell et al., 2017; Zahi, Mahir, Azanmasso, Lmidmani, & El Fatimi, 2016). Early symptoms of PSD increase the risk of major depression onset at 6 months post-stroke, the stage of recovery where the risk of disability and death by suicide may reach as high as 70%–90% (Lewin-Richter, Volz, Jobges, & Werheid, 2015). In other words, the morbidity and mortality risks of PSD equal or exceed the morbidity and mortality risks of mild-to-moderate stroke. This is due in large part to the effects of early-stage PSD on prognosis and quality of life outcomes (Bartoli et al., 2013; Koositamongkol, Sindhu, Pinyopasakul, Nilanont, & Redman, 2013; Schulte-Altedorneburg & Bereczki, 2014).

PSD complicates the recovery of speech and motor functions and decreases the ability and desire to participate in rehabilitation, to socialize, and to "rejoin" life (Dwyer Hollender, 2014; Towfighi et al., 2017). Neurobiological findings show that early-stage PSD may increase the 1-year risk of stroke recurrence by as high as 49%, even with treatment with antidepressant medications (Yuan et al., 2012). Moreover, early-stage PSD increases the risk of chronic depression. A retrospective study found that 68.7% of patients diagnosed with chronic PSD also

[1]PhD, RN, Associate Professor, School of Nursing, Wenzhou Medical University, Wenzhou, Zhejiang, PRC • [2]PhD, RN, Professor, School of Nursing, University of Wisconsin-Madison, Madison, Wisconsin, USA • [3]PhD, Professor, School of Nursing, University of Wisconsin-Madison, Madison, Wisconsin, USA • [4]BSN, RN, Supervisor Nurse, Neurological Department, The First Affiliated Hospital of Wenzhou Medical University, Wenzhou, Zhejiang, PRC • [5]MD, Professor, Neurological Department, The First Affiliated Hospital of Chongqing Medical University, Chongqing, PRC • [6]Contributed equally as first author.

had early PSD symptoms (Shi et al., 2016). Also, early-stage PSD at 6 and 12 months has been shown to be associated with stroke-related mortality at 12 and 24 months post-stroke (Lewin-Richter et al., 2015). In recognition of the clinical risks of early-stage PSD, clinicians are now expected to identify and effectively manage early-stage PSD symptoms (Schneider & Schneider, 2012). However, because both outcomes are poorly understood (Robinson & Jorge, 2015), few patients with acute stroke are likely to receive timely and effective assessment and management. The central problem is the lack of screening tools specifically developed to detect symptoms of early-stage PSD in patients with acute stroke.

Background

Several clinical assumptions decrease the probability that any symptoms of PSD are adequately assessed during the first 30 days post-stroke. First, clinicians who are confident in the treatment imperative to prioritize physical symptoms during the acute post-stroke stage are less likely to treat symptoms of depression (Li, 2016). Second, proper mental healthcare services often are not available or accessible to hospital patients. Third, studies show that the prognosis and emotions of patients during the acute stage may be unstable, thereby increasing the probability that any findings from a psychological assessment may not be reliable or stable. Although these observations cannot be dismissed, they incorrectly assume that early symptoms of PSD in the patients with acute stroke are clinically less important and have negligible risk of severe morbidity and mortality. Study findings have shown that assessing early symptoms of PSD when assessing the physical symptoms of mild-to-moderate stroke may decrease the risk of PSD and major depression onset at 6 months.

Most of the related research in the literature are studies of late-onset symptoms of depression in recovering patients with stroke who meet diagnostic criteria for major depression, or major depression is reconceptualized, using lower scores, as a milder form of the illness (Li, Oakley, Li, & Luo, 2018). The aim of these assessments is thus primarily to detect symptoms of major depression or dysthymic depression in patients with a history of stroke. In contrast, this study addresses clinical problems related to assessing, detecting, and managing PSD as a unique condition on the depression spectrum, with early-stage PSD defined as the onset of symptoms and somatic signs in the acute (first 30 days) post-stroke stage (Li et al., 2016). Early-stage patients are more likely to show symptoms of depression with vegetative state and impaired social skills related to psychological dysfunctions (Tateno, Kimura, & Robinson, 2002), whereas major depression is a state of depressed mood characterized by slow thinking and less activity. Time frame, the important distinction between PSD and major depression, complicates the assessment of early-stage PSD (Li, 2016). The 2-week time frame for assessing and diagnosing symptoms of major depression is a better fit with preexisting or prestroke symptoms of depression than early-onset symptoms of PSD within a few days post-stroke (Shi et al., 2015).

The PSD measure in this study was developed (Li et al., 2018), and preliminary psychometric testing was conducted (Li et al., 2016) of a revised version of the Early Symptom Measurement of Post-Stroke Depression (ESM-PSD) using separate samples of hospitalized patients with stroke who were 7–30 days post-stroke. The ESM-PSD, designed for use as an assessment tool, has been shown to have acceptable internal reliability (total Cronbach's α = .93, domains = .82–.90) and discriminant validity in patients with acute stroke. The specific aim of this study was to use the Hamilton Rating Scale for Depression-24 (HAMD-24) to evaluate the concurrent criterion validity and scoring of the ESM-PSD in hospitalized patients with acute stroke. Acceptable evidence of ESM-PSD concurrent criterion validity and clinically relevant scoring would allow the testing of the validity and reliability of the ESM-PSD to assess and detect early-stage PSD in hospitalized patients with early-stage stroke and to compare ESM-PSD scores with 3-month, 6-month, and 9-month follow-up assessments of symptoms of major depression.

Methods

Sample

Purposive recruitment methods were used over a period of 6 months from March to August in 2015 to develop a qualified sample of adult patients with stroke newly admitted to a general hospital in southeast China. Eligible male and female patients were 18 years old or older, had a primary admission diagnosis of mild or moderate stroke as confirmed by computed tomography and magnetic resonance images, and were between 7 and 30 days post-stroke at the time of interview. Patients were not eligible if their primary admission diagnosis was severe or critical stroke as confirmed by computed tomography and magnetic resonance images: if they were seriously ill or in need of intensive care; if their current symptoms included severe aphasia, attention impairment, or cognitive impairment; or if either the patient or a close family member has been diagnosed with any form of mental disorder. All eligible patient volunteers (N = 144) were invited to take part in the study. Five appeared too uncomfortable to continue shortly after starting and were withdrawn by a qualified member of the research team. The final analytic sample included 139 patients with early-stage stroke.

Procedures

All of the study procedures were reviewed and approved by the appropriate university institutional review board (Approval No. 2015-14). All of the recruitment and safety protocols were performed by trained members of the research team. Patient eligibility was confirmed by chart review prior to first patient contact. Individual, face-to-face interviews were conducted with the eligible patients, all of whom provided written consent. All of the study measures were read aloud to the participants, who responded by speaking their answers. Each participant was reassured that he or she could withdraw from the study at any time for any reason without question and that the interviewer could end the interview and withdraw the participant from the study if, at any time, the patient appeared fatigued or uncomfortable.

Measures

Background

Participant background items included age, number of days post-stroke, gender, marital status, live with family members (yes, no), total completed years of education, monthly household income, current employment status, residential district (urban, rural), religious beliefs (yes, no), medical coverage/payments (yes, no), and family member is the primary caregiver post-stroke (yes, no).

Post-stroke depression

The ESM-PSD was developed in a sample of patients with acute stroke (mean = 11.07 days post-stroke; Li et al., 2016). This measure includes 26 items and the following six symptom domains: (a) *low* (e.g., I feel life is meaningless), (b) *dull* (e.g., My mind is not as clear as usual), (c) *guilt* (e.g., I feel I am a burden on my family), (d) *emotional* (e.g., I get angry more easily than usual), (e) *wakefulness* (e.g., I need more time than before to fall asleep), and (f) *nervous* (e.g., I worry excessively about my physical health). Respondents are asked to rate their symptom frequency during the last 7 days on a 5-point scale: 0 = *never*, 1 = *rarely*, 2 = *sometimes*, 3 = *often*, and 4 = *always*. All of the responses are summed, and the possible score range is 0–104. The ESM-PSD has acceptable construct validity and internal reliability.

Clinical depression

The HAMD-24 is the most commonly used depression scale worldwide (Aben, Verhey, Lousberg, Lodder, & Honig, 2002). In this study, HAMD-24 was selected as the criterion-related variable for several reasons. First, HAMD-24 has been widely used in validation studies of new measures (Bagby, Ryder, Schuller, & Marshall, 2004). Second, clinical psychiatrists tend to use the 17-item HAMD to assess the treatment of patients in China (Zheng et al., 1988), whereas researchers needing greater specificity use the 24-item HAMD for clinical studies of stroke-related depression (Yue, 2017). Third, healthcare professionals use the 24-item HAMD when assessments of symptom severity must cover all symptom domains: anxiety/somatic, weight loss, cognition, day–night change, psychomotor retardation, sleep disorders, and desperation. Lastly, although the Beck Depression Inventory has been reported by some researchers as more suitable than HAMD-24 for screening depression in patients with stroke (Berg, Lönnqvist, Palomäki, & Kaste, 2009), HAMD-24 has shown higher specificity in the same patient group (Berg et al., 2009). For the above reasons, the HAMD-24 was selected as the criterion-related variable in this study. The HAMD-24 may be used with either a three-item or five-item response scale. In addition, total HAMD-24 scores may be used to define clinically relevant symptom levels: < 8 = *no depression*, 8–19 = *mild depression*, 20–34 = *moderate depression*, and ≥ 35 = *severe depression* (Pan et al., 2017; Zhu et al., 2015). The HAMD-24 is not sensitive to administrative error and has acceptable interrater reliability and internal reliability (Cronbach's α = .88–.99, $p < .01$). The empirical authenticity coefficient, an indicator of assessment accuracy for clinically relevant symptom severity, is .92 (Sun, Li, Yu, & Li, 2017). In this study, the HAMD-24 interrater reliability coefficient is .83. Each participant was administered the HAMD-24 twice by two respective researchers, with the final HAMD-24 score for each participant calculated as the mean of these two scores.

Statistical Analysis

SPSS Statistics Version 23.0 (IBM, Inc., Armonk, NY, USA) was used to perform all of the analyses in this study. To describe the sample, the total frequencies and percentages for all background items were calculated. Means and standard deviations were used to statistically characterize all of the symptom domains in the ESM-PSD and the HAMD-24. Cronbach's alpha coefficients were used to estimate the internal measurement consistency of all of the symptom domains and total scores (Houser, 2013). Pearson bivariate correlations were used to estimate the size and direction of all of the associations among the related symptom domains and total scores. Cutoff scores for the HAMD-24 were accepted as clinically relevant levels of depression symptom severity. The receiver operating characteristic (ROC) curve for the ESM-PSD on the HAMD-24 was used to define clinically relevant cutoff scores for the ESM-PSD. Parabola estimation methods (Simpson) were used to calculate the area under the curve, sensitivity (*Se*), total score specificity points (*Sp*), and the Youden index [*Se* + *Sp* − 1] (Moon, Jin, Jin, & Lee, 2017). The best cutoff points for the total ESM-PSD score based on the maximum Youden index, sensitivity, and specificity were adopted (Maggino et al., 2019). The discriminate validity of the ESM-PSD scores were explored using three HAMD-24 reference points (8, 24, and 35) to identify the participants with no depression, with mild-to-moderate depression, and with moderate-to-severe depression. One-way analysis of variance (ANOVA) was employed to further confirm the diagnostic ability of the cutoff scores of HAMD-24 and ESM-PSD to distinguish the different levels of depression. The Kappa coefficient is a test of the degree of coincidence between the cutoff scores for the two measures. The Kappa coefficient value ranges from [−1 to 1], with higher values associated with a higher degree of measurement consistency. Kappa coefficients greater than .75 indicate good measurement consistency, whereas those less than .40 indicate poor measurement consistency (Tang, Hu, Zhang, Wu, & He, 2015).

Results

Participants

Background characteristics for the final sample ($N = 139$) are presented in Table 1. The mean age of the sample was 64.24 years (SD = 12.44), and the mean number of post-stroke days was 11.99 (SD = 7.68). Most participants were male (64.7%), married (85.6%), and living with family (92.8%), and most had completed between 6 and 16 years of education (71.9%). Few rated their monthly household income as high (n = 20, 14.4%). Less than a quarter were retired (20.1%), most lived in rural districts (66.2%), less than half were religious or held religious beliefs (31.7%), and most (66.9%) had medical coverage that paid approximately 70% of their medical and hospital costs.

Early Symptom Measurement of Post-Stroke Depression and Hamilton Rating Scale for Depression-24 Internal Consistency

The Cronbach's alpha coefficients for the domains of the ESM-PSD in patients with acute stroke ranged from .78 to .90 (Table 2). These estimates met the preliminary criteria in this study for acceptable measurement reliability (≥ .70; Houser, 2013; Santos, 1999). Except for the single-item domains, similar evidence was found in this study for the domain internal consistency of the HAMD-24 (Cronbach's α = .76–.79). The Cronbach's alpha for the HAMD-24 domains that failed to reach .70 were as follows: psychomotor retardation (four items) = .26, sleep disorders (three items) = .52, desperation (three items) = .69, weight loss (one item), and day–night change (one item).

TABLE 1.
Demographic Characteristics of the Participants (N = 139)

Variable	*M*	*SD*
Age (years)	64.24	12.44
Average number of days post-stroke	11.99	7.68
	n	%
Male	90	64.7
Married	119	85.6
Living with family members	129	92.8
Educated	100	71.9
High monthly income (more than 5,000 RMB)[a]	20	14.4
Retired	28	20.1
Living in rural area	92	66.2
Having religious beliefs	44	31.7
Medical payment	93	66.9
Primary caregivers: family members	117	84.2

[a]Chinese currency.

Early Symptom Measurement of Post-Stroke Depression Concurrent Criterion Validity

Pearson bivariate correlation coefficients (Table 3) estimated concurrent criterion validity by comparing ESM-PSD and HAMD-24 items (Coronado et al., 2016; DeSimone, Harms, Vanhove, & Herian, 2017). Meaningful comparisons are able to be made because the HAMD-24 is a well-established, clinical interview approach that is used to assess depression symptom severity or change in depression symptom severity in clinically populations and is used routinely to test criterion validity in new measures (Kang et al., 2013). The correlation coefficient for total ESM-PSD and HAMD-24 scores was found to be positive and statistically significant ($r = .689, p < .05$). In addition, the correlation coefficient for ESM-PSD and HAMD-24 domain scores were positive and statistically significant, ranging from .197 to .772 ($p < .05$). Four ESM-PSD scores (*low, wakefulness, nervous, total*) correlated positively with six HAMD-24 scores. Two ESM-PSD scores (*dull, guilt*) positively correlated with all but one HAMD-24 domain (*day–night change*). One ESM-PSD score (*emotional*) positively correlated with all but one HAMD-24 domain (*retardation*).

Three Early Symptom Measurement of Post-Stroke Depression Cutoff Scores Determined Using the Receiver Operating Characteristic Curve

Post-stroke patients with or without symptoms

An HAMD-24 cutoff score of 8 was used as the reference point to explore which potential ESM-PSD cutoff score is able to best discriminate between post-stroke patients with and without depression. The sensitivity, specificity, Youden index, and ROC curve of the ESM-PSD total scores are presented in Table 4, with an HAMD-24 cutoff score of 8 used as the reference point. An ESM-PSD score of 14.5 corresponds with the maximum Youden index (0.811), with a corresponding sensitivity and specificity of 94.4% and 86.7%, respectively. For this ESM-PSD score, the area under the ROC curve is 0.941 (95% CI [0.893, 0.989]). An ESM-PSD cutoff score of 14.5 was then used to divide the sample of post-stroke patients into two groups. An independent-sample t test of the mean ESM-PSD scores for both groups showed statistically significant differences, $t(117.280) = 20.375$, $p < .001$, between post-stroke patients with no symptoms of depression ($M = 5.26, SD = 3.91$) and post-stroke patients with symptoms of depression ($M = 38.94, SD = 15.30$). These results support that an ESM-PSD cutoff score of 14.5 distinguishes between post-stroke patients with or without early-stage PSD.

TABLE 2.

Descriptions and Cronbach's Alpha of the Early Symptoms Measurement of Post-Stroke Depression (ESM-PSD) and the Hamilton Rating Scale for Depression-24 (HAMD-24) Domains (N = 139)

ESM-PSD					HAMD-24				
Domain	Item	*M*	*SD*	Cronbach's α	Domain	Item	*M*	*SD*	Cronbach's α
Low	5	6.34	4.02	.78	Anxiety/somatic	6	4.92	2.69	.79
Dull	3	4.16	2.85	.84	Cognition disorder	6	2.56	2.71	.76
Guilt	4	4.39	3.57	.86	Retardation	4	8.06	5.28	.26
Emotional	4	5.37	5.17	.86	Sleep disorders	3	2.89	2.09	.52
Wakefulness	5	7.58	5.08	.89	Desperation	3	2.99	2.06	.69
Nervous	5	6.27	3.80	.80	Weight loss	1	0.50	0.61	–
Total	26	34.10	18.52	.90	Day–night change	1	0.30	0.56	–
					Total	24	17.09	8.91	.76

Post-stroke patients with mild or moderate symptoms

An HAMD-24 cutoff score of 20 was used as the reference point to explore potential ESM-PSD cutoff scores to discriminate between post-stroke patients with mild symptoms and post-stroke patients with moderate symptoms. The sensitivity, specificity, Youden index, and ROC curve of the ESM-PSD total scores using an HAMD-24 cutoff of 20 are presented in Table 4. An ESM-PSD total score of 25.5 corresponds with the maximum Youden index (0.595), with a corresponding sensitivity and specificity of 92.3% and 67.2%, respectively. For this ESM-PSD score, the area under the ROC curve is 0.858 (95% CI [0.795, 0.921]). Next, we used an ESM-PSD cutoff score of 25.5 to divide the post-stroke patients into two groups. An independent-sample *t*-test comparison of subgroup means showed statistically significant symptom differences, $t(137) = 14.251$, $p < .001$, between post-stroke patients with mild symptoms ($M = 14.15$, $SD = 8.47$) and post-stroke patients with moderate symptoms ($M = 44.29$, $SD = 13.16$). These results support using an ESM-PSD cutoff score of 25.5 to distinguish post-stroke patients with mild depressive symptoms from post-stroke patients with moderate depressive symptoms.

Post-stroke patients with moderate or severe symptoms

An HAMD-24 cutoff score of 35 was used as the reference point to explore ESM-PSD cutoff scores to distinguish post-stroke patients with moderate symptoms from post-stroke patients with severe symptoms. The sensitivity, specificity, Youden index, and ROC curve of the ESM-PSD total scores using an

TABLE 3.

Pearson Correlations of Early Symptom Measurement of Post-Stroke Depression (ESM-PSD) and the Hamilton Rating Scale for Depression-24 (HAMD-24) Domains (N = 139)

	ESM-PSD						
Domain	Low	Dull	Guilt	Emotional	Wakefulness	Nervous	Total
HAMD-24							
Anxiety/somatic	.546**	.462**	.493**	.341**	.466**	.523**	.615**
Cognition disorder	.460**	.317**	.448**	.376**	.461**	.377**	.544**
Retardation	.248**	.350**	.231**	.091	.248**	.321**	.311**
Sleep disorder	.408**	.290**	.326**	.431**	.573**	.367**	.549**
Desperation	.660**	.535**	.621**	.523**	.572**	.604**	.772**
Weight loss	.323**	.238**	.289**	.249**	.421**	.259**	.400**
Day–night change	.302**	.082	.130	.209*	.197*	.214*	.259**
Total	.576**	.510**	.521**	.407**	.572**	.560**	.689**

*$p < .05$. **$p < .01$.

TABLE 4.

The Raw Score, Sensitivity, Specificity, and Youden Index of the Early Symptom Measurement of Post-Stroke Depression (ESM-PSD) According to Hamilton Rating Scale for Depression-24 (HAMD-24) Cutoffs (N = 139)

ESM-PSD Raw Scores	Sensitivity	Specificity	Youden Index	ROC Curve
HAMD-24 cutoff 8				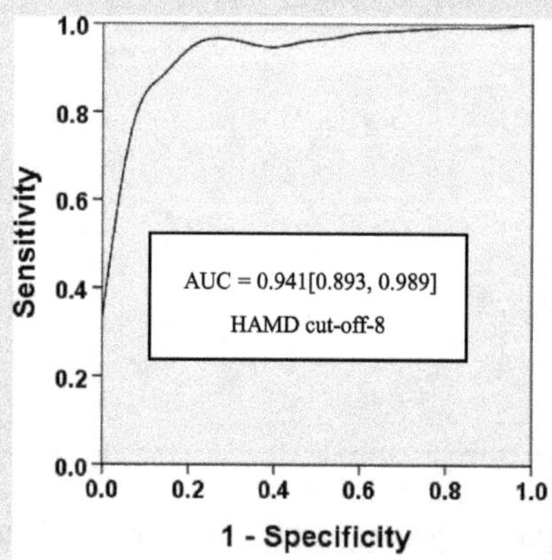 Diagonal segments are produced by ties.
4.6	0.976	0.400	0.376	
5.5	0.968	0.467	0.435	
6.5	0.968	0.533	0.501	
7.5	0.952	0.533	0.485	
8.5	0.952	0.600	0.552	
9.5	0.944	0.600	0.544	
11.5	0.944	0.800	0.744	
14.5	0.944	0.867	0.811	
16.5	0.911	0.867	0.778	
17.0	0.903	0.867	0.770	
17.5	0.895	0.867	0.762	
18.2	0.887	0.867	0.754	
18.7	0.879	0.867	0.746	
19.1	0.863	0.867	0.730	
19.6	0.855	0.867	0.722	
HAMD-24 cutoff 20				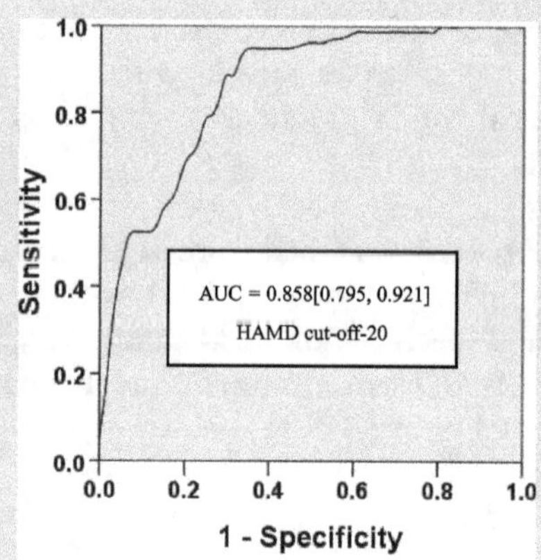 Diagonal segments are produced by ties.
21.1	0.962	0.492	0.454	
21.6	0.962	0.508	0.470	
22.5	0.949	0.557	0.506	
23.2	0.949	0.574	0.523	
23.4	0.949	0.590	0.539	
23.7	0.949	0.607	0.556	
24.5	0.949	0.639	0.588	
25.5	0.923	0.672	0.595	
26.2	0.885	0.689	0.574	
26.7	0.885	0.705	0.590	
27.0	0.872	0.721	0.593	
27.5	0.859	0.721	0.580	
28.5	0.821	0.721	0.542	
29.5	0.808	0.721	0.529	
30.1	0.795	0.721	0.516	
HAMD-24 cutoff 35				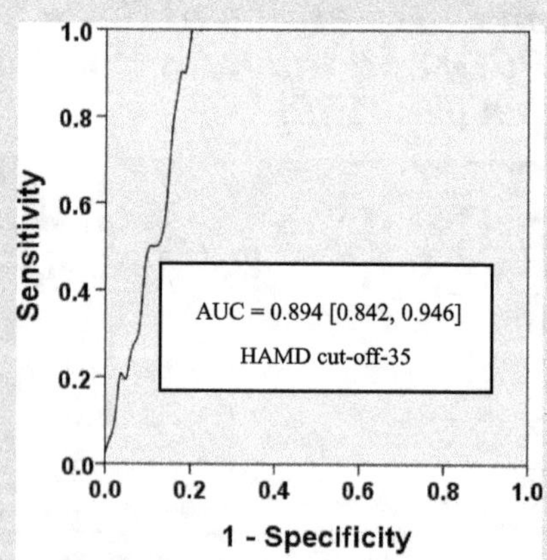 Diagonal segments are produced by ties.
39.5	1.000	0.714	0.714	
40.5	1.000	0.739	0.739	
41.5	1.000	0.748	0.748	
42.7	1.000	0.756	0.756	
43.2	1.000	0.765	0.765	
43.7	1.000	0.773	0.773	
44.5	1.000	0.782	0.782	
45.5	1.000	0.798	0.798	
46.2	0.900	0.815	0.715	
46.7	0.900	0.824	0.724	
47.5	0.850	0.832	0.682	
48.5	0.800	0.840	0.640	
49.5	0.600	0.857	0.457	
50.5	0.500	0.882	0.382	
52.0	0.500	0.891	0.391	

Note. ROC = receiver operating characteristic; AUC = area under the curve.

HAMD-24 cutoff score of 35 are presented in Table 4. A total ESM-PSD score of 45.5 corresponds to the maximum Youden index (0.798), with a corresponding sensitivity and specificity of 100.0% and 79.8%, respectively. For this ESM-PSD score, the area under the ROC curve is 0.894 (95% CI [0.842, 0.946]). This ESM-PSD score divides the post-stroke patients into two groups. An independent-sample *t* test, $t(97.781) = 14.717$, $p < .001$, showed statistically significant differences between post-stroke patients with moderate depressive symptoms ($M = 24.51$, $SD = 12.57$) and post-stroke patients with severe depressive symptoms ($M = 54.80$, $SD = 10.65$). These results show that an ESM-PSD cutoff score of 45.5 distinguishes between post-stroke patients with moderate depressive symptoms and severe depressive symptoms.

Mean Differences Between Depression Severity Levels of Hamilton Rating Scale for Depression-24 and Early Symptom Measurement of Post-Stroke Depression

The one-way ANOVA results showed significant differences between the different depression levels divided by the cutoff scores of HAMD-24 and ESM-PSD (Table 5). Furthermore, post hoc results revealed that the depression levels divided by the cutoff scores of HAMD-24 and ESM-PSD were significantly different from the other groups. This result indicates that the cutoff scores of ESM-PSD determined by the cutoff scores of HAMD-24 distinguish different levels of depression adequately.

In summary, we used the ROC curve to evaluate the specificity, sensitivity, and Youden index of the ESM-PSD cutoff scores (Tables 4 and 5). The ESM-PSD cutoff scores showed the expected correspondence with mild–moderate–severe HAMD-24 symptoms with high area under the curve evidence. Furthermore, the one-way ANOVA confirmed significant differences between different levels of depression and thus proved the effectiveness of ESM-PSD cutoff scores in distinguishing different levels of PSD.

Clinical Agreement in the Early Symptom Measurement of Post-Stroke Depression and the Hamilton Rating Scale for Depression-24

The Kappa coefficient for the ESM-PSD and HAMD-24 was .454 ($p < .001$). This level of agreement is lower than the accepted criteria of .75 because a moderate level of statistically significant agreement reflects accurately the similarities and differences between two diagnostic measures in a sample of acute post-stroke patients assessed for symptoms of early-stage PSD. Although both of the scales measure negative changes in thought and mood, the ESM-PSD further measures the attribution of these negative changes to "acute post-stroke" as the underlying condition.

Discussion

In a sample of hospital patients who were, on average, less than 2 weeks post-stroke, we examined ESM-PSD internal consistency, concurrent criterion validity, and cut-off scores. Accepted statistical tests show the ESM-PSD total score, and six domains have acceptable levels of internal consistency and, using the HAMD-24 as the gold standard, acceptable criterion validity, as a measure of clinically relevant symptoms of early-stage PSD in the patients with acute stroke. As described in the Results section, some HAMD-24 domains did not reach the .70 criteria for internal consistency: psychomotor retardation = .26, sleep disorders = .52, and desperation = .69. These findings may be expected given that HAMD-24 items are designed primarily to identify major depression. Patients with stroke experiencing early-stage PSD are unlikely to have symptoms of psychomotor retardation, hypersomnia, or desperation. Thus, these were the three domains of the HAMD-24 that showed relatively low internal consistency in the participants. Early-stage PSD is distinct from major depression, yet PSD has been shown to increase the risk of late-onset major depression, suicidality, and limited functional recovery. Therefore, the level of the correlations and explanatory

TABLE 5.

Early Symptom Measurement of Post-Stroke Depression (ESM-PSD) Cutoff Value According to the Hamilton Rating Scale for Depression-24 (HAMD-24) Cutoff Value Using the Receiver Operating Characteristic (ROC) Model (N = 139)

	HAMD-24							ESM-PSD (ROC)						
Depression Level	Cutoff	*n*	%	*M*	*SD*	*F*	*p*	Cutoff	*n*	%	*M*	*SD*	*F*	*p*
No	0	17	12.2	5.30	2.11	312.219	<.001	0	20	14.4	5.26	3.91	259.673	< .001
Mild	8	38	27.3	14.06	3.21			14.5	27	19.4	20.73	3.16		
Moderate	19	64	46.0	25.39	4.41			25.5	48	34.5	34.65	5.77		
Severe	35	20	14.4	41.99	5.66			45.5	44	31.7	54.80	10.65		

relationships between the ESM-PSD and HAMD-24 were as expected.

The strong, positive correlation ($r = .689$) found for ESM-PSD and HAMD-24 total scores is evidence of concurrent criterion validity, whereas the interesting domain correlations that were found suggest areas of measurement where the similarity between these two measures end. The ESM-PSD *low* domain positively correlated with all of the domains of the HAMD-24. This finding suggests that, in acute post-stroke patients, the *low* domain of the ESM-PSD may measure an early-stage core symptom of PSD or subclinical major depression. The ESM-PSD *dull* domain positively correlated with all domains of the HAMD-24, except for the HAMD-24 *day–night change* domain. The ESM-PSD screens patients with acute stroke for early symptoms of stroke-related depression. In earlier item development research, neither patients nor experts recommended the experience of *day–night change* as an early symptom of PSD (Li et al., 2018). The ESM-PSD *guilt* domain and *emotional* domain positively correlated with the HAMD-24 *desperation* domain. Stroke-related guilt appears to be a common experience among patients with acute stroke. It is possible that this domain addresses a second early-stage core symptom of PSD. The ESM-PSD *wakefulness* and *nervous* domains were positively correlated with all of the HAMD-24 domains. Sleep changes and excessive biopsychosocial arousal and worry are symptoms commonly used to diagnose major depression. However, in the acute post-stroke patient, these symptoms may reflect understandable sense of alarm in response to a health event such as stroke.

In this study, the ROC model was used to define ESM-PSD cutoff scores because this method of analysis allows evaluation of the clinical relevance of these scores. Based on the results, it is recommended that these cutoff scores be used to assess newly admitted, acute post-stroke patients who do not require intensive care. The aim of this research was to develop a measure that is able to detect early symptoms of stroke-related depression in post-stroke patients early enough for the patient to receive prompt psychological care to reduce the risk of stroke-related major depression, suicidality, and impaired psychosocial functioning. According to the cutoff scores defined by the ROC curve, 80% of the participants met the criteria for early-stage PSD (Table 5), a rate that reflects the PSD incidence rates found in other studies. Although the immediate management of the physical symptoms of stroke is still the treatment priority, the depression-related morbidity and mortality associated with mild-to-moderate stroke makes PSD a second, but equal, priority. The lower Kappa coefficient (.454) for ESM-PSD and HAMD-24 is expected because, whereas the HAMD-24 measures general depression, the ESM-PSD measures disease-specific depression for patients with stroke. Furthermore, the lower Kappa coefficient for the two measures indicates that the disease-specific depression in patients with stroke as measured by ESM-PSD is different from general depression as measured by HAMD-24. Therefore, the development of ESM-PSD is required urgently to assess early-stage stroke-related depression accurately. Further research will help determine whether the ESM-PSD measures specific early symptoms of clinical depression in patients with acute stroke or early symptoms of PSD that increase the risk of clinical depression within 6 months (Berg et al., 2009; Meng et al., 2017; Yang et al., 2013).

Research shows that high HAMD-24 scores ($OR = 2.38$, 95% CI [1.61, 3.50], $p < .001$) independently predict increased risk of PSD (Meng et al., 2017). Three scales, including the Center for Epidemiological Studies Depression Scale, the HAMD-24, and the Patient Health Questionnaire-9, are currently regularly used to screen post-stroke patients for PSD, although each appears to be an unsatisfactory screen for case finding (Meader, Moe-Byrne, Llewellyn, & Mitchell, 2014; Rogers, 2017). This limitation is critical. PSD screens must be clinically effective, meaning that a screen must generate a score that may be used to decide when preventive interventions are needed. The findings of this study suggest that an ESM-PSD score of 14.5 shows treatment levels of early-stage PSD.

Limitations

A major limitation of this study was the use of HAMD-24 cutoff scores as the gold standard for determining clinically relevant cutoffs for the ESM-PSD. However, the HAMD-24 is a recognized interview screen for depression in both clinical and research populations. A different depression screen may yield a different ESM-PSD cutoff score, although it is unlikely that the symptom level associated with that score would differ significantly. To further test the clinical relevance of the ESM-PSD cutoff scores, future research has already been planned to cross-validate the ESM-PSD cutoff scores according to diagnostic results by the clinical specialists (Lam et al., 2017).

Conclusion

The major findings of this study permit the researchers to proceed with planned studies of measurement invariance in a similar sample of U.S. patients with acute stroke and a 3-, 6-, and 9-month follow-up comparison tests of ESM-PSD score as a predictor of increased risk for depressive illness.

Relevance to Clinical Practice

The clinical relevance of this study is the finding that the ESM-PSD is able to detect the early symptoms of PSD in patients with acute stroke at clinically relevant levels of symptom severity. Nurses who recognize dysphoric emotional distress in a newly admitted post-stroke patient are more likely to act on their clinical observation by screening the patient for ESM-PSD if an accurate, easy-to-use assessment tool is available.

Acknowledgments

The authors acknowledge the following agencies who provided financial support to this study: the National Natural Science

Foundation of China (Grant Number 71804134), the Natural Science Foundation of Zhejiang Province (Grant Number LQ18G030006), the Project of Humanities and Social Sciences from the Ministry of Education in China (Grant Number 18YJCZH078), the Wenzhou Science and Technology Bureau (Grant Number Y20180054), and the Health Commission of Zhejiang Province (Grant Number 2020KY631).

Author Contributions

Study conception and design: JL, YLuo
Data collection: YLi
Data analysis and interpretation: RLB
Drafting of the article: JL
Critical revision of the article: LDO

References

Aben, I., Verhey, F., Lousberg, R., Lodder, J., & Honig, A. (2002). Validity of the Beck Depression Inventory, Hospital Anxiety and Depression Scale, SCL-90, and Hamilton Depression Rating Scale as screening instruments for depression in stroke patients. *Psychosomatics, 43*(5), 386–393. https://doi.org/10.1176/appi.psy.43.5.386

Bagby, R. M., Ryder, A. G., Schuller, D. R., & Marshall, M. B. (2004). The Hamilton Depression Rating Scale: Has the gold standard become a lead weight? *The American Journal of Psychiatry, 161*(12), 2163–2177. https://doi.org/10.1176/appi.ajp.161.12.2163

Bartoli, F., Lillia, N., Lax, A., Crocamo, C., Mantero, V., Carrà, G., ... Clerici, M. (2013). Depression after stroke and risk of mortality: A systematic review and meta-analysis. *Stroke Research and Treatment,* 2013, Article ID 862978. https://doi.org/10.1155/2013/862978

Berg, A., Lönnqvist, J., Palomäki, H., & Kaste, M. (2009). Assessment of depression after stroke: A comparison of different screening instruments. *Stroke, 40*(2), 523–529. https://doi.org/10.1161/strokeaha.108.527705

Coronado, P. J., Sanchez-Borrego, R., Ruiz, M. A., Baquedano, L., Sánchez, S., Argudo, C., ... Rejas, J. (2016). Psychometric attributes of the Cervantes short-form questionnaire for measuring health-related quality of life in menopausal women. *Maturitas, 84,* 55–62. https://doi.org/10.1016/j.maturitas.2015.10.013

DeSimone, J. A., Harms, P. D., Vanhove, A. J., & Herian, M. N. (2017). Development and validation of the Five-by-Five Resilience Scale. *Assessment, 24*(6), 778–797. https://doi.org/10.1177/1073191115625803

Dwyer Hollender, K. (2014). Screening, diagnosis, and treatment of post-stroke depression. *The Journal of Neuroscience Nursing, 46*(3), 135–141. https://doi.org/10.1097/jnn.0000000000000047

Gao, Q. (2015). *The incidence and correlated factors of acute post-stroke depression* (Unpublished master's thesis). Jilin University, PRC. (Original work published in Chinese)

Houser, J. (2013). *Nursing research: Reading, using and creating evidence* (3rd ed.). Burlington, MA: Jones & Bartlett Learning.

Kang, H. J., Stewart, R., Kim, J. M., Jang, J. E., Kim, S. Y., Bae, K. Y., ... Yoon, J. S. (2013). Comparative validity of depression assessment scales for screening poststroke depression. *Journal of Affective Disorders, 147*(1–3), 186–191. https://doi.org/10.1016/j.jad.2012.10.035

Koositamongkol, S., Sindhu, S., Pinyopasakul, W., Nilanont, Y., & Redman, R. W. (2013). Factors influencing functional recovery in patients with acute ischemic stroke. *Collegian, 20*(4), 207–213. https://doi.org/10.1016/j.colegn.2012.09.002

Lam, S. C., Yeung, C. C. Y., Chan, J. H. M., Lam, D. W. C., Lam, A. H. Y., Annesi-Maesano, I., & Bousquet, J. (2017). Adaptation of the score for allergic rhinitis in the Chinese population: Psychometric properties and diagnostic accuracy. *International Archives of Allergy Immunology, 173*(4), 213–224. https://doi.org/10.1159/000477727

Lewin-Richter, A., Volz, M., Jobges, M., & Werheid, K. (2015). Predictivity of early depressive symptoms for post-stroke depression. *The Journal of Nutrition, Health & Aging, 19*(7), 754–758. https://doi.org/10.1007/s12603-015-0540-x

Li, J. (2016). *Development of the post-stroke early screening tool and its preliminary application* (Unpublished doctoral dissertation). Chongqing Medical University, PRC. (Original work published in Chinese)

Li, J., Oakley, L. D., Brown, R. L., Li, Y., Ye, M., & Luo, Y. (2016). Early Symptom Measurement of Post-Stroke Depression (PSD). *Journal of Affective Disorders, 197,* 215–222. https://doi.org/10.1016/j.jad.2016.03.038

Li, J., Oakley, L. D., Li, Y., & Luo, Y. (2018). Development and initial validation of a clinical measure to assess early symptoms of post-stroke depression in the acute stroke patient. *Journal of Clinical Nursing, 27*(3–4), 784–794. https://doi.org/10.1111/jocn.14099

Maggino, L., Malleo, G., Bassi, C., Allegrini, V., Beane, J. D., Beckman, R. M., ... Vollmer, C. M. Jr. (2019). Identification of an optimal cut-off for drain fluid amylase on postoperative day 1 for predicting clinically relevant fistula after distal pancreatectomy: A multi-institutional analysis and external validation. *Annals of Surgery, 269*(2), 337–343. https://doi.org/10.1097/SLA.0000000000002532

Meader, N., Moe-Byrne, T., Llewellyn, A., & Mitchell, A. J. (2014). Screening for poststroke major depression: A meta-analysis of diagnostic validity studies. *Journal of Neurology, Neurosurgery and Psychiatry, 85*(2), 198–206. https://doi.org/10.1136/jnnp-2012-304194

Meng, G., Ma, X., Li, L., Tan, Y., Liu, X., Liu, X., & Zhao, Y. (2017). Predictors of early-onset post-ischemic stroke depression: A cross-sectional study. *BMC Neurology, 17*(1), Article number 199. https://doi.org/10.1186/s12883-017-0980-5

Mitchell, A. J., Sheth, B., Gill, J., Yadegarfar, M., Stubbs, B., Yadegarfar, M., & Meader, N. (2017). Prevalence and predictors of post-stroke mood disorders: A meta-analysis and meta-regression of depression, anxiety and adjustment disorder. *General Hospital Psychiatry, 47,* 48–60. https://doi.org/10.1016/j.genhosppsych.2017.04.001

Moon, K. J., Jin, Y., Jin, T., & Lee, S. M. (2017). Development and validation of an automated delirium risk assessment system (auto-DelRAS) implemented in the electronic health record system. *International Journal of Nursing Studies, 77,* 46–53. https://doi.org/10.1016/j.ijnurstu.2017.09.014

Pan, S., Liu, Z. W., Shi, S., Ma, X., Song, W. Q., Guan, G. C., ... Lv, Y. (2017). Hamilton Rating Scale for Depression-24 (HAM-D24) as a novel predictor for diabetic microvascular complications in Type 2 diabetes mellitus patients. *Psychiatry Research, 258*, 177–183. https://doi.org/10.1016/j.psychres.2017.07.050

Robinson, R. G., & Jorge, R. E. (2015). Post-stroke depression: A review. *The American Journal of Psychiatry, 173*(3), 221–231. https://doi.org/10.1176/appi.ajp.2015.15030363

Rogers, S. C. (2017). Poststroke depression screening: An executive summary. *The Journal of Neuroscience Nursing, 49*(2), 66–68. https://doi.org/10.1097/jnn.0000000000000270

Santos, J. R. A. (1999). Cronbach's alpha: A tool for assessing the reliability of scales. *Journal of Extension, 37*(2), 1–5. Retrieved from http://www.joe.org/joe/1999april/tt3.php

Schneider, M. A., & Schneider, M. D. (2012). Recognizing poststroke depression. *Nursing, 42*(12), 60–63. https://doi.org/10.1097/01.NURSE.0000422646.06254.1c

Schulte-Altedorneburg, M., & Bereczki, D. (2014). Post-stroke depression. *Orvosi Hetilap, 155*(34), 1335–1343. https://doi.org/10.1556/oh.2014.29968 (Original work published in Hungarian)

Shi, Y. Z., Xiang, Y. T., Yang, Y., Zhang, N., Wang, S., Ungvari, G. S., ... Wang, C. (2015). Depression after minor stroke: Prevalence and predictors. *Journal of Psychosomatic Research, 79*(2), 143–147. https://doi.org/10.1016/j.jpsychores.2015.03.012

Shi, Y. Z., Xiang, Y. T., Yang, Y., Zhang, N., Wang, S., Ungvari, G. S., ... Wang, C. X. (2016). Depression after minor stroke: The association with disability and quality of life—A 1-year follow-up study. *International Journal of Geriatric Psychiatry, 31*(4), 421–427. https://doi.org/10.1002/gps.4353

Sun, X. Y., Li, Y. X., Yu, C. Q., & Li, L. M. (2017). Reliability and validity of depression scales of Chinese version: A systematic review. *Zhonghua Liu Xing Bing Xue Za Zhi, 38*(1), 110–116. https://doi.org/10.3760/cma.j.issn.0254-6450.2017.01.021 (Original work published in Chinese)

Tang, W., Hu, J., Zhang, H., Wu, P., & He, H. (2015). Kappa coefficient: A popular measure of rater agreement. *Shanghai Archives of Psychiatry, 27*(1), 62–67. https://doi.org/10.11919/j.issn.1002-0829.215010 (Original work published in Chinese)

Tateno, A., Kimura, M., & Robinson, R. G. (2002). Phenomenological characteristics of poststroke depression: Early- versus late-onset. *The American Journal of Geriatric Psychiatry, 10*(5), 575–582. https://doi.org/10.1097/00019442-200209000-00011

Towfighi, A., Ovbiagele, B., El Husseini, N., Hackett, M. L., Jorge, R. E., Kissela, B. M., ... Williams, L. S. (2017). Poststroke depression: A scientific statement for healthcare professionals from the American Heart Association/American Stroke Association. *Stroke, 48*(2), e30–e43. https://doi.org/10.1161/STR.0000000000000113

Yang, S. R., Hua, P., Shang, X. Y., Hu, R., Mo, X. E., & Pan, X. P. (2013). Predictors of early post ischemic stroke apathy and depression: A cross-sectional study. *BMC Psychiatry, 13*(1), 164. https://doi.org/10.1186/1471-244X-13-164

Yuan, H. W., Wang, C. X., Zhang, N., Bai, Y., Shi, Y. Z., Zhou, Y., ... Wang, Y. J. (2012). Poststroke depression and risk of recurrent stroke at 1 year in a Chinese cohort study. *PLOS ONE, 7*(10), e46906. https://doi.org/10.1371/journal.pone.0046906

Yue, Y. (2017). *The study of evaluation, diagnostic criteria, risk prediction, and biomarkers for post-stroke depression* (Unpublished doctoral dissertation). Dongnan University, PRC. (Original work published in Chinese)

Zahi, S., Mahir, L., Azanmasso, H., Lmidmani, F., & El Fatimi, A. (2016). Anxiety and depression after stroke: Report of 64 cases. *Annals of Physical and Rehabilitation Medicine, 59S*, e76. https://doi.org/10.1016/j.rehab.2016.07.178

Zhang, Y., Zeng, L., & Liu, J. (2015). Analysis of the incidence of early depression and its influencing factors after stroke. *Chinese Journal of Modern Nervous Diseases, 15*(3), 203–208. (Original work published in Chinese)

Zheng, Y. P., Zhao, J. P., Phillips, M., Liu, J. B., Cai, M. F., Sun, S. Q., & Huang, M. F. (1988). Validity and reliability of the Chinese Hamilton Depression Rating Scale. *The British Journal of Psychiatry, 152*(5), 660–664. https://doi.org/10.1192/bjp.152.5.660

Zhu, G., Yin, Y., Xiao, C. L., Mao, R. J., Shi, B. H., Jie, Y., & Wang, Z. W. (2015). Serum DHEAS levels are associated with the development of depression. *Psychiatry Research, 229*(1–2), 447–453. https://doi.org/10.1016/j.psychres.2015.05.093

22

Effects of Environmental Crude Oil Pollution on Newborn Birth Outcomes: A Retrospective Cohort Study

Chinemerem ELEKE[1]* • Sabinah Obele NGBALA-OKPABI[2] • Daprim OGAJI[3] • Ifeyinwa S. AGU[4] • Esther N. BEMPONG-ELEKE[5]

ABSTRACT

Background: The World Health Organization encourages countries to improve birth outcomes to reduce rates of neonatal mortality and morbidity.

Purpose: This study was designed to examine the effect of environmental crude oil pollution on newborn birth outcomes in Rivers State, Nigeria.

Methods: A retrospective cohort design was used to examine the effects of exposure to oil pollution on birth outcomes using facility-based records. K-Dere (an oil-polluted community) served as the exposure group, whereas birth records from Iriebe served as the comparison group. A sample size of 338 systematically selected birth records was examined (169 records for each arm of the study). A data extraction sheet was used for data collection. Data were analyzed using descriptive and inferential statistics at $p < .05$.

Results: The risk of preterm birth was significantly higher in the exposed group (16% vs. 7.7%, relative risk = 2.08, 95% CI [1.11, 3.89], $p = .018$). At 6 weeks after birth, newborns in the exposed group weighed significantly less (4.64 ± 0.82 vs. 4.85 ± 0.92 kg, $p = .032$) and reported significantly higher incidence of morbidity compared with the newborns in the comparison group (relative risk = 3.03, 95% CI [2.20, 4.19], $p < .001$).

Conclusions: The oil-polluted area examined in this study was found to have a higher risk of preterm birth, a slower rate of newborn growth, and a higher rate of newborn morbidity than the non-oil-polluted area at 6 weeks after birth. Stakeholders should sustain efforts to remediate the environment in polluted regions and prevent oil pollution. Future research should investigate the mechanisms of the observed toxicological effects and the targeted protection of vulnerable groups in oil-polluted communities.

KEY WORDS:
birth, newborn, environment, pollution.

Introduction

Newborn birth outcomes are a crucial community midwifery concern, as adverse birth events remain one of the leading causes of morbidity and mortality in newborns worldwide (World Health Organization, 2020). About 7% of newborns in developed countries and 16% in developing countries are affected by low birth weight (Lamichhane et al., 2015). About 5%–18% of births are preterm births (Seabrook et al., 2019). In addition, 37% of all births in developing countries result in neonatal death (Oghenetega, Ojengbede, & Ana, 2020). These challenges have resulted in a greater focus on ensuring healthy living and well-being for all individuals, especially pregnant women. This focus is captured in Sustainable Development Goal 3, which is a target statement put together by the United Nations aimed at motivating countries toward reducing mortality in neonates and children under 5 years old to below 25 per 1,000 live births (World Health Organization, 2020).

Pregnancy is considered to be a period when the health of a mother and her developing fetus (unborn child) is particularly vulnerable to the effects of natural and chemical catastrophes (Harville et al., 2017). Pregnancy is a unique life-changing period for both the pregnant woman and her fetus. Certain physiological, physical, and emotional changes occur during pregnancy as the woman interacts with her environment. This has drawn the attention of researchers to examine the environments in which pregnant women live in search of possible environmental pollutants that may be etiologies for adverse newborn outcomes such as preterm birth, low birth weight, and congenital defects (Casey et al., 2018).

Environmental pollution is the release of typically harmful substances into the environment (Dunlap, 2018). Possible sources of environmental pollution include coal, diesel traffic,

[1]*MSN, RM, RN, Lecturer, Faculty of Clinical Sciences, Department of Nursing, University of Port Harcourt, Choba, Nigeria* • [2]*MSN, RM, RN, Researcher, Africa Centre of Excellence in Public Health and Toxicology Research, University of Port Harcourt, Choba, Nigeria* • [3]*PhD, MBBS, Centre Leader and Research Coordinator, Africa Centre of Excellence in Public Health and Toxicology Research, University of Port Harcourt, Choba, Nigeria* • [4]*MSN, RM, RN, Lecturer, Department of Nursing Sciences, Abia State University, Uturu, Nigeria* • [5]*BSN, RN, Research Assistant, Home Health Services, Amedisys, Worcester, USA.*

generator use, petrol traffic, particulate matter, and crude oil extraction processes, among others (Janitz et al., 2019). Most of the world's environmental pollutants may be traceable to hydrocarbon-related compounds and activities. Fossil-fuel-related environmental pollution is directly related to the worldwide, insatiable demand for energy from natural gas and crude oil (Balise et al., 2016). The need for energy from crude oil has led to increased use of conventional, unconventional, and clandestine crude oil processing methods (Walker Whitworth et al., 2018). Clandestine crude oil processing, which refers to the illegal extraction of crude oil, is often performed using unconventional means. Clandestine oil processing and poor pipeline maintenance have been identified as causes of a noninsignificant percentage of oil spills in the roughly 70,000 crude-oil-producing communities around the world (Oghenetega, Ana, et al., 2020). The Niger Delta region in Nigeria has been cited as a region experiencing gross environmental pollution from oil spills caused by clandestine crude oil processing (Bruederle & Hodler, 2019).

Onshore crude oil spills may lead to irreparable environmental degradation and pose hazards to human and environmental health (Atubi, 2015). Nigeria is the second largest crude oil producer in Africa. Much of Nigeria's crude oil deposits are located in the Niger Delta region. Crude oil spills have had a significant impact on essential community resources in the Niger Delta. Communities in River State, especially those in Ogoniland like K-Dere and B-Dere, have been worst hit by the deleterious impact of environmental crude oil pollution (Yakubu, 2017). These communities have had their farmlands, playgrounds, rivers, and drinking water pol luted by crude oil spills (Digha et al., 2017). Pregnant women and their newborns residing in these oil-polluted communities are vulnerable to the possible effects of these pollutants through ingestion, contact, and inhalation (Bové et al., 2019). Bové et al. found evidence that ingested fossil-fuel hydrocarbon pollutants are toxic to human cells and are able to reach the fetal side of the placenta in women who are pregnant. Therefore, the health impact of oil spills and the resultant environmental pollution on newborn birth outcomes require closer and more-rigorous examination.

The impact on newborn birth outcomes of crude-oil-spill-related environmental pollution has been copiously studied outside Africa in recent decades (Apergis et al., 2019). One study conducted by Janitz et al. (2019) in Oklahoma, USA, found no significant association between an area's oil-producing status and risk of birth defects. However, another study by Apergis et al. conducted in the same state found an association between the proximity of a mother's residence to crude oil fracking wells and risk of negative birth outcomes. Furthermore, Walker Whitworth et al. (2018) found a significant association between the proximity of a mother's residence to areas of unconventional crude oil exploration and preterm births in the Barnett Shale area of Texas, USA. Casey et al. (2018) found a significant decrease in preterm births that correlated with reduced crude oil processing in California, USA. Willis and Hystad (2019) found no association between city air pollutant exposure and risk of adverse birth outcomes in Portland, Oregon, USA. In addition, McKenzie et al. (2014) found a significant association between the density and proximity of natural gas wells within a 16-km radius of maternal residence and the prevalence of congenital defects in Colorado, USA. Few studies on the effects of crude-oil-related environmental pollution on newborn birth outcomes have been conducted in Nigeria. A pivotal study by Bruederle and Hodler (2019) found an association between onshore crude oil spills and an increase in neonatal death in Nigeria's Niger Delta region. The paucity of studies focusing on oil-producing regions outside the United States justifies the need for more studies on this issue in other countries. This study was designed to investigate the effect of environmental crude oil pollution on newborn birth outcomes in registered births in Rivers State, Nigeria.

Methods

Design

A retrospective cohort design based on birth records was used for this study. The area of study was Rivers State in Southern Nigeria's Niger Delta region. Rivers State is home to several crude-oil-producing communities. Moreover, onshore crude oil spills occur regularly in many of these communities, in part because of clandestine and conventional crude oil processing (Bruederle & Hodler, 2019). The most environmentally polluted communities in this state are in the Ogoniland area (Digha et al., 2017). Thus, K-Dere, about 52 km southeast of Port Harcourt City in the Gokana local government area in Ogoniland, Rivers State, was selected as the target exposed community in this study. K-Dere is a rural community with a population mostly engaged as farmers, petty traders, and artisans. It has one comprehensive primary health center (K-Dere Comprehensive Primary Health Centre [K-Dere PHC]), which serves a population of about 3,180 women of childbearing age within a 15-km radius. K-Dere PHC offers a broad spectrum of maternity services to mothers and community training services to midwifery students at the University of Port Harcourt.

Iriebe in the Obio/Akpor local government area in Rivers State was chosen as the comparison community. Iriebe lies about 25 km northeast of Port Harcourt City and about 41 km northwest of the K-Dere community. Iriebe is widely considered to be the least environmentally polluted region in Rivers State after Port Harcourt City. It is a semiurban area with a population mostly engaged as petty traders, artisans, and farmers. It has one primary health center (Iriebe Comprehensive Primary Health Centre [Iriebe PHC]), which serves about 2,205 women of childbearing age within a 5.2-km radius. Iriebe PHC offers a broad spectrum of maternity services to mothers and community training services to medical students at the University of Port Harcourt.

The birth records for the above two PHCs comprise case notes kept by clinicians that contain activity and event records maintained between childbirth and the first 6 weeks of follow-up. Information on background maternal characteristics, gestation, spontaneity of labor, mode of birth, birth complications, reported morbidity, and treatments administered are all documented in the birth records.

The research team considered K-Dere and Iriebe PHCs to be highly similar in terms of skill mix, quality of maternity care, and service administration and thus suitable for comparison. The status of K-Dere as a predominantly oil-spill-polluted community and Iriebe as a community largely unaffected by oil spill issues allowed the researchers to treat residents of the former as the exposure group and those of the latter as the comparison group.

Target Population

The target population for the study was the 3,088 recorded births in K-Dere and Iriebe PHCs (1,698 in K-Dere and 1,390 in Iriebe) covering a period of 5 years (2015–2019).

Sample Size Determination

A total sample size of 338 was used in the study. The minimum sample size was calculated using Cochran's (1977) sample size formula for studies involving proportion, mathematically stated as $n_s = \{[Z^2_{1-\alpha/2} \times P(1 - P)] \div d^2\}$ where n_s is the minimum sample size, $Z_{1-\alpha/2}$ is the Type 1 error at $p < 5\% = 1.96$, P is the prevalence of first parity preterm birth in mothers living in exposed areas relative to reference areas at 12.5% (Bruederle & Hodler, 2019), and d is precision = 0.05 (Charan & Biswas, 2013). A minimum required sample size of 169 birth records was calculated for each group. The total sample size of 338 is double the minimum sample size for each arm. The sample size of 169 birth records represented approximately 10% of the birth records for the study period in K-Dere PHC and approximately 12% of the birth records for the study period in Iriebe PHC.

Sampling Technique

A systematic sampling technique was utilized to select birth records for this study. The point of random origin "6" was generated using Microsoft Excel Statistical Package 2007 (Microsoft Inc., Redmond, WA, USA). The sampling interval was determined by dividing the total number of records in each of the facilities (1,698 in K-Dere and 1,390 in Iriebe) by 169, which generated systematic intervals of 10 and 8 for K-Dere and Iriebe, respectively. One hundred sixty-nine birth records were selected from registered childbirths at each PHC facility between January 2015 and December 2019.

Instrument for Data Collection

A data extraction sheet designed by the research team was used for data collection.

Validity of the instrument

To ensure face validity, the instrument was reviewed by five nursing and midwifery research experts in the Department of Nursing, University of Port Harcourt, Nigeria. These experts examined the instrument for font size, character, organization, brevity, and conformity with operationalized outcome variables. Identified areas of temporal ambiguity were corrected.

For content validity, the corrected instrument was resubmitted to another set of five research experts from the Maternal and Child Health Unit, Faculty of Clinical Sciences, University of Port Harcourt. To measure the suitability of the data extraction sheet items in measuring the intended outcome variables, these five experts were requested to score each item on the data extraction sheet dichotomously as relevant or not relevant. Analysis of the score data generated an item validity index (agreement between raters) score $\geq .8$ and a content validity index score of .917. Following Polit and Beck (2012), a content validity index value > .8 was considered valid.

Reliability of the instrument

The interrater reliability was not examined because only one member of the research team was tasked with data collection using the instrument, whereas another member of the research team was tasked with confirming the correctness of the collected data.

Ethical Considerations

The protocol used in this study was reviewed for ethical quality and approved by the Research Ethics Committee, Office of Research Management and Development, University of Port Harcourt (approval number: UPH/CEREMAD/REC/MM68/020). Administrative permission was also obtained from the Rivers State Primary Health Care Management Board, which has oversight responsibilities for the comprehensive primary health centers. The birth records of participants were kept anonymous throughout the period of data collection. All collected data were protected and used only for the approved academic purpose.

Data Collection

Data were collected during the month of March 2020. Systematically selected birth records were scrutinized for birth outcome parameters in the most recent birth. Data were extracted using the data extraction sheet designed by the research team. The outcome variables extracted were gestation at birth, labor onset, mode of birth, birth status, birth weight, newborn weight at 6 weeks, and morbidity at 6 weeks.

Operational Definition of Terms

Gestation at birth was operationalized as preterm (< 37 weeks) or term (37–40 weeks). Labor onset was operationalized as spontaneous or assisted labor. Mode of birth was operationalized as spontaneous vaginal birth or assisted birth. Birth status was operationalized as live birth or stillbirth. Birth weight was operationalized as low birth weight (< 2.5 kg) or normal birth weight ($\geq$ 2.5 kg). Newborn weight at 6 weeks was operationalized as recorded weight (in kilograms) of the unclothed newborn at 6 weeks. Morbidity at 6 weeks was operationalized as the recorded clinical symptoms of a newborn during postnatal clinical examinations performed within 6 weeks after birth.

Data Analysis

Categorical, discrete, and continuous data were collected. Descriptive statistics were used to summarize nominal (categorical), interval (discrete), and ratio (continuous) data. The hypotheses were tested using the *F* test to compare the mean scores for discrete and continuous data between groups. Chi-square, Fisher exact, and relative risk tests were used to compare categorical frequencies between groups. All hypotheses were tested at a 5% level of significance.

Results

The exposed group (K-Dere) was similar to the comparison group (Iriebe) in terms of age, previous pregnancies, parity status, and previous births ($p > .05$). Nonetheless, the exposed group differed from the comparison group in terms of occupation (Fisher's exact test = 45.32, $p < .001$). The exposed group included fewer civil servants (1.8%) than the comparison group (12.4%). The background sociodemographic characteristics of the participants are summarized in Table 1.

A significant difference between the exposed group and the comparison group was found in terms of preterm birth incidents (16.0% vs. 7.7%, $p = .018$). The exposed group had a 108% higher incidence of preterm births than the comparison group (relative risk = 2.08, 95% CI [1.11, 3.89], $p = .018$). Nonetheless, onset of labor, mode of birth, birth status, and birth weight were similar between the two groups ($p > .05$). Data on newborn birth outcomes are summarized in Table 2.

Data on newborn morbidity at 6 weeks after birth are summarized in Table 3. Further data analysis revealed significant differences between the exposed and comparison groups with respect to newborn weight and morbidity within 6 weeks of birth. At 6 weeks after birth, the newborns in the exposed group weighed significantly less than those in the comparison group (4.64 ± 0.82 vs. 4.85 ± 0.92 kg, $p = .032$). In addition, morbidity within 6 weeks of birth was 203% more likely for newborns in the exposed group than in the comparison group (relative risk = 3.03, 95% CI [2.20, 4.19], $p < .001$).

Discussion

This study found that the exposed group experienced 2 times more preterm births than the comparison group. This finding suggests that residing in crude-oil-polluted areas such as K-Dere greatly increases the risk of experiencing preterm birth. Preterm births in K-Dere were 16.0%, whereas those

Table 1

Sociodemographic Characteristics of Participants (Mothers; N = 338)

Variable	K-Dere (*n* = 169)		Iriebe (*n* = 169)		χ^2	*p*
	n	%	*n*	%		
Age (years)					2.07 [a]	.355
15–24	39	23.1	30	17.8		
25–34	112	66.3	115	68.0		
35–44	18	10.6	24	14.2		
Occupation					39.89 [a]	< .001*
Trader	106	62.7	124	73.4		
Farmer	42	24.9	6	3.6		
Housewife	10	5.8	12	7.0		
Hairdresser	5	3.0	3	1.8		
Civil servant	3	1.8	21	12.4		
Seamstress	3	1.8	3	1.8		
Previous pregnancies (times)					0.20 [a]	.903
1–3	134	79.3	135	79.9		
4–6	32	18.9	32	18.9		
7–9	3	1.8	2	1.2		
Parity status					1.13	.288
Primipara	47	27.8	56	33.1		
Multipara	122	72.2	113	66.9		
Previous births (times)					0.20 [a]	.903
1–3	134	79.3	135	79.9		
4–6	32	18.9	32	18.9		
7–9	3	1.8	2	1.2		

[a] Fisher statistic.

*$p < .05$.

Table 2
Newborn Birth Outcomes in Public Health Care Facilities in K-Dere and Iriebe (N = 338)

Variable	K-Dere (n = 169)		Iriebe (n = 169)		Fisher	p	Relative Risk	95% CI
	n	%	n	%				
Duration of pregnancy					5.56	.018*	2.08	[1.11, 3.89]
Preterm (< 37 weeks)	27	16.0	13	7.7				
Term (37–40 weeks)	142	84.0	156	92.3				
Labor onset								
Spontaneous onset	169	100.0	169	100.0				
Mode of birth								
Spontaneous vaginal birth	169	100.0	169	100.0				
Birth status					1.83	.371		
Live birth	168	99.4	165	97.6				
Stillbirth	1	0.6	4	2.4				
Birth weight [a]					3.65	.056		
Normal (> 2.5 kg)	145	85.8	153	90.5				
Low (≤ 2.5 kg)	23	13.6	12	7.1				

[a] Missing data.
*$p < .05$.

in Iriebe were only 7.7%. This finding is supported by Walker Whitworth et al. (2018) who found a relationship between unconventional gas development activity and preterm birth levels in Texas, USA, showing that pregnant women in areas of crude oil exploration activities faced a 20% higher risk of experiencing preterm birth ($p < .01$). The similarity in findings between this study and Whitworth et al.'s study may be related to the similarity in study design used. Retrospective cohorts nested from recorded births were used in both Whitworth et al.'s study and this study. Furthermore, the finding of higher preterm birth risk found in this study was in line with Casey et al. (2018) who studied the effect of coal and oil power plant retirements in California, USA, on preterm births in nearby populations. They found a reduction in preterm birth risk of 5%–7% in areas where crude oil plants had been shut down and retired. The findings of Casey et al. suggest that a threshold of 5% or fewer preterm births is obtainable in the absence of crude oil and hydrocarbon activities and may

Table 3
Newborn Morbidities at 6 Weeks After Birth in K-Dere and Iriebe (N = 338)

Variable	K-Dere (n = 168)		Iriebe (n = 165)		F	χ^2	p	Relative Risk	95% CI
	n	%	n	%					
Weight (mean and *SD*)	4.64	0.82	4.85	0.92	4.64		.032*	3.03	[2.20, 4.19]
Feeding						0.49	.484		
Exclusive breastfeeding	51	30.4	56	33.9					
Breastfeeding + water	117	69.6	109	66.1					
Morbidity						22.57 [a]	< .001*		
None identified	63	37.5	131	79.4					
Catarrh	12	7.1	1	0.6					
Cough and catarrh	24	14.3	14	8.5					
Boils and rashes	36	21.4	3	1.8					
Diarrhea	13	7.7	–	–					
Fever	14	8.3	16	9.7					
Cough, catarrh, boils, rashes, and fever	6	3.6	–	–					
Morbidity reclassified						60.08 [a]	< .001*		
No signs and symptoms present	63	37.5	131	79.4					
Signs and symptoms were present	105	62.5	34	20.6					

[a] Fisher statistic.
*$p < .05$.

increase to 7% if crude oil activities are introduced nearby (within 0–10 km of residence). Nevertheless, this finding contrasts with that of Willis and Hystad (2019) who studied the relationship between hazardous air pollutants and adverse birth outcomes in Portland, Oregon, USA, and found no consistent association between hydrocarbon-based air pollutants and preterm births. This divergence in findings may be explained by the focus in this study on crude oil environmental pollution, which includes farmland and water-source contamination and flaring. Willis and Hystad considered hydrocarbon air pollutants from traffic and industrial sources only. The difference in scope between this study and that of Willis and Hystad may account for the difference in results.

In this study, living in the crude-oil-polluted K-Dere area was found to be associated with a significantly increased risk of slower newborn growth rate, with body weight at 6 weeks after birth significantly lower in the exposed group than in the comparison group. This finding is supported by Bruederle and Hodler (2019) who found in a study on the impact of oil spills on infant mortality in Nigeria that pregnancies in crude-oil-polluted areas faced a significantly higher risk of negative developmental health effects in neonates and infants. The similarity in findings between this study and that of Bruederle and Hodler may be explained by both studies being conducted in the Niger Delta region. This finding was also supported by Atubi (2015) who found in a study on the effects of oil spillage on human health in nine Niger Delta communities in Delta State, Nigeria, that crude-oil-related pollution had negative effects on humans. Ingested hydrocarbon pollutants expressed in maternal breast milk may have been directly responsible for the observed slower infant growth. This assertion was supported by Digha et al. (2017) who noted in a study carried out in the Niger Delta in Nigeria that oil pollution has massively contaminated water sources, fishing areas, and livelihoods and may have contaminated the food chain.

The results of this study found that residing in the crude-oil-polluted area of K-Dere increased the risk of 6-week newborn morbidity by over 200%. This finding echoes that of Apergis et al. (2019) who found in a study on fracking and infant mortality in Oklahoma, USA, that residing within 0–10 km of crude oil processing plants was associated with negative infant health and survival indices. This finding was further buttressed by Bruederle and Hodler (2019) who found that residing near areas of oil exploration increased infant mortality by 3.8%, which effectively doubled the expected threshold. The similarity in findings between this study and Apergis et al.'s study may reflect that mostly singleton births were selected in each of the studies. The selection of singletons for assessment helps preserve participant homogeneity and the reproducibility of findings.

Limitations

This study was affected by one major limitation. The records-based retrospective cohort design utilized did not control for several potentially confounding variables, including maternal practice of adequate nutrition in pregnancy, maternal utilization of antenatal services, occupation, and compliance with prenatal drug prescriptions. This limitation may affect the validity of the conclusions. Thus, future studies may consider using a randomized controlled trial approach to improve the validity of results.

Conclusions

Pregnancies in environments affected by crude oil pollution face increased risks of preterm birth, slower newborn growth, and newborn morbidity within 6 weeks of birth. Stakeholders should lobby policymakers to promptly clean up crude-oil-polluted regions. In addition, crude oil wells should be relocated to locations that are at least 40 km distant from residential clusters, as supported by empirical studies such as Apergis et al. (2019) and Casey et al. (2018).

Author Contributions

Study conception and design: SON-O, DO, CE
Data collection: SON-O, CE
Data analysis and interpretation: All authors
Drafting of the article: All authors
Critical revision of the article: CE, SON-O, ISA, ENB-E

References

Apergis, N., Hayat, T., & Saeed, T. (2019). Fracking and infant mortality: Fresh evidence from Oklahoma. *Environmental Science and Pollution Research, 26*(31), 32360–32367. https://doi.org/10.1007/s11356-019-06478-z

Atubi, A. O. (2015). Effects of oil spillage on human health in producing communities of Delta State, Nigeria. *European Journal of Business and Social Sciences, 4*(8), 14–30.

Balise, V. D., Meng, C. X., Cornelius-Green, J. N., Kassotis, C. D., Kennedy, R., & Nagel, S. C. (2016). Systematic review of the association between oil and natural gas extraction processes and human reproduction. *Fertility and Sterility, 106*(4), 795–819. https://doi.org/10.1016/j.fertnstert.2016.07.1099

Bové, H., Bongaerts, E., Slenders, E., Bijnens, E. M., Saenen, N. D., Gyselaers, W., Van Eyken, P., Plusquin, M., Roeffaers, M. B. J., Ameloot, M., & Nawrot, T. S. (2019). Ambient black carbon particles reach the fetal side of human placenta. *Nature Communications, 10*(1), Article No. 3866. https://doi.org/10.1038/s41467-019-11654-3

Bruederle, A., & Hodler, R. (2019). Effect of oil spills on infant mortality in Nigeria. *PNAS, 116*(12), 5467–5471. https://doi.org/10.1073/pnas.1818303116

Casey, J. A., Karasek, D., Ogburn, E. L., Goin, D. E., Dang, K., Braveman, P. A., & Morello-Frosch, R. (2018). Retirements of coal and oil power plants in California: Association with reduced preterm birth among populations nearby. *American Journal of Epidemiology, 187*(8), 1586–1594. https://doi.org/10.1093/aje/kwy110

Charan, J., & Biswas, T. (2013). How to calculate sample size for different study designs in medical research. *Indian Journal of Psychological Medicine, 35*(2), 121–126. https://doi.org/10.4103/0253-7176.116232

Cochran, W. G. (1977). *Sampling techniques* (3rd ed.). John Wiley & Sons.

Digha, O. N., Ambah, B., & Jacob, E. N. (2017). The effects of crude oil spillage on farmland in Gokana local government area of Rivers State. *European Journal of Basic and Applied Sciences, 4*(1), 76–96.

Dunlap, K. (2018). *Research review of air pollution and fetal development* (pp. 1–5). https://cleanaircarolina.org/wp-content/uploads/2018/08/Air-Pollution-and-Fetal-Development-Final-2018.pdf

Harville, E. W., Shankar, A., Zilversmit, L., & Buekens, P. (2017). Self-reported oil spill exposure and pregnancy complications: The GROWH study. *International Journal of Environmental Research and Public Health, 14*(7), Article 692. https://doi.org/10.3390/ijerph14070692

Janitz, A. E., Dao, H. D., Campbell, J. E., Stoner, J. A., & Peck, J. D. (2019). The association between natural gas well activity and specific congenital anomalies in Oklahoma, 1997–2009. *Environment International, 122*, 381–388. https://doi.org/10.1016/j.envint.2018.12.011

Lamichhane, D. K., Leem, J. H., Lee, J. Y., & Kim, H. C. (2015). A meta-analysis of exposure to particulate matter and adverse birth outcomes. *Environmental Analysis Health and Toxicology, 30*, Article No. e2015011. https://doi.org/10.5620/eht.e2015011

McKenzie, L. M., Guo, R., Witter, R. Z., Savitz, D. A., Newman, L. S., & Adgate, J. L. (2014). Birth outcomes and maternal residential proximity to natural gas development in rural Colorado. *Environmental Health Perspectives, 122*(4), 412–417. https://doi.org/10.1289/eph.1306722

Oghenetega, O. B., Ana, G. R. E. E., Okunlola, M. A., & Ojengbede, O. A. (2020). Oil spills, gas flaring and adverse pregnancy outcomes: A systematic review. *Open Journal of Obstetrics and Gynecology, 10*(1), 187–199. https://doi.org/10.4236/ojog.2020.1010016

Oghenetega, O. B., Ojengbede, O. A., & Ana, G. R. E. E. (2020). Perception determinants of women and healthcare providers on the effects of oil pollution on maternal and newborn outcomes in the Niger Delta, Nigeria. *International Journal of Women's Health, 12*, 197–205. https://doi.org/10.2147/IJWH.S235536

Polit, D. F., & Beck, C. T. (2012). *Nursing research: Generating and assessing evidence for nursing practice* (9th ed.). Lippincott Williams & Wilkins.

Seabrook, J. A., Smith, A., Clark, A. F., & Gilliland, J. A. (2019). Geospatial analyses of adverse birth outcomes in southwestern Ontario: Examining the impact of environmental factors. *Environmental Research, 172*, 18–26. https://doi.org/10.1016/j.envres.2018.12.068

Walker Whitworth, K., Kaye Marshall, A., & Symanski, E. (2018). Drilling and production activity related to unconventional gas development and severity of preterm birth. *Environmental Health Perspectives, 126*(3), Article 037006. https://doi.org/10.1289/EHP2622

Willis, M., & Hystad, P. (2019). Hazardous air pollutants and adverse birth outcomes in Portland, OR. *Environmental Epidemiology, 3*(1), Article e034. https://doi.org/10.1097/EE9.0000000000000034

World Health Organization. (2020). *Newborns: Improving survival and well-being*. Author. https://www.who.int/news-room/fact-sheets/detail/newborns-reducing-mortality

Yakubu, O. H. (2017). Addressing environmental health problems in Ogoniland through implementation of United Nations environment program recommendations: Environmental management strategies. *Environments, 4*(2), Article 28. https://doi.org/10.3390/environments4020028

23

The Association Between Traditional Chinese Medicine Body Constitution Deviation and Essential Hypertension: A Case–Control Study

Yung-Cheng LIAO[1] • Li-Li CHEN[2*] • Hsiao-Chiao WANG[3,7] • Jui-Shan LIN[4] • Tin-Kwang LIN[5] • Shu-Chuan Amy LIN[6]

ABSTRACT

Background: The prevention and treatment of hypertension is valued globally. The World Health Organization advocates combining traditional medicines in the prevention and treatment of diseases. Traditional Chinese medicine (TCM) assumes that diseases originate from the attenuation of one's body constitution. A few studies have found that hypertension is correlated with TCM body constitution. However, body constitution is also affected by living environment. Therefore, investigating the correlation between deviations in body constitution and essential hypertension in different living environments is necessary to provide the basis for using TCM in combination with conventional Western medicine to prevent and treat hypertension.

Purpose: The aim of this study was to explore the association between TCM body constitution deviation and essential hypertension.

Methods: A case–control study was designed. Participants were selected from the outpatient clinics and neighboring communities of a regional teaching hospital in southern Taiwan. The study included 210 hypertension and 210 nonhypertension cases. Blood pressures were measured using an electronic sphygmomanometer to confirm the presence or absence of hypertension. The TCM Body Constitution Questionnaire, demographic datasheet, and hypertension-related factors questionnaire were used to collect data.

Results: A higher proportion of patients with body constitution deviation were found in the hypertension group than the nonhypertension group. The proportions of patients with Yin-Xu, Yang-Xu, and stasis constitution were 44.8%, 32.4%, and 30.6%, respectively, in the hypertension group and 28.6%, 25.2%, and 19.6%, respectively, in the nonhypertension group. After performing univariate analysis, the results showed significant differences between the two groups in terms of average body mass index; emotional traits of anger, worry, and fear; hyperlipidemia; hyperuricemia; Yin-Xu constitution; and stasis constitution. However, the multivariate analysis revealed having a Yin-Xu constitution to be a risk factor of essential hypertension after adjusting for age, gender, body mass index, emotional traits, drinking habit, hyperlipidemia, and hyperuricemia.

Conclusions/Implications for Practice: The results suggest that Yin-Xu and stasis constitutions are respectively associated with essential hypertension. The findings offer a valuable reference to governments and healthcare professionals to prevent the risk of essential hypertension. Screening and healthcare measures for TCM Yin-Xu or stasis constitution may be included in related prevention plans to minimize public exposure to the risk factors of essential hypertension.

KEY WORDS:
essential hypertension, traditional Chinese medicine (TCM), Yin-Xu (Yin deficiency) constitution, Yang-Xu (Yang deficiency) constitution, stasis constitution.

Introduction

Hypertension is a common disease and major risk factor for coronary ischemia, stroke, renal failure, and mortality (Williams et al., 2018; World Health Organization, 2019). In 2018, hypertension was the eighth most common cause of death in Taiwan (Health Promotion Administration, Ministry of Health and Welfare, Taiwan, ROC, 2020). According to the World Health Organization, 40% of the world's population over the age of 25 years (about one billion people) had hypertension in 2008, with 1.56 billion people expected to experience hypertension worldwide by 2025. Approximately eight million people die each year from hypertension-related diseases (Williams et al., 2018). The prevalence of hypertension is on the rise (Fryar et al., 2017; Health Promotion Administration, Ministry of Health and Welfare, Taiwan,

[1]*MS, RN, NP, Department of Nursing, Buddhist Tzu Chi General Hospital, Chia-Yi, Taiwan* • [2]*PhD, RN, Professor, School of Nursing, College of Health Care, China Medical University, Taichung, Taiwan, and Department of Nursing, China Medical University Hospital, Taichung, Taiwan* • [3]*PhD, RN, Assistant Professor, School of Nursing, College of Health Care, China Medical University, Taichung, Taiwan, and Department of Nursing, China Medical University Hospital, Taichung, Taiwan* • [4]*PhD, MD, Attending Physician, Department of Chinese Medicine, Tri-Service General Hospital, Taipei, Taiwan* • [5]*PhD, MD, Director, Department of Cardiology, Buddhist Tzu Chi General Hospital, Chia-Yi, Taiwan* • [6]*PhD, RN, NP, Director, Department of Nursing, National Yang Ming Chiao Tung University Hospital, Yilan, Taiwan, and Assistant Professor, School of Nursing, National Yang Ming Chiao Tung University, Taipei, Taiwan; and* [7]*Contributed equally as the corresponding author.*

ROC, 2017), and reducing the prevalence of hypertension is a worldwide health goal (World Health Organization, 2016). Therefore, the prevention and treatment of this disease are challenges for healthcare professionals worldwide.

Studies have shown the risk factors of essential hypertension to include genetics, gender, age, body mass index (BMI), socioeconomic status, eating habits, smoking, drinking, stress, emotional state, hyperlipidemia, and hyperuricemia, among others (Lu et al., 2015; H. C. Wang et al., 2012; World Health Organization, 2019; Yang et al., 2012; Zekewos et al., 2019). However, the cause of hypertension remains unknown in most cases (Bolívar, 2013). Further investigation is needed, because pinpointing the risk factors of this disease will aid in its prevention and treatment.

Body constitution, which refers to the fundamental components that constitute a human being, includes the total expression of physiological, psychological, and pathological traits (Su et al., 2008; Q. Wang, 2012). In addition, body constitution may reflect the state of balance between the yin and the yang and their related functions (Su et al., 2008). Su et al. defined body constitution as the physiologic state maintained by the dynamic interaction of energy (yang) and materials (yin) within the body. Body constitution deviation is defined as an imbalance in the consumption of yin and yang (L. L. Chen et al., 2009; Su et al., 2008). Having a "Yang-Xu constitution" implies that the energy needed to maintain bodily functions has diminished, which may be expressed in subjective symptoms such as fatigue, shortness of breath, chills, and loose stools (Su et al., 2008). Having a "Yin-Xu constitution" implies that the materials needed to perform or maintain body function have diminished, which may result in subjective symptoms such as thirst, hot flushes, and hard stools (J. D. Lin, Chen, et al., 2012; J. S. Lin et al., 2012). Having a "stasis constitution" implies that the dynamic interaction between yin and yang has slowed down and is less efficient, which may lead to subjective symptoms such as dizziness, chest tightness, or numbness in the limbs (J. D. Lin, Lin, et al., 2012). Traditional Chinese medicine (TCM) experts have suggested a correlation between body constitution and the occurrence and progression of disease and that individuals with unbalanced body constitutions are susceptible to certain pathogenic factors and related diseases (Su et al., 2008; Sun et al., 2018; Q. Wang, 2012). Implementation of appropriate care measures such as emotional management, exercise, suitable lifestyle, and living environment after detection of body constitution deviation and in accordance with body-constitution deviation type may reduce the occurrence and recurrence of disease (Shen et al., 2010; Q. Wang, 2012; Q. Wang et al., 2018). Therefore, this study was developed to explore the relationship between type of body constitution deviation and essential hypertension. The findings are provided as a reference for preventing essential hypertension.

In recent years, the World Health Organization has advocated a combination of traditional medical measures to prevent and treat diseases (World Health Organization, 2013). TCM is commonly combined with conventional Western medicine to treat hypertension in Chinese around Asia and in Chinese populations elsewhere in the world (Fan et al., 2019; J. Wang & Xiong, 2013). Only a few studies in Mainland China have correlated essential hypertension with phlegm wetness, Yin-Xu, blood stasis, and qi deficiency body constitution (Y. Li et al., 2017; Zhu et al., 2017). However, other studies have shown that living environment may affect body constitution status and subsequently affect the physical response to pathogenic factors of diseases (L. Li et al., 2019). Additional studies are required among Chinese populations in areas outside Mainland China to elucidate the relationship between TCM body constitution and hypertension. No research on the relationship between type of body constitution deviation and essential hypertension has been conducted in Taiwan. Therefore, this study was developed to explore the association between TCM body constitution deviation and essential hypertension among residents in Taiwan. The result of this study provides empirical evidence to help governments and healthcare professionals plan healthcare strategies to prevent essential hypertension.

Methods

Study Design and Participants

Study design and setting

A case–control study design and a purposive sampling strategy were adopted. The participants were selected from the cardiac clinic of a regional hospital and the community health checkup program in a neighboring community in southern Taiwan. Physicians confirmed the presence/absence of essential hypertension during regular patient health checkups.

Estimation of sample size

A pilot study comprising 29 patients with essential hypertension and 29 without hypertension was conducted to select cases meeting the inclusion conditions. The results were used to calculate the number of participants needed and the Cronbach's α values for the questionnaire. When comparing the average body constitution scores, the difference in stasis was the smallest between the hypertension and nonhypertension groups, which were 26.03 ± 8.72 and 23.03 ± 7.46, respectively. G*Power 3.1 statistical software was used to calculate the sample size needed for *t* test. Setting the α error probability to .05 and the power (1 – β error probability) to 0.95, 384 participants were required. The number of required participants was increased by 10% to 420 to account for possible participant attrition during the study.

Sample

The inclusion criteria for the hypertension group included the following: (a) diagnosis of essential hypertension by a physician or in the two measurements (taken at an interval of 30 minutes) at the time of recruitment and (b) systolic blood pressure of ≥ 140 mmHg or diastolic blood pressure of ≥ 90 mmHg (the Seventh Report of the Joint National Committee criteria for diagnosing hypertension). The inclusion criteria for the nonhypertension group included the following: (a) the absence of hypertension confirmed by a physician and blood pressure readings at the time of recruitment of < 140 mmHg (systolic) and < 90 mmHg (diastolic). The participants in both groups were all between 20 and 80 years old. All of the participants could communicate, were willing to participate, and signed consent forms. The exclusion criteria for both groups were as follows: the presence of other chronic diseases, severe acute illness within the past 3 months, continued use of drugs that affect blood pressure, and pregnancy. From August 2014 to July 2015, 210 participants with hypertension and 210 participants without hypertension were recruited (Table 1). Because age and gender affect TCM body constitution and blood pressure (National Health Bureau, Department of Health, Executive Yuan, Taiwan, ROC, 2011; Sun et al., 2018), the

Table 1

Distribution and Chi-Square Test of Basic Attribute Data and Related Factors in the Hypertension and Nonhypertension Groups (N = 420)

Item	Total (*N* = 420)		Hypertension (*n* = 210)		Nonhypertension (*n* = 210)		χ^2	*p*
	n	%	*n*	%	*n*	%		
Employed							1.11	.293
No	132	31.4	61	29.0	71	33.8		
Yes	288	68.6	149	71.0	139	66.2		
Late sleeper (after midnight)							0.09	.769
No	201	47.9	99	47.2	102	48.6		
Yes	219	52.1	111	52.8	108	51.4		
Exercise							0.01	.919
Irregular	153	36.4	77	36.6	76	36.2		
Regular (30 minutes or more)	267	63.6	133	63.4	134	63.8		
Salty foods							1.76	.185
No	352	83.8	171	81.4	181	86.2		
Yes	68	16.2	39	18.6	29	13.8		
Fried foods							0.78	.377
No	112	26.7	60	28.6	52	24.8		
Yes	308	73.3	150	71.4	158	75.2		
Smoking habit							0.46	.496
No	382	91.0	189	90.0	193	92.0		
Yes	38	9.0	21	10.0	17	8.0		
Drinking habit							2.97	.085
No	364	86.7	176	83.8	188	89.6		
Yes	56	13.3	34	16.2	22	10.4		
Hyperlipidemia							13.17	< .001
No	375	89.3	176	83.8	199	94.8		
Yes	45	10.7	34	16.2	11	5.2		
Hyperuricemia							6.27	.012
No	386	91.9	186	88.6	200	95.2		
Yes	34	8.1	24	11.4	10	4.8		
Yin-Xu constitution							11.85	.001
No	266	63.3	116	55.2	150	71.4		
Yes	154	36.7	94	44.8	60	28.6		
Yang-Xu constitution							2.61	.106
No	299	71.2	142	67.6	157	74.8		
Yes	121	28.8	68	32.4	53	25.2		
Stasis constitution							5.67	.017
No	317	75.5	148	70.4	169	80.4		
Yes	103	24.5	62	30.6	41	19.6		

participants were first stratified by presence or absence of hypertension and then by gender and age. The age interval of each stratum was 20 years, as recommended by the National Surveillance Definitions for Hypertension in the United States (Fryar et al., 2017). In accordance with the stratification conditions, the number of participants with and without hypertension in each group was selected as 1:1 using purposive sampling. However, as cases of essential hypertension among younger-aged individuals are less common, only 10 younger participants (< 40 years old) were recruited, with five assigned to each group, respectively.

Measurements

A questionnaire survey method was used in this study. The measurement tools used were structured questionnaires and included the TCM Body Constitution Questionnaire (BCQ; L. L. Chen et al., 2009; J. D. Lin, Chen, et al., 2012; J. D. Lin, Lin, et al., 2012; J. S. Lin et al., 2012; Su et al., 2008), the Five Emotions Questionnaire (M. H. Wang, 1995), and a demographics and hypertension-related factors datasheet. The published versions of the BCQ and the Five Emotions Questionnaire were used with permission from the original authors. In addition, blood pressure was measured twice at recruitment using an electronic sphygmomanometer to determine the case grouping.

Traditional Chinese medicine Body Constitution Questionnaire

The BCQ developed by Su et al.'s research team in Taiwan (L. L. Chen et al., 2009; J. D. Lin, Chen, et al., 2012, J. D. Lin, Lin, et al., 2012; J. S. Lin et al., 2012; Su et al., 2008) was used to measure TCM body constitution deviation. In the study questionnaire used in this study, the concepts of yang and yin were used in their broadest sense, with yang including the function of qi, yin including the function of blood, and stasis including the function of phlegm dampness (J. D. Lin, Lin, et al., 2012; Su et al., 2008). The BCQ comprised three parts, as follows: assessment of Yin-Xu constitution (BCQ−; 19 questions including blood deficiency), assessment of Yang-Xu constitution (BCQ+; 19 questions including qi deficiency), and assessment of stasis constitution (BCQ_S; 16 questions including phlegm dampness). Some questions were shared by the three scales, and the total number of questions in the BCQ was 44. The questionnaire was completed by the participants, based on their perceived intensity or frequency of physical symptoms during the past month. A 5-point Likert scale was used for scoring, as follows: 1 = *not at all/never*, 2 = *slightly/occasional*, 3 = *moderate/half of the time*, 4 = *severe/very often*, and 5 = *very severe/always*. The score for each BCQ was calculated separately, with the scores for BCQ− (BCQ to assess Yin-Xu) ranging from 19 to 95, those for BCQ+ (BCQ to assess Yang-Xu) ranging from 19 to 95, and those for BCQ_S (BCQ to assess stasis) ranging from 16 to 80. A higher score on the BCQ−, BCQ+, or BCQ_S was interpreted to indicate, respectively, a more pronounced Yin-Xu, Yang-Xu, or stasis constitution (L. L. Chen et al., 2009; J. D. Lin, Lin, et al., 2012; J. S. Lin et al., 2012), and the total score of each BCQ was used in this study to indicate whether the participant had a Yin-Xu, Yang-Xu, or stasis constitution. Participants with a total BCQ− score $\geq$ 29.5 were categorized as having a Yin-Xu constitution, participants with a total BCQ+ score $\geq$ 30.5 were categorized as having a Yang-Xu constitution, and participants with a total BCQ_S score $\geq$ 26.5 were categorized as having a stasis constitution (L. L. Chen et al., 2009; J. D. Lin, Lin, et al., 2012; J. S. Lin et al., 2012).

Using the BCQ− to assess Yin-Xu constitution (J. D. Lin, Chen, et al., 2012; J. S. Lin et al., 2012) earned a Cronbach's α value of .85 and a retest reliability intraclass correlation coefficient (ICC) value of .91. Using the BCQ+ to assess Yang-Xu constitution (L. L. Chen et al., 2009; J. D. Lin, Lin, et al., 2012; Su et al., 2008) earned a Cronbach's α value of .88 and a retest reliability ICC value of .91. Using the BCQ_S to assess stasis constitution (J. D. Lin, Lin, et al., 2012) earned a Cronbach's α value of .88 and a retest reliability ICC value of .92. The Cronbach's α values of the BCQ−, BCQ+, and BCQ_S pilot studies were .85, .86, and .86, respectively.

Five Emotions Questionnaire

The Five Emotions Questionnaire developed by M. H. Wang was used in this study to measure anger, joy, worry, sadness, and fear. Participants used the questionnaire, with five questions related to each emotion, to self-assess their emotional state during the past month (M. H. Wang, 1995). Approval was given by the original author to change the scale from a 4-point scale to a 5-point Likert scale. Each question was scored as follows: 1 = *not at all*, 2 = *occasionally*, 3 = *half of the time*, 4 = *often*, and 5 = *always*. The total possible score for each emotion category ranged from 5 to 25 points, with higher scores associated with a higher likeliness of occurrence of the associated emotional tendency (M. H. Wang, 1995). This study tested the Cronbach's α values of anger, joy, worry, sadness, and fear as .68, .72, .57, .87, and .75, respectively.

Demographics and hypertension-related factors questionnaire

This questionnaire gathered data on the basic demographics, blood pressure values, hypertension-related lifestyles, personal habit factors (i.e., staying up late, smoking, drinking, eating unhealthy foods, and regular exercise), and disease factors (i.e., hyperlipidemia or hyperuricemia) of participants. Questions regarding habits and disease factors were binary yes/no answers. Regular exercise referred to performing at least 30 minutes of continuous exercise, and staying up late referred to going to sleep after midnight. Two TCM physicians and three nursing experts were asked to check the applicability and relevance of the question contents. The expertise of nursing experts included TCM nursing and adult nursing. The content validity index value was 1, indicating that all of the questions were applicable, although the wording of some questions required modification.

Electronic sphygmomanometer

Blood pressure was measured using an electronic sphygmomanometer (UDEX-Twin; Elquest Corporation, Inc., Chiba, Japan) to confirm the hypertension status of each participant. The sphygmomanometer was certified under international standards and was maintained and calibrated to regularly ensure numerical accuracy. The measurement range of the sphygmomanometer was 10–285 mmHg, and the error value was ± 3 mmHg.

Data Collection and Analysis

This study was approved by the institutional review board (No. B10303010). All of the questionnaires were collected by the same researcher, who had received prior training. Blood pressure readings were taken by another researcher to increase the consistency of the data collection process. Both were registered nurses with clinical experience. The data collection sites were the outpatient waiting area and the community activity center of a regional teaching hospital in southern Taiwan. Eligible patients were invited to participate in the study and, if willing, were asked to provide written informed consent. After an explanation of the study process and participant rights, the participants completed the questionnaires. If participants were unable to fill out the questionnaires independently, the researcher recorded their answers for them. All of the participants had their blood pressure measured once, respectively, before and after completing the questionnaire to determine the presence or absence of hypertension.

Statistical analysis was performed using SPSS Statistics 22.0 software (IBM, Inc., Armonk, NY, USA). A chi-square test, an independent *t* test, and a multivariate logistic regression were used to analyze the influence of the presence or absence of hypertension by TCM body constitution, the five emotions, and demographic/hypertension-related factors. The p value was arbitrarily set at .05 to test the hypothesis based on Type I error ($\alpha = .05$), as the results of univariate analysis may be biased by other variables and the pseudo-association between independent variables may confound the "true" difference between two groups. Because the p value and search for significance level may be used as decision criteria (Dahiru, 2008; Greenland et al., 2016), the borderline level of significance was reset in this study to .10 ($\alpha = .1$), making the test of significance in the univariate analysis less stringent to include the variables of weak evidence against null effect in multivariate logistic regression analysis for adjusting the important confounders.

Results

The study recruitment period was between August 2014 and July 2015. Four hundred forty questionnaires were completed by participants who met the criteria for inclusion. Questionnaires from individuals with no history of hypertension and for whom hypertension was detected in only one of the measurements were excluded. Four hundred twenty (95%) of the completed questionnaires (210 in the hypertension group and 210 in the nonhypertension group) were valid and included in the analysis. The hypertension group included 138 participants (65.7%) from the community and 72 (34.3%) from the cardiology outpatient department of the target hospital. The nonhypertension group included 180 participants (85.7%) from the community and 30 (14.3%) who were family members accompanying outpatients at the hospital.

Distribution and Analysis of Demographics, Lifestyle, Five Emotions, and Traditional Chinese Medicine Body Constitution Status in Patients With/Without Hypertension

The data regarding the demographics, lifestyle, five emotions, and TCM body constitution status of the participants are shown in Tables 1 and 2. For participants in the hypertension and nonhypertension groups, respectively, the mean ages were 59.68 ± 11.27 years (range: 27–80 years) and 58.14 ± 10.32 years (range: 26–80 years), the systolic blood pressure readings at the second measurement were 141.64 ± 17.43 and 118.43 ± 10.39 mmHg, the diastolic blood pressure readings were 84.67 ± 10.97 and 73.68 ± 7.81 mmHg, the percentages having Yin-Xu constitutions were 44.8% and 28.6%, the percentages having Yang-Xu constitutions were 32.4% and 25.2%, and the percentages having stasis constitutions were 30.6% and 19.6%. The hypertension group had higher mean emotional and life-stress scores than the nonhypertension group. Moreover, the proportions of participants with hyperlipidemia, hyperuricemia, and Yin-Xu, Yang-Xu, and stasis constitutions in the hypertension group were higher than those in the nonhypertension group. Chi-square tests and independent *t* tests were performed on factors affecting the presence or absence of essential hypertension, with results showing statistically significant differences between the two groups ($p < .05$) in terms of BMI; drinking habit; hyperlipidemia or hyperuricemia; the emotional traits of anger, worry, and fear; and having a Yin-Xu or stasis body constitution (Tables 1 and 2). However, the lifestyle was similar between the two groups ($p > .05$).

Correlation Between Traditional Chinese Medicine Body Constitution Deviation and Essential Hypertension

The variables with a p value < .1 in the univariate analysis results were included in the multivariate logistic regression analysis to adjust for interfering factors. The factors affecting the presence or absence of essential hypertension are summarized in Table 3, with results showing statistically significant differences between the two groups in terms of age, BMI, hyperlipidemia, and Yin-Xu constitution ($p < .05$). After adjusting for the

Table 2

Distribution and Independent t Test of Basic Attribute Data and Related Factors in the Hypertension and Nonhypertension Groups (N = 420)

Item	Total (*N* = 420)		Hypertension (*n* = 210)		Nonhypertension (*n* = 210)		χ^2	*p*
	Mean	*SD*	Mean	*SD*	Mean	*SD*		
Age (years)	58.91	10.82	59.68	11.27	58.14	10.32	−1.463	.144
Body mass index (Kg/m^2)	24.32	3.27	25.27	3.44	23.36	2.78	−6.251	< .001
Life stress	0.72	0.77	0.76	0.81	0.68	0.72	−1.082	.280
Five Emotions Questionnaire								
Anger score	7.92	2.72	8.39	3.00	7.46	2.33	−3.547	< .001
Joy score	10.14	3.33	10.21	3.28	10.07	3.39	−0.453	.650
Worry score	9.11	3.07	9.45	3.27	8.76	2.82	−2.317	.021
Sadness score	7.60	2.78	7.75	2.93	7.44	2.60	−1.143	.254
Fear score	6.63	2.14	6.93	2.43	6.32	1.77	−2.963	.003
Body Constitution Questionnaire								
Yin-Xu constitution score	28.79	6.78	30.13	7.73	27.45	5.37	−4.120	< .001
Yang-Xu constitution score	28.30	7.36	29.49	8.32	27.11	6.06	−3.360	.001
Stasis constitution score	23.02	6.22	24.26	7.19	21.78	4.76	−4.178	< .001

other variables, the odds of hypertension were shown to increase by an average of 1.03 times for every 1-year increase in age and 1.25 times for every 1 kg/m^2 of BMI increase. Furthermore, the odds of hypertension in those with a history of hyperlipidemia were found to be 2.63 times higher than in those without this history, and the odds of hypertension in those with Yin-Xu constitution were found to be 2.15 times than in those without Yin-Xu. This indicates that, after adjusting for demographics and other related factors, the risk of developing hypertension is higher in those with Yin-Xu constitution than in those without Yin-Xu.

Discussion

This study found BMI; having hyperlipidemia or hyperuricemia; having the emotional traits of anger, worry, or fear; and having a Yin-Xu or stasis constitution to be correlated with essential hypertension. After adjusting for other potential

Table 3

Factors Related to Hypertension, as Revealed by Multivariate Logistic Regression (N = 420)

Item	*B*	*SE*	Wald Value	*p*	*OR*	95% CI
Gender (female = 0)	−0.35	0.24	2.16	.141	0.71	[0.44, 1.12]
Age	0.03	0.01	8.00	.005	1.03	[1.01, 1.05]
BMI	0.22	0.04	32.43	< .001	1.25	[1.16, 1.35]
Drinking (no = 0)	0.35	0.35	0.97	.324	1.42	[0.71, 2.84]
Hyperlipidemia (no = 0)	0.97	0.39	6.20	.013	2.63	[1.23, −5.62]
Hyperuricemia (no = 0)	0.49	0.44	1.23	.268	1.63	[0.69, 3.87]
Anger	0.09	0.06	2.46	.117	1.10	[0.98, 1.23]
Worry	−0.02	0.05	0.10	.753	0.99	[0.90, 1.08]
Fear	0.06	0.06	0.97	.326	1.07	[0.94, 1.21]
Yin-Xu (no = 0)	0.76	0.35	4.88	.027	2.15	[1.09, 4.23]
Yang-Xu (no = 0)	−0.53	0.35	2.24	.135	0.59	[0.30, 1.18]
Stasis (no = 0)	0.13	0.35	0.14	.708	1.14	[0.58, 2.24]
Constant	−8.42	1.36	38.30	< .001	0.00	

Note. *SE* = standard error; *OR* = odds ratio; CI = confidence interval; BMI = body mass index. Nagelkerke R^2 = .231; χ^2 = 79.808 ($p < .001$).

variables, having a Yin-Xu constitution was identified as a risk factor for essential hypertension. This finding provides empirical evidence for governments and healthcare professionals to enact measures to prevent essential hypertension. The results suggest that the TCM BCQ may be used to screen people with Yin-Xu and stasis constitutions, with the results used to provide appropriate conditioning body-constitution care measures to reduce exposure to the risk factors of essential hypertension.

The scales of three TCM body constitution types developed by Su et al. were used in this study (L. L. Chen, et al., 2009; J. D. Lin, Chen, et al., 2012; Lin, Lin, et al., 2012; J. S. Lin et al., 2012; Su et al., 2008), with the results showing the proportions of people with Yin-Xu, Yang-Xu, and stasis constitutions were higher in the hypertension group than in the nonhypertension group. This finding is similar to the results of previous studies (Cen & Liu, 2016; Wu et al., 2009; Zhu et al., 2017) that used the scales of nine TCM body constitution types developed by Q. Wang et al. (2006). Furthermore, the results of this study indicate that those with TCM body constitution deviations are more prone to essential hypertension than those without body constitution deviations, which is consistent with the theory that disease occurrence is correlated with body constitution deviation (Sun et al., 2018).

Further analysis in this study showed both having a Yin-Xu constitution and having a stasis constitution to be correlated with essential hypertension. In addition, the stasis constitution measurement in this study included phlegm dampness (J. D. Lin, Lin, et al., 2012). Therefore, the result of this study is similar to that of Zu et al. (2013), which showed that Yin-Xu, phlegm dampness, and blood stasis influence the prevalence of hypertension. Moreover, this study also compared the body constitution differences between prehypertension and healthy individuals, finding that Yin-Xu, phlegm-dampness, and blood stasis constitution influence prehypertension. Yin-Xu produces internal heat that disturbs the orifices, causing hyperactivity of the yang, which is one of the main risk factors for hypertension (H. J. Chen & Dung, 2014). Phlegm dampness blocks the meridians and turns into heat, which disturbs the orifices and causes hypertension. In addition, retention of phlegm and fluid causes poor blood circulation, resulting in stasis, which may aggravate hypertension (H. J. Chen & Dung, 2014; J. Wang & Xiong, 2012).

As some of the risk factors of essential hypertension could not be controlled in this study, a multivariate logistic regression model was employed to adjust for the potentially interfering factors. The results of this model showed only Yin-Xu constitution as associated with essential hypertension, which differs partially from the findings of previous studies (Cen & Liu, 2016; Y. Li et al., 2017; Wu et al., 2009; Zhu et al., 2017). This difference may be because a different body constitution questionnaire and classifications were used, the living environments of participants were significantly different, and related interfering factors may not have been included in the multivariate logistic regression model analysis. The body-constitution classifications and measurement questions used in previous studies differed from those used in this study (Cen & Liu, 2016; Y. Li et al., 2017; Wu et al., 2009; Zhu et al., 2017). In addition, previous studies may have included different interfering factors in the multivariate regression model analysis to adjust for the effects of other variables (Cen & Liu, 2016; Y. Li et al., 2017; Wu et al., 2009).

The stratified sampling approach used in this study excluded some potential research subjects and utilized multivariate regression model analysis to adjust for confounding factors and to reduce error (Portney & Watkins, 2009). It has been reported that, as body constitution distribution differs by gender and age group, gender and age are correlated with the occurrence of essential hypertension (National Health Bureau, Department of Health, Executive Yuan, Taiwan, ROC, 2011; Williams et al., 2018). Therefore, this study used stratified sampling so that the two groups were similar in terms of gender and age to adjust for the potential interference of these two variables on the relationship between TCM constitution deviation and essential hypertension. Moreover, the sources of subjects for the two groups were similar, which may have reduced case-selection-related errors (Portney & Watkins, 2009). Blood pressure was measured twice at recruitment to improve the accuracy of participant groupings. To avoid the influence of chronic diseases other than hyperlipidemia and hyperuricemia on TCM body constitution distribution (S. C. A. Lin et al., 2017; Zhu et al., 2017), individuals with other chronic diseases were excluded.

However, the participants in this study had already developed the disease, which may have influenced the results. In other words, although this study found Yin-Xu constitution as correlated with essential hypertension, it is impossible to judge the order of occurrence of Yin-Xu constitution and essential hypertension. Longitudinal design studies that incorporate the BCQ into the follow-up study plan of the National Health Interview Survey (Health Promotion Administration, Ministry of Health and Welfare, Taiwan, ROC, 2017) are needed to further explore the causality between Yin-Xu and essential hypertension.

Limitations

Nearly half of the participants in this study were over 60 years old. Elderly individuals may be more likely to miss questions and may be less clear about their own disease status than younger individuals (Tsai et al., 2007). Thus, recall bias may have been an unavoidable limitation in this study. Some of the participants in the hypertension and nonhypertension groups (3.3% and 2.9%, respectively) required assistance with recording their answers because of their visual deterioration or illiteracy. This process may not completely avoid errors in data collection. However, the average ages of the participants in the two groups were similar. Thus, these errors may be expected to be consistent between the two groups. To further reduce error, the study process and recruitment criteria were explained in detail. Blood pressure was measured before and after the questionnaire was completed to improve the accuracy of subject grouping. The interviewer's manual was prepared before implementation of the study to maintain consistency and to reduce data collection errors. Because the participants had no other chronic diseases and as there were significantly fewer patients with hypertension below the age of 40 years, the results of this study should not be inferred to patients with hypertension with other comorbidities or to patients with hypertension less than 40 years old.

Conclusions

The results of this study established the empirical data necessary to confirm a correlation between TCM body constitution deviation and essential hypertension. The results suggest that TCM Yin-Xu and stasis constitutions are associated with essential hypertension. After adjusting for BMI, drinking habit, hyperlipidemia status, hyperuricemia status, emotional traits, and other potential confounding factors, Yin-Xu constitution was found to be a risk factor for the development of essential hypertension. These empirical data may be used as a basis to combine TCM methods in the prevention of essential hypertension. They also provide a reference for governments and healthcare professionals to screen and plan TCM Yin-Xu constitution healthcare strategies to reduce public/patient exposure to the risk factors of essential hypertension.

Acknowledgments

The authors would like to thank the study participants for their participation and the China Medical University (CMU103-S-32) and Buddhist Dalin Tzuchi General Hospital (DTCRD104-E-05), Taiwan, for their funding support.

Author Contributions

Study conception and design: YCL, LLC, JSL
Data collection: YCL, TKL, SCAL, HCW
Data analysis and interpretation: LLC, YCL, HCW
Drafting of the article: LLC, YCL, HCW
Critical revision of the article: LLC, HCW

References

Bolívar, J. J. (2013). Essential hypertension: An approach to its etiology and neurogenic pathophysiology. *International Journal of Hypertension, 2013*, Article ID 547809. https://doi.org/10.1155/2013/547809

Cen, Y. Z., & Liu, X. X. (2016). The relationship between TCM constitutions and primary hypertension in community elderly people. *Guangming Journal of Chinese Medicine, 31*(24), 3537–3539. (Original work published in Chinese)

Chen, H. J., & Dung, G. Y. (2014). A discussion on TCM physique and hypertension. *Clinical Journal of Chinese Medicine, 2*(11), 54–56. (Original work published in Chinese)

Chen, L.-L., Lin, J.-S., Lin, J.-D., Chang, C.-H., Kuo, H.-W., Liang, W.-M., & Su, Y.-C. (2009). BCQ+: A body constitution questionnaire to assess Yang-Xu. Part II: Evaluation of reliability and validity. *Forschende Komplementärmedizin, 16*(1), 20–27. https://doi.org/10.1159/000197770

Dahiru, T. (2008). P-value, a true test of statistical significance? A cautionary note. *Annals of Ibadan Postgraduate Medicine, 6* (1), 21–26. https://doi.org/10.4314/aipm.v6i1.64038

Fan, H., Lu, F., Yang, A., Dong, Y., Liu, P., Wang, Y., & Wang, Y. (2019). A review on the nonpharmacological therapy of traditional Chinese medicine with antihypertensive effects. *Evidence-Based Complementary and Alternative Medicine, 2019*, Article ID 1317842. https://doi.org/10.1155/2019/1317842

Fryar, C. D., Ostchega, Y., Hales, C. M., Zhang, G., & Kruszon-Moran, D. (2017). Hypertension prevalence and control among adults: United States, 2015–2016. *NCHS Data Brief, 289*, 1–8.

Greenland, S., Senn, S. J., Rothman, K. J., Carlin, J. B., Poole, C., Goodman, S. N., & Altman, D. G. (2016). Statistical tests, *p* values, confidence intervals, and power: A guide to misinterpretations. *European Journal of Epidemiology, 31*(4), 337–350. https://doi.org/10.1007/s10654-016-0149-3

Health Promotion Administration, Ministry of Health and Welfare, Taiwan, ROC. (2017). *National health interview survey*. https://www.hpa.gov.tw/Pages/List.aspx?nodeid=106 (Original work published in Chinese)

Health Promotion Administration, Ministry of Health and Welfare, Taiwan, ROC. (2020, March 2). *Statistics of causes of death in Taiwan, 2018*. https://www.mohw.gov.tw/cp-16-48057-1.html (Original work published in Chinese)

Li, L., Yao, H., Wang, J., Li, Y., & Wang, Q. (2019). The role of Chinese medicine in health maintenance and disease prevention: Application of constitution theory. *The American Journal of Chinese Medicine, 47*(3), 495–506. https://doi.org/10.1142/S0192415X19500253

Li, Y., Li, X.-H., Huang, X., Yin, L., Guo, C.-X., Liu, C., He, Y.-M., Liu, X., & Yuan, H. (2017). Individualized prevention against hypertension based on traditional Chinese medicine constitution theory: A large community-based retrospective, STROBE-compliant study among Chinese population. *Medicine, 96*(46), Article e8513. https://doi.org/10.1097/MD.0000000000008513

Lin, J.-D., Chen, L.-L., Lin, J.-S., Chang, C.-H., Huang, Y.-C., & Su, Y.-C. (2012). BCQ–: A body constitution questionnaire to assess Yin-Xu. Part I: Evaluation of reliability and validity. *Forschende Komplementärmedizin, 19*(5), 234–241. https://doi.org/10.1159/000343580

Lin, J.-D., Lin, J.-S., Chen, L.-L., Chan, C.-H., Huang, Y.-C., & Su, T.-C. (2012). BCQs: A body constitution questionnaire to assess stasis in traditional Chinese medicine. *European Journal of Integrative Medicine, 4*(4), e379–e391. https://doi.org/10.1016/j.eujim.2012.05.001

Lin, J.-S., Chen, L.-L., Lin, J.-D., Chang, C.-H., Huang, C.-H., Mayer, P. K., & Su, Y.-C. (2012). BCQ–: A body constitution questionnaire to assess Yin-Xu. Part II: Evaluation of reliability and validity. *Forschende Komplementärmedizin, 19*(6), 285–292. https://doi.org/10.1159/000346060

Lin, S.-C. A., Chu, P.-Y., Chen, L.-L., Su, Y.-C., & Wang, S.-M. (2017). The prevalence rate of deviations in body constitutions and related factors in follow-up stage breast cancer patients—A nationwide study. *Complementary Therapies in Medicine, 32*, 49–55. https://doi.org/10.1016/j.ctim.2017.03.013

Lu, Y., Lu, M., Dai, H., Yang, P., Smith-Gagen, J., Miao, R., Zhong, H., Chen, R., Liu, X., Huang, Z., & Yuan, H. (2015). Lifestyle and risk of hypertension: Follow-up of a young pre-hypertensive cohort. *International Journal of Medical Sciences, 12*(7), 605–612. https://doi.org/10.7150/ijms.12446

National Health Bureau, Department of Health, Executive Yuan, Taiwan, ROC. (2011). 2007 survey on the prevalence of hypertension, hyperglycemia and hyperlipidemia in Taiwan. https://bit.ly/3t5RUrX

Portney, L. G., & Watkins, M. P. (2009). Exploratory research: Observational designs. In L. G. Portney & M. P. Watkins (Eds.), *Foundations of clinical research: Applications to practice* (3rd ed., pp. 282–286). Pearson.

Shen, C. Z., Pang, S. M.-C., Kwong, E. W.-Y., & Cheng, Z. Q. (2010). The effect of Chinese food therapy on community dwelling Chinese hypertensive patients with Yin-deficiency. *Journal of Clinical Nursing, 19*(7–8), 1008–1020. https://doi.org/10.1111/j.1365-2702.2009.02937.x

Su, Y.-C., Chen, L.-L., Lin, J.-D., Lin, J.-S., Huang, Y.-C., & Lai, J.-S. (2008). BCQ+: A body constitution questionnaire to assess Yang-Xu. Part I: Establishment of a first final version through a Delphi process. *Forschende Komplementärmedizin, 15*(6), 327–334. https://doi.org/10.1159/000175938

Sun, Y., Zhao, Y., Xue, S. A., & Chen, J. (2018). The theory development of traditional Chinese medicine constitution: A review. *Journal of Traditional Chinese Medical Sciences, 5*(1), 16–28. https://doi.org/10.1016/j.jtcms.2018.02.007

Tsai, A. C.-H., Liou, J.-C., & Chang, M.-C. (2007). Interview to study the determinants of hypertension in older adults in Taiwan: A population based cross-sectional survey. *Asia Pacific Journal of Clinical Nutrition, 16*(2), 338–345. https://doi.org/10.6133/apjcn.2007.16.2.20

Wang, H.-C., Liu, Y.-C., Huang, C.-H., & Weng, H.-C. (2012). Analysis hypertension hypertriglyceridemia and hyperglycemia from medical employee in a medical center in Southern Taiwan. *Chinese Journal of Occupational Medicine, 19*(1), 39–48. https://doi.org/10.30027/CJOM.201201.0005 (Original work published in Chinese)

Wang, J., & Xiong, X. (2012). Control strategy on hypertension in Chinese medicine. *Evidence-Based Complementary and Alternative Medicine, 2012*, Article ID 284847. https://doi.org/10.1155/2012/284847

Wang, J., & Xiong, X. (2013). Evidence-based Chinese medicine for hypertension. *Evidence-Based Complementary and Alternative Medicine, 2013*, Article ID 978398. https://doi.org/10.1155/2013/978398

Wang, M.-H. (1995). The relationship between the five organs and the five emotions as described in the "Yellow Emperor's Classic of Internal Medicine". *China Medical College Journal, 4*, 123–130. (Original work published in Chinese)

Wang, Q. (2012). Individualized medicine, health medicine, and constitutional theory in Chinese medicine. *Frontiers of Medicine, 6*(1), 1–7. https://doi.org/10.1007/s11684-012-0173-y

Wang, Q., Bai, M., Yang, Y., Liang, X., Sun, P., Han, J., Fan, T., & Yuan, C. (2018). Application of TCM constitution in lifetime health maintenance. *Journal of Traditional Chinese Medical Sciences, 5*(1), 6–15. https://doi.org/10.1016/j.jtcms.2018.02.006

Wang, Q., Zhu, Y.-B., Xue, H.-S., & Li, S. (2006). Primary compiling of constitution in Chinese medicine questionnaire. *Chinese Journal of Clinical Rehabilitation, 10*(3), 12–14. (Original work published in Chinese)

Williams, B., Mancia, G., Spiering, W., Agabiti Rosei, E., Azizi, M., Burnier, M., Clement, D. L., Coca, A., de Simone, G., Dominiczak, A., Kahan, T., Mahfoud, F., Redon, J., Ruilope, L., Zanchetti, A., Kerin, M., Kjeldsen, S. E., Kreutz, R., Laurent, S., ... Desormais, I. (2018). 2018 ESC/ESH guidelines for the management of arterial hypertension: The task force for the management of arterial hypertension of the European Society of Cardiology (ESC) and the European Society of Hypertension (ESH). *European Heart Journal, 39*(33), 3021–3104. https://doi.org/10.1093/eurheartj/ehy339

World Health Organization. (2013). *WHO Traditional Medicine Strategy: 2014–2023*. https://www.who.int/publications-detail/who-traditional-medicine-strategy-2014-2023

World Health Organization. (2016). *Global NCD target: Reduce high blood pressure*. https://www.who.int/publications/i/item/global-ncd-target-reduce-high-blood-pressure

World Health Organization. (2019). *Hypertension*. https://www.who.int/news-room/fact-sheets/detail/hypertension

Wu, H. d., Wang, Q., & Dong, J. (2009). Multiple logistic regression analysis on constitutional factors of hypertension. *Journal of Beijing University of Traditional Chinese Medicine, 16*(5), 12–13. (Original work published in Chinese)

Yang, T., Chu, C.-H., Bai, C.-H., You, S.-L., Chou, Y.-C., Hwang, L.-C., Chien, K.-L., Su, T.-C., Tseng, C.-H., & Sun, C.-A. (2012). Uric acid concentration as a risk marker for blood pressure progression and incident hypertension: A Chinese cohort study. *Metabolism: Clinical and Experimental, 61*(12), 1747–1755. https://doi.org/10.1016/j.metabol.2012.05.006

Zekewos, A., Egeno, T., & Loha, E. (2019). The magnitude of hypertension and its risk factors in southern Ethiopia: A community based study. *PLOS ONE, 14*(8), Article e0221726. https://doi.org/10.1371/journal.pone.0221726

Zhu, Y., Shi, H., Wang, Q., Wang, Y., Yu, X., Di, J., Zhang, X., Li, Y., Li, T., & Yan, H. (2017). Association between nine types of TCM constitution and five chronic diseases: A correspondence analysis based on a sample of 2,660 participants. *Evidence-Based Complementary and Alternative Medicine, 2017*, Article ID 9439682. https://doi.org/10.1155/2017/9439682

Zu, J., Chen, G. H., Zhong, J. H., & Huo, R. (2013). Preliminary study on the Chinese medicine constitutional characteristics in the prehypertension. Journal of Emergency in Traditional Chinese Medicine, *22*(8), 1328–1329. (Original work published in Chinese)

The Process of Developing Resilience in Patients With Burn Injuries

Jing HAN[1,5] • Xue-Ping ZHOU[2,5] • Jun-E LIU[3]* • Peng YUE[4] • Li GAO[4]

ABSTRACT

Background: Patients with burn injuries resulting in visible disabilities may face negative emotional experiences during rehabilitation. Understanding the development of resilience in these patients may help those who are seeking methods to better adapt to their new situation.

Purpose: This study aimed to explore the development of resilience in patients with burns during their convalescence.

Methods: Ten patients with burn injuries who were convalescing in a general hospital in China were recruited and enrolled as participants. Data were collected using recorded, semistructured in-depth interviews and analyzed following the principles of grounded theory.

Results: The development of resilience in patients with burns included five stages of "black hole," "introspection," "integration," "practice," and "growth." Both internal and external protective factors were identified. The internal protective factors included hope, sincerity, will, belief, and curiosity, and the external protective factor was mutual relationships that reflected the qualities of caring, support, sharing, commitment, and intimacy.

Conclusions: Resilience was achieved gradually over several progressive steps through the five stages (black hole, introspection, integration, practice, and growth). The results of this research may provide insights and support to patients who seek to improve their adaptation to new situations.

Key Words:
burn, resilience, psychological rehabilitation, grounded theory.

Introduction

Patients with burn injuries have experienced a traumatic event that may lead to multiple psychological problems (Dunpath, Chetty, & Van Der Reyden, 2014). For example, during the discharge rehabilitation stage (3 months after injury), patients may feel shame or inferiority in interpersonal relationships, and these feelings may develop into posttraumatic stress disorder (PTSD; Dunpath et al., 2014). Although patients with burn injuries return to society once their physical ailments have been treated, postdischarge psychological rehabilitation determines how they manage the challenges of their new lives. PTSD affects approximately 30% of patients with burns (Cakir, Terzi, Abaci, & Aker, 2015; Van Loey, van de Schoot, & Faber, 2012) and may be caused by clinical symptoms such as itching, pain, ulceration, and contracture. Some burned patients adapt well to life after injury (Dahl, 2013; Waqas et al., 2016) after addressing the traumatic events that led to PTSD and related symptoms. Successful adaptation indicates that these individuals have tried to cope with the event and process the traumatic information, a process that is considered integral to the development of resilience (Endfield, 2012; Kornhaber, Bridgman, McLean, & Vandervord, 2016).

Resilience is a multifaceted concept that is characterized by a dynamic process involving the interaction between the intrapsychic and social factors of risk and protection (Garcia-Dia, DiNapoli, Garcia-Ona, Jakubowski, & O'Flaherty, 2013). Resilience may be defined as "the human ability to adapt in the face of tragedy, trauma, adversity, hardship, and ongoing significant life stressors" (Newman, 2005). In Richardson's Resiliency Model (Richardson, 2002), although an individual initially experiences balanced biopsychospiritual homeostasis, stressors (e.g., adverse life events) may begin to interact with personal protective factors and lead to system collapse and reintegration. The four possible outcomes when protective factors are insufficient to withstand a stressor include resilient reintegration, reintegration back to homeostasis, reintegration with loss, and dysfunctional reintegration. Resilience influences the effective adaptation and mental health of individuals facing stressors, promoting personal development (Wanberg & Banas, 2000), improving mental health (Friborg, Barlaug, Martinussen, Rosenvinge, & Hjemdal, 2005), and predicting negative psychological symptoms after trauma (Campbell-sills, Cohan, & Stein, 2006).

Studies have shown a relationship between resilience and burn injury. Quantitative interviews have found that resilience exerts positive effects immediately after a burn occurs

[1]*MSN, RN, Doctoral Student, School of Nursing, Capital Medical University, Beijing, PRC* • [2]*MSN, RN, Psychological Counselor, School of Nursing, Capital Medical University, Beijing, PRC* • [3]*PhD, RN, Professor, School of Nursing, Capital Medical University, Beijing, PRC* • [4]*PhD, RN, Associate Professor, School of Nursing, Capital Medical University, Beijing, PRC* • [5]*Contributed equally.*

and may predict psychological symptoms after the injury (Wang & Chen, 2007). Moreover, the positive effects of resilience may occur in the process of self-reconstruction after a burn injury (Lau & van Niekerk, 2011). Cross-sectional surveys have found a significant correlation between the psychological resilience of burned patients and their subjective well-being (He, Cao, Feng, Guan, & Peng, 2013) and found that self-esteem and family support predicted resilience in patients with burns (Jang, Park, Chong, & Sok, 2017). However, there are few studies on the process of developing resilience in patients with burns. Some researchers have suggested that studying the development of resilience may help in understanding the phenomenon of resilience and ultimately foster occupational adaptation in patients (Lopez, 2011; Xi, Zuo, & Wu, 2012). This study examines the development of resilience among patients with burn injuries and the related factors of influence, with the intent to help nurses provide more effective support.

The aim of this study was to explore resilience development in patients who have suffered a burn injury.

Methods

Design and Participants

This study applied grounded theory because of the focus of this theoretical approach on processes and theory generation (Chen, 2000). Ten patients with burns in visible areas that were associated with cicatricial contracture or dysfunction who were convalescing in a general hospital in China were recruited from the comprehensive department of burn and orthopedics. Six men and four women, from 19 to 44 years old, participated in the study; five were married, four were single, and one was divorced; and nine of the 10 participants had completed at least high school. The burn areas covered from 16% to 50% of their bodies.

Ethical Considerations

This study was approved by the Ethics Committee of Capital Medical University (2010SY24) and adhered to the committee's ethical guidelines. All recruits volunteered to participate and signed an informed consent. Codes were used to ensure participant anonymity and confidentiality.

Data Collection

This study was conducted from November 2012 to February 2013. Posters providing information about the study were placed in the burn ward, and patients interested in participating were asked to contact the researcher. The in-depth interviews were conducted in a quiet place using a semistructured guide with six questions (based on a literature review and the aims of the study). Example questions included (a) "When you felt stress after your burn experience, what did you do?", (b) "What were your feelings during the convalescence period?", and (c) "If you could, what changes would you make next?". All interviews were tape-recorded and transcribed verbatim within 24 hours. Each participant received a printed interview transcript to ensure that the recorded information accurately reflected meaning. The printed copies were returned 3 days later, and no changes were made to the original transcripts.

One of the researchers, the nurse who had regular care responsibilities for the participants and had thus developed relationships of mutual trust, conducted the interviews. Data collection and analysis were conducted concurrently. On the basis of each data analysis experience, the researchers developed concepts, categories, and preliminary theories that were applied to subsequent in-depth interviews. This helped ensure that the rich data collection procedure generated reliable results.

Data Analysis

All data were analyzed using grounded theory methods, which involved coding, making constant comparisons, and writing memos. Two authors performed independent coding, which consisted of opening coding, axis coding, and selecting coding (Charmaz, 2006). Throughout the process, the results were discussed in regular group meetings and compared continually to refine the different concept categories and identify relationships among these categories. Written memos and self-reflection occurred continually during the research period.

Rigor

Credibility, dependability, conformability, and transferability were used to evaluate the rigor of the qualitative research (Streubert & Carpenter, 2010). As previously discussed, interviews were tape-recorded and transcripts were checked by each participant to ensure credibility. The audit trail, which involved the interview guide, audio recordings, field notes, and data analysis process, was clearly detailed. Two researchers carried out the initial coding independently, and weekly meetings involving five researchers helped establish dependability and conformability. In addition to the primary researcher, four researchers who were experienced in burn care were involved in the analysis of data. To ensure transferability, secondary interviews with the participants about the preliminary results and detailed descriptions based on the data were completed.

Results

The process of developing resilience was represented using a circular framework (Figure 1) after an analysis based on grounded theory. This process involved five closely related stages of resilience generation, with five internal and five external protective factors. These five stages, defined as black hole, introspection, integration, practice, and growth, were placed on the periphery of the circular resilience framework diagram. The five internal protective factors were hope, sincerity, will, belief, and curiosity, whereas the five external protective factors were caring, supportive, sharing, committed,

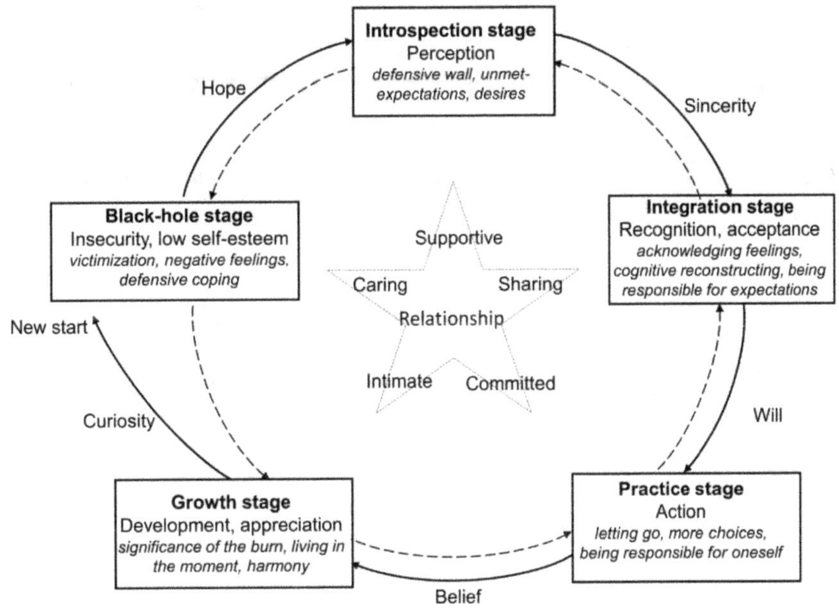

Figure 1. The process of developing resilience in patients with burns.

and intimate relationships. The five parts of the cyclical process shared dynamic and interactive relationships, and the development of each stage, facilitated by internal and external protective factors, occurred in an open, spiraling, and upward direction. The participants might repeat the cycle multiple times, incorporating additional experiences as they returned to each stage. Every cycle led to more experience and increased freedom; for example, the arrow emerging from the growth stage led to a more developed state rather than a return to the original black hole stage. However, the order of the cycle is not simple or linear; connections among the stages are indicated by arrows pointing in opposite directions. The solid outer ring represents protective factors that promote the development of resilience, and the dotted inner ring indicates regression. The dotted star in the middle of the diagram shows that resilience is based on interpersonal relationships that lead to several changes, each of which corresponds to one of the five stages in the periphery, ultimately leading to the emergence of the protective factors of resilience on the outer ring.

The Process of Developing Resilience

Black hole stage

The black hole, representing the psychological dilemma faced by the patient with burn injury, is typified by a lost sense of security and low self-esteem caused by victimization, negative feelings, and defensive coping.

"Victimization" refers to a patient's self-perception of his or her own identity and situation. The patient self-perceives as a "burned patient" who has experienced serious physical and psychological harm and thus assumes the role of a victim. Victimization is a manifestation of low self-esteem: "*The burn left me with nothing and makes me nothing. What can I do from now on? There is nothing I can do. I rely on others to take care of me in my daily life and will depend on others to realize my dreams.*" (A)

"Negative feelings" primarily include fear, anxiety, anger, and depression. During this stage, participants directly experienced negative feelings (e.g., low self-esteem and poor sense of security) but may not be aware of the underlying reasons: "*I always feel anxious when I think about gains and losses, speculate about what others say and do, get angry without rhyme or reason, and want to decide or control something. I wear a lot of clothes, even a hat in the ward. Sometimes I think that maybe I would feel most comfortable living in a desert.*" (E)

"Defensive coping" refers to reactive and unconscious behaviors undertaken by a participant to survive, self-protect, and achieve desires. Each defensive coping style represents an attitude toward survival and manifests low self-esteem. In this study, defensive coping was exhibited in four ways:

1. Placating (nonassertive): Participants suppressed their feelings, such as sadness, disappointment, and anger; were nonassertive; and avoided being disagreeable. Thus, participants avoided conflict and concerns over how others perceived them. "*My wife took me to visit many plastic surgeons, hoping that I could recover better. Actually, I don't want to go out. I hate being talked about. But she thought it would be good for me, and so I cooperated with her.*" (D)
2. Blaming: Participants thought, "*It's all my fault, and I have to change first.*" (A, B, C, F). The participants also blamed themselves for feeling guilty: "*I just think of myself over and over again. I should care not only about my own thoughts but also about the needs of others.*" (B, C)
3. Denying: Emotions may manifest in physical symptoms: "*Even I don't like this (my) face. So, I never look in the mirror, never go out, never want to stay with someone*

else. I don't want others to see how I look and find fault, and I don't want people to see my self-abasement." (H)

4. Super reasoning: Participants disregarded their own and others' feelings and focused only on the current situation. For example, when a doctor asked one participant if the process of changing her wound dressings was overly painful, she replied: "*The pain is bearable.*" (G)

Introspection stage

Introspection refers to the process by which participants understood their inner world by developing perceptive abilities. The main feature of this stage is perception, and participants in this stage reflected on topics such as defensive wall construction, unmet expectations, and desires.

Defensive wall: The participants in this study referred to walls that they had built around their hearts because they were victims. Participants maintained this wall using survivalist attitudes and holding limited expectations to resist pressures from the outside world and to protect themselves. (a) "Survivalist attitude" consisted of a series of communication styles that were used to develop a sense of security and that may reflect inner desires. The consequences of participants exhibiting survivalist attitudes included separating from their true selves, alienating others, and strengthening the perception of their role as a victim, thereby continuously experiencing negative feelings: "*After introspection, I found that I had adopted many behaviors just to avoid hurt and to survive. But I didn't know why I did that (adopted these behaviors). In fact, in the end, these methods didn't make me feel better.*" (E); (b) "Limiting beliefs" are trauma-inspired ideas that prevented the participants from becoming successful and happy. Participants stated that their feelings were often affected by limiting beliefs, which hampered their understanding of the true nature of certain situations and engendered feelings of low self-esteem: "*I always had some beliefs before, such as 'I am worthless, I don't deserve to be happy, I always cause trouble for my family.' I used to feel that my thoughts were right, and I was like a person with a limited outlook, right? Because of those thoughts, I did a lot of harm to myself and others. As result, I felt I was never good enough and like I was driven to a dead end.*" (A)

Unmet expectations: Participants often expected others to satisfy their desires, and when these were unmet, they experienced negative feelings or developed a survivalist attitude: "*In the beginning, my doctor said plastic surgery could change my appearance. You know, this kind of surgery can only save life but can't improve one's appearance. So, I didn't want to acknowledge the doctor, as he made me very disappointed. My poor treatment of my doctor also reflected my unwillingness to accept the reality and my counting on him to resolve all of these [disappointments]. However, in the course of treatment and rehabilitation, my doctors and nurses provided professional care and psychological support for me. Later, I opened my heart to communicate my feelings and expectations sincerely with them, and now I have accepted myself.*" (B)

"Desires" are often hidden and were conveyed in participant expectations of others and their situation. After asking themselves why others had so many expectations, the participants realized that they also had many desires that had been buried through their survivalist attitudes: "*In the past, I always made every effort to meet my desires, and [now] it is others who meet my desires. When [my desires] fail to be met, I feel pain and blame others. But I couldn't see all this before.*" (E)

Integration stage

Integration is the process by which patients assimilate their experiences to create a new self. The main features of integration are recognition and acceptance, which come from acknowledging feelings, cognitive restructuring, and taking responsibility for expectations.

"Acknowledging feelings" refers to recognizing and accepting one's feelings after realizing that they are an interpretation of perceptions: "*My pain is not someone else's fault, but my choice. The pain is actually a revelation for me, telling me that there is trouble. However, the feeling itself is not a problem, as it guides me to see where the problem is. I just need to follow its guidance in order to solve the problem.*" (E)

"Cognitive restructuring" refers to restructuring restrictive beliefs as positive beliefs: "*I grew to believe that one good turn deserves another. But why did I get burned? What did I do wrong to suffer such retribution? I was stuck in such confusion and was unable to extricate myself. Later, I began to realize that this was just my idea, not a fact. Actually, this world is always unpredictable, and whatever happens is normal. The key is how we face these things.*" (C)

"Being responsible for one's expectations" refers to participants' recognition that their expectations of others and their situation resulted from their inner desires and that they must accept and take responsibility for their expectations: "*The closer people were to me, the more I wanted them to follow my ideas to do this and that. After understanding that these were all just my requirements and thoughts, I realized that all these were normal. The reason I had requirements of others lies in the fact that I couldn't accept myself. Even failing to accept myself generates a lot of self-dissatisfaction. So, I disagreed with [the people close to me] and blamed them for many irrational behaviors.*" (F)

Practice stage

The practice stage refers to when participants practiced and maintained new skills. The main characteristic of this stage is action, namely, letting go, accepting more choices, and taking responsibility for oneself.

"Letting go" means that, once participants perceived, recognized, and accepted that they were still strongly influenced by experiential feelings and behavioral patterns, they could work on setting these feelings and patterns aside to realize the freedom of living in the moment: "*Every time fear wells up, I have a dialogue with it to see what it wants to say and what makes me afraid. If I no longer firmly hold it, it will be gone soon, and I will feel very relaxed and pleasant. At the same time, I no longer worry or fear, so I can do enjoyable things.*" (F)

"Accepting more choices" refers to becoming empowered and free to acknowledge more choices. After removing defensive walls and letting negative feelings go, participants perceived opportunity for more choices at every turn: "*I believe that only by learning to love yourself first can you love others. When I treat myself well instead of asking family members to do things for me, the distance between family members and me grows smaller. This distance was so wide once, and I was so dissociated from myself.*" (B)

"Taking responsibility for oneself" meant that participants took ownership of their behaviors, feelings, expectations, desires, and choices to become empowered to take responsibility for their own lives. The participant who experienced an electrical burn during work described her accident during this stage: "*It's not anyone's fault, and I have the ability to let it go.*" (G)

Growth stage

During the growth stage, participants gained positive power and an appreciation for life after struggling with their dilemmas. The main features of this stage include development and appreciation, as reflected in defining the significance of the burn, living in the moment, and achieving harmony.

"Significance of the burn" refers to participants finding new significance in their burn injury and themselves and consisted of three levels: (a) changing one's perception: "*The burn was just an event, and the problem is not the event but how I judge it and why I judge it. When I really feel and accept it (the event), the problem disappears. The event seems to have left me for a long time and is now just a life experience.*" (I); (b) believing in the significance of the burn: "*I no longer escape or resist. It's like I was imprisoned after being burned and it was very painful. Now, I don't want to be immersed in the pain of the burn anymore and have come to believe that the burn has brought me some positive things.*" (D); and (c) significance of life: "*The burn gave me a new life. It doesn't mean that I like the burn. I regard the burn as a guide for life, guiding me to learn to appreciate and be grateful in my life's path. It is just the beginning, not the end.*" (F)

"Living in the moment" refers to the realization of a peaceful, devoted, and free state of life through acceptance of misfortune and discarding previous fantasies: "*As I like writing, I kept writing at home, completely focusing on writing and feeling the peace of the pen touching the paper. I like myself in that moment, I feel alive. Then I find that I'm able to do this every time, more and more easily.*" (E)

"Harmony" refers to participants experiencing an existential state after becoming more complete. Harmony reflects a communicative attitude that respects the self, others, and situations: "*I can be increasingly true to myself, neither hurting others nor deprecating myself, which is not difficult, as all that is needed is just mutual respect and love.*" (B, J)

Protective Factors

Internal protective factors

"Hope" represents a cognitive state in which participants realized their situation and chose to achieve challenging objectives. In this study, hope was generated in the participants and by caring relationships: "*It seems that my daughter was never disturbed by my injury. Her attitude encouraged me to move forward instead of being pessimistic. You have to get over it.*" (C) Hope motivated the participants to move from the black hole stage into the introspection stage.

"Sincerity" means sharing and expressing oneself or having honest reservations. In this study, the more a participant shared with and expressed to others, the more open and compassionate they were to themselves: "*I admitted that I was often angry because I was afraid no one liked me anymore. I'm afraid because I'm not confident. I found that when I have the courage to expose myself, there will be no problem.*" (B) Sincerity motivated the participants to move from the introspection stage into the integration stage.

"Will" reflects self-belief in one's behavior that translates self-perceptions and feelings into desired practice: "*I can stay at home as long as I want. But I want to go outside to face my life.*" (J) Will motivated the participants to move from the integration stage into the practice stage.

"Belief" represents an inner belief that life will continue. In this study, the depth of this belief related positively to the encouragement that participants received to be actively involved in recovery: "*Whatever it is going to be, it is better than anything I can imagine.*" (B) Belief motivated the participants to move from the practice stage into the growth stage.

"Curiosity" represents open-mindedness about the unknown in terms of a participant's individuality and about everything that will happen: "*I have no so-called aims or plans. Just let me live like a three-year-old, curious kid.*" (F) Curiosity helped participants progress into the upward spiral.

External protective factors

Caring relationships: In the black hole stage, participants needed to receive care from others and find comfort in this care. The participants in this study gained a sense of security from their caring relationships: "*I feel I am just a dead dog. I have to be taken care of. Thank God that my family members are always there. It makes me feel warm and safe.*" (A)

Supportive relationships: In the introspection stage, participants perceived abundant love, acceptance, and support in their relationships, which provided significant additional encouragement and strength: "*I am sure that I am still loved and supported by my family, merely through my observation with no analysis or judgement.*" (I)

"Sharing relationships" were established based on the self-recognition, self-acceptance, and self-expression of participants during the integration stage: "*I feel relaxed when I tell others how my mind suffered from the burn. One day my husband told me how sad and helpless he felt when I got injured and he cried. That moment, I felt his strong love and was moved by him. I hugged him with assurance and belief.*" (A)

"Committed relationships" were established by trusting during the practice stage and involved self-commitment from the participants, rather than commitment provided at the behest of others: "*Being together with persons I trust, I can better accept myself, no matter what is being done. I drive myself willingly to real life.*" (H)

"Intimate relationships" resulted in deeper mutual understanding and more sharing. In the growth stage, both people in the relationship were able to commit and share moments of their lives to establish an intimate relationship: "*I believe I can love again. I feel love in my intimate relationship, and it can cure anything.*" (G)

Discussion

The participants in this study achieved resilience through a gradual process. Although causal factors and injury severities were not the same, the development of resilience in the 10 participants always involved the five stages identified in the previous discussion: black hole, introspection, integration, practice, and growth. The development of resilience is one of change and transformation. A process represents the way to change, which is the core of developing mental resilience. Many small changes experienced by participants contributed to the development of resilience. The cycle through the five stages may need to be repeated many times before a major transformation occurs. This finding supplements and supports the reintegration process that is described in Richardson's Resiliency Model (Richardson, 2002), which provides a framework for understanding the individual experience of system collapse and reintegration without giving details of the process of resilience development. This study described the full process of resilience development and clearly defined the specific events of system collapse and reintegration and internal change. This information may assist medical staff and families to understand the experiences of patients with burn injury and provide targeted support during the different processes.

Changes during the resilience development process involve adaptations from consciousness to behavior at the three levels of consciousness, interpersonal relationships, and life direction. Individual transformation occurs at every stage. During the black hole period, one participant (G) regularly complained that she was a victim. However, through continuous growth, her self-responsibility improved. During the introspection stage, she was aware that her mindset was the reason why she perceived herself as a victim; during the integration stage, she told herself to face the burn, although doing so was psychologically painful; during the practice stage, she believed that the burn was no one's fault and that she had the ability to let her negative thoughts about it go; and during the growth stage, she discovered the significance of the burn and found its benefits and gained strength from it. Other participants experienced similar feelings and changes. Participant B regularly blamed his wife during the black hole stage; with self-responsibility and continuous growth during the introspection and integration stages, he faced his unmet expectations and took responsibility for them; during the practice stage, he perceived more choices before blaming others and learned to love himself; and during the growth stage, he experienced harmony in understanding that he and his wife respected and loved each other. This finding regarding behaviors, emotions, and cognition at each stage may assist medical staff to understand the changes that patients with burn injury undergo during the development of resilience.

In this study, the internal protective factors were the participants' core resources of hope, sincerity, will, belief, and curiosity, whereas the external protective factors were the participants' relationship resources of caring, supportive, sharing, intimate, and committed relationships. Although these factors affected each stage of resilience development, there were essential protective factors at critical junctions, such as hope and caring relationships in the black hole stage. Interactive relationships between internal and external protective factors promote mental resilience. This is consistent with the findings of Luthar, Cicchetti, and Becker (2000) in that resilience is affected by the interaction between protective factors and the environment. Resilience is promoted when protective factors are enhanced and supported (Quezada, González, & Mecott, 2016). However, the findings of this study differ from Connor and Davidson's five factors: sense of control, spirituality, perseverance, positive acceptance of change, and strong interpersonal relationships (Connor & Davidson, 2003). Prior studies have shown that the protective factors underlying resilience may differ between different populations with different living conditions, cultural backgrounds, and sociodemographic characteristics (Manzano-García & Ayala Calvo, 2013; Sexton, Byrd, & von Kluge, 2010; Wu, Tan, & Liu, 2017). Moreover, Ungar pointed out that protective factors are specific to each patient's environment, which is a significant consideration when working to understand the development of resilience in different cultural systems (Ungar, 2008). In China, inner resources and relationship resources are major factors affecting the development of psychological resilience in burned patients. The findings of this study may help healthcare providers provide better and more effective psychological support to Chinese patients with burn injury.

Implications

On the basis of the characteristics of the five stages of resilience, opportunities to promote the development of resilience in different stages are discussed here to provide guidance for practitioners. The black hole stage is based on thoughts and caring relationships. Therefore, practitioners should provide constant care during this stage to establish a secure environment in which patients may develop their resources and nurture hope. During the introspection stage, practitioners should work to establish a relationship with patients and gain their trust, offering a reliable and supportive environment to improve their cognitive abilities. During the integration stage, practitioners should actively listen when patients share information, even when they find that their patients are trapped in a defensive mode or hold harmful beliefs. During the practice stage, practitioners should assess whether patients have made their choices and are ready to put these choices into action and then provide their patients with an open, accepting, and sharing environment. During the growth stage, practitioners should provide a platform to allow patients to achieve their desires.

Limitations

Several limitations of this study should be considered when interpreting the results. This study recruited only those participants who were willing to discuss their feelings about their burn injury and treatment. Thus, patients who were not sufficiently communicative may have held opinions and thoughts on the process of resilience that differed significantly from the sample. Although interviews are the most commonly used method of data collection in grounded theory studies, observation and documents should also be used for data enrichment and triangulation to further bolster the validity of results.

Conclusion and Recommendations

Five stages of the development of resilience were introduced in this study. The essential aspects of resilience were discussed thoroughly by the participants, who were all burned patients currently undergoing treatment in a hospital. The findings may provide helpful insight and support patients seeking to adapt to new situations. In addition, it is recommended that medical staff, patient families, and survivors who have succeeded in achieving resilience share their experiences to help those who are still struggling to adapt and to face future challenges.

Acknowledgments

This research was funded by the Importation and Development of High-Caliber Talents Project of Beijing Municipal Institutions (Grant no. CIT&TCD20140328).

Author Contributions

Study conception and design: JEL, XPZ
Data collection: XPZ, PY
Data analysis and interpretation: XPZ, PY, LG, JEL
Drafting of the article: XPZ, JH
Critical revision of the article: JH, JEL

References

Cakir, U., Terzi, R., Abaci, F., & Aker, T. (2015). The prevalence of post-traumatic stress disorder in patients with burn injuries, and their quality of life. *International Journal of Psychiatry in Clinical Practice, 19*(1), 56–59. https://doi.org/10.3109/13651501.2014.981545

Campbell-sills, L., Cohan, S. L., & Stein, M. B. (2006). Relationship of resilience to personality, coping, and psychiatric symptoms in young adults. *Behaviour Research and Therapy, 44*(4), 585–599. https://doi.org/10.1016/j.brat.2005.05.001

Charmaz, K. (2006). *Constructing grounded theory: A practical guide through qualitative analysis* (1st ed.). London, England: Sage.

Chen, X. M. (2000). *Qualitative research in social sciences.* Beijing, PRC: Educational Science Publishing House.

Connor, K. M., & Davidson, J. R. (2003). Development of a new resilience scale: The Connor–Davidson Resilience Scale (CD-RISC). *Depression & Anxiety, 18*(2), 76–82. https://doi.org/10.1002/da.10113

Dahl, O. (2013). *Memories of pain, adaptation to life and early identification of stressors in patients with burns.* Stockholm, Sweden: Karolinska Institutet.

Dunpath, T., Chetty, V., & Van Der Reyden, D. (2014). The experience of acute burns of the hand—Patients perspectives. *Disability and Rehabilitation, 37*(10), 892–898. https://doi.org/10.3109/09638288.2014.948129

Endfield, G. H. (2012). The resilience and adaptive capacity of social–environmental systems in colonial Mexico. *Proceedings of the National Academy of Sciences of the United States of America, 109*(10), 3676–3681. https://doi.org/10.1073/pnas.1114831109

Friborg, O., Barlaug, D., Martinussen, M., Rosenvinge, J. H., & Hjemdal, O. (2005). Resilience in relation to personality and intelligence. *International Journal of Methods in Psychiatric Research, 14*(1), 29–42. https://doi.org/10.1002/mpr.15

Garcia-Dia, M. J., DiNapoli, J. M., Garcia-Ona, L., Jakubowski, R., & O'Flaherty, D. (2013). Concept analysis: Resilience. *Archives of Psychiatric Nursing, 27*(6), 264–270. https://doi.org/10.1016/j.apnu.2013.07.003

He, F., Cao, R., Feng, Z., Guan, H., & Peng, J. (2013). The impacts of dispositional optimism and psychological resilience on the subjective well-being of burn patients: A structural equation modelling analysis. *PLoS ONE, 8*(12), e82939. https://doi.org/10.1371/journal.pone.0082939

Jang, M. H., Park, J., Chong, M. K., & Sok, S. R. (2017). Factors influencing resilience of burn patients in South Korea. *Journal of Nursing Scholarship, 49*(5), 478–486. https://doi.org/10.1111/jnu.12311

Kornhaber, R., Bridgman, H., McLean, L., & Vandervord, J. (2016). The role of resilience in the recovery of the burn-injured patient: An integrative review. *Chronic Wound Care Management and Research, 3,* 41–50. https://doi.org/10.2147/CWCMR.S94618

Lau, U., & van Niekerk, A. (2011). Restorying the self: An exploration of young burn survivors' narratives of resilience. *Qualitative Health Research, 21*(9), 1165–1181. https://doi.org/10.1177/1049732311405686

Lopez, A. (2011). Posttraumatic stress disorder and occupational performance: Building resilience and fostering occupational adaptation. *Work, 38*(1), 33–38. https://doi.org/10.3233/WOR-2011-1102

Luthar, S. S., Cicchetti, D., & Becker, B. (2000). The construct of resilience: A critical evaluation and guidelines for future work. *Child Development, 71*(3), 543–562. https://doi.org/10.1111/1467-8624.00164

Manzano-García, G., & Ayala Calvo, J. C. (2013). Psychometric properties of Connor–Davidson resilience scale in a Spanish sample of entrepreneurs. *Psicothema, 25*(2), 245–251. https://doi.org/10.7334/psicothema2012.183

Newman, R. (2005). APA's resilience initiative. *Professional Psychology: Research and Practice, 36*(3), 227–229. https://doi.org/10.1037/0735-7028.36.3.227

Quezada, L., González, M. T., & Mecott, G. A. (2016). Explanatory model of resilience in pediatric burn survivors. *Journal of Burn Care & Research, 37*(4), 216–225. https://doi.org/10.1097/BCR.0000000000000261

Richardson, G. E. (2002). The metatheory of resilience and resiliency. *Journal of Clinical Psychology, 58*(3), 307–321. https://doi.org/10.1002/jclp.10020

Sexton, M. B., Byrd, M. R., & von Kluge, S. (2010). Measuring resilience in women experiencing infertility using the CD-RISC: Examining infertility-related stress, general distress, and coping styles. *Journal of Psychiatric Research, 44*(4), 236–241. https://doi.org/10.1016/j.jpsychires.2009.06.007

Streubert, H. J., & Carpenter, D. R. (2010). *Qualitative research in nursing: Advancing the humanistic imperative* (5th ed.). New York, NY: Lippincott Williams & Wilkins.

Ungar, M. (2008). Resilience across cultures. *The British Journal of Social Work, 38*(2), 218–235. https://doi.org/10.1093/bjsw/bcl343

Van Loey, N. E., van de Schoot, R., & Faber, A. W. (2012). Posttraumatic stress symptoms after exposure to two fire disasters: Comparative study. *PLoS ONE, 7*(7), e41532. https://doi.org/10.1371/journal.pone.0041532

Wanberg, C. R., & Banas, J. T. (2000). Predictors and outcomes of openness to changes in a reorganizing workplace. *Journal of Applied Psychology, 85*(1), 132–142. https://dx.doi.org/10.1037/0021-9010.85.1.132

Wang, S. Y., & Chen, S. H. (2007). *Associations of sense of self, resilience and posttraumatic stress symptoms among burn patients* (Master's thesis). National Taiwan University, Taipei, Taiwan, ROC. https://doi.org/10.6342/NTU.2007.00229

Waqas, A., Naveed, S., Bhuiyan, M. M., Usman, J., Inam-UL-Haq, A., & Cheema, S. S. (2016). Social support and resilience among patients with burn injury in Lahore, Pakistan. *Cureus, 8*(11), e867. https://doi.org/10.7759/cureus.867

Wu, L., Tan, Y., & Liu, Y. (2017). Factor structure and psychometric evaluation of the Connor–Davidson resilience scale in a new employee population of China. *BMC Psychiatry, 17*(1), 49. https://doi.org/10.1186/s12888-017-1219-0

Xi, J. Z., Zuo, Z. H., & Wu, W. (2012). Approaches to research on resilience. *Advances in Psychological Science, 20*(9), 1426–1447. https://doi.org/10.3724/SP.J.1042.2012.01426

25

Factors Associated With Blood Pressure Classification in Korean University Students: A Descriptive Survey

Eun-Ju CHOI[1] • Ae Kyung CHANG[2] • Jin Yi CHOI[3]*

ABSTRACT

Background: The prevalence of hypertension in young adults has increased. Hypertension is known to be a leading contributor to many diseases.

Purpose: The study aimed to identify factors influencing blood pressure (BP) classification in university students and to establish a basis for the prevention and management of hypertension in young adults.

Methods: Four hundred three university students in South Korea were analyzed to determine the factors that influence BP classification. Data were analyzed using the chi-square test, analysis of variance, and multinomial logistic regression.

Results: The reference group for the logistic regression analysis included students with normal BP. The odds of being male and of having an overweight or obese body mass index were significantly higher in the prehypertension group than in the normal BP group. The odds of regular (≥ 6 months) exercise habits, having subcutaneous and borderline visceral fat types, and social support were significantly lower in the prehypertension group than in the normal BP group. The odds of being male, being overweight or obese, and having more exercise barriers were significantly higher in the hypertension group than in the normal BP group. The odds of having a high or low economic status were higher and lower in the hypertension group, respectively. Finally, the odds of having subcutaneous or borderline visceral fat types and a vigorous physical activity level were significantly lower in the hypertension group than in the normal BP group.

Conclusions: Interventions that address the factors related to BP in young adults are necessary to prevent the occurrence and progression of hypertension in young adults.

Key Words:
blood pressure, university student.

Introduction

Blood pressure (BP), which may be categorized as normal, prehypertensive, and hypertensive, may increase because of a diverse set of factors, which include age, gender, weight, and diet. The global prevalence of prehypertension is 25%–50%, and the risk of progression to hypertension within 5 years is high. Particularly, 22%–50% of patients with prehypertension develop hypertension (Egan & Stevens-Fabry, 2015). The prevalence rates of hypertension in adults aged 30–39 years in South Korea are 16.9% and 3.3% in men and women, respectively (Korea Centers for Disease Control & Prevention, 2017). However, the prevalence rate of hypertension in adults aged 18–29 years has not been reported in South Korea. In the United States, the prevalence rate of hypertension in adults aged 18–40 years is 7.3%, with the prevalence higher among men than women and the prevalence increasing rapidly (over four-fold) after the age 40 years (Yoon, Carroll, & Fryar, 2015). Compared with middle-aged and elderly individuals, young adults have a low level of knowledge and awareness regarding the treatment and management of hypertension, which increases their risk of cardiovascular disease and stroke (Benjamin et al., 2017; De Venecia, Lu, & Figueredo, 2016).

Prehypertension and hypertension may be major factors contributing to cardiovascular death in adults (Egan & Stevens-Fabry, 2015; Viera & Hawes, 2016). Hypertension is associated with an increased likelihood of obesity in adults, changes in lifestyle, increased uric acid levels, higher concentrations of triglycerides in the blood, and higher resting heart rate (Ashman, Rui, & Schappert, 2016; Cheng, Medlow, & Steinbeck, 2016; De Venecia et al., 2016). Because of the rising prevalence of hypertension and prehypertension in young adults, research is needed on the prevention and management of this issue in this group (Cheng et al., 2016; Egan & Stevens-Fabry, 2015; Korea Centers for Disease Control & Prevention, 2017; Zhang & Moran, 2017). However, most studies on hypertension have been conducted on the older adults or on adults older than 40 years. Comparatively little research has been done on this issue in young adults.

Compared with middle-aged and elderly individuals, fewer young, hypertensive patients (aged 18–44 years) engage in the

[1]PhD, Assistant Professor, Department of Physical Education, Daegu Catholic University, Gyeongsan, Republic of Korea • [2]PhD, RN, Associate Professor, College of Nursing Science, Kyung Hee University, Seoul, Republic of Korea • [3]PhD, RN, Associate Professor, Department of Nursing, Konkuk University, Chungju, Republic of Korea.

treatment or management of hypertension, and they tend to have lower hypertension awareness (Ashman et al., 2016; Wang et al., 2014; Yoon et al., 2015). Young adults must cope with obesity, psychological stresses in adapting to college life, anxiety, and depression (Bruno et al., 2016; De Venecia et al., 2016). As they become independent of parental influence at the age of 19 years or older, they may face difficulties in managing their lifestyle habits, leading to increased drinking, smoking, and inappropriate eating behaviors that negatively influence cardiovascular health and ultimately increase the prevalence of hypertension (Benjamin et al., 2017; Lee et al., 2014). Hence, the prevalence of hypertension, as well as associated secondary complications and concomitant diseases, has been shown to rapidly increase among middle-aged and elderly individuals (Ashman et al., 2016; De Venecia et al., 2016; Yoon et al., 2015).

The primary intervention that is currently used to manage BP is the correction of lifestyle habits through increased physical activity and dietary control (Gabb et al., 2016). However, young adults differ in terms of physical condition, physical activities, diet, drinking habits, and various physiological factors from their elderly and middle-aged adult peers (Mucci et al., 2016). People are most physically active during young adulthood, and physical activity decreases after 30 years old, resulting in reduced muscle mass and increased body fat. Hence, the prevalence of hypertension is higher among individuals who are 30 years and older (Korea Centers for Disease Control & Prevention, 2017; Shin & Ok, 2012).

Therefore, identifying hypertension risk factors according to BP classifications is necessary to prevent the onset and progression of hypertension in university students. This descriptive survey study was conducted to identify the related risk factors by BP classification in university students and to establish a basis for preventing and managing hypertension in young adults.

Methods

Participants

The participants in this study were university students aged 20–35 years (classified as young adults) who understood the study objectives, volunteered to participate, and were able to complete a self-report survey. We obtained institutional review board approval (IRB: CBNU-2015-0088) and informed consent from all of the participants before data collection. The participants ($N = 420$) were recruited via convenience sampling from three universities in three cities in South Korea (Seoul, Daejeon, and Cheongju). Young adults were recruited through posters placed in university lecture rooms and on bulletin boards. The minimum sample size was estimated using G*Power 3.1 (Kiel University, Kiel, Germany) based on a medium effect size (0.15), a significance level of .05, and a statistical power of 0.80. The estimated minimum sample size was 376. Four hundred twenty subjects were recruited to allow for dropouts. Four hundred twenty surveys were returned between September and October 2016, of which 17 were excluded because of incomplete responses, leaving 403 for inclusion in the final analysis.

Demographic Characteristics

The participants were classified into normal BP, prehypertensive, and hypertensive groups by measuring BP once after a 5-minute rest period. Sociodemographic characteristics, including age, gender, economic status, stress level, subjective health status, smoking status, drinking status, sleep duration (hours), visceral fat level, and body mass index (BMI), were examined. Subjective health status was measured on a 5-point scale. Stress level was measured using the Korean version of the Brief Encounter Psychosocial Instrument (Hur et al., 1996). The Cronbach's α of the Korean version of the Brief Encounter Psychosocial Instrument was .80 at the time of its development and .816 in this study.

BMI was classified as underweight (< 18.5 kg/m^2), healthy weight (18.5–24.9 kg/m^2), overweight (25–29.9 kg/m^2), or obese (≥ 30 kg/m^2 or more; WHO Expert Consultation, 2004). Visceral fat, measured using a body composition analyzer (Inbody 720; Biospace Co., Seoul, South Korea) that employed bioelectric impedance analysis, was classified into several types, including subcutaneous, balanced, borderline, visceral obese, and excessively visceral obese.

Physical Activity

Physical activity characteristics included physical activity level, exercise habits, self-efficacy in exercise, social support for physical activity, exercise-related decision making (exercise benefits and factors that impede exercise), and physical activity planning adjustment. Physical activity level was measured using the International Physical Activity Questionnaire and classified as light, moderate, or vigorous based on scoring and classification systems (IPAQ Research Committee, 2005). Exercise habits were examined using the Stage of Readiness to Exercise Questionnaire. Those participants who exercised were categorized into three groups according to whether they exercised regularly for ≥ 6 months or for < 6 months, and all others were categorized into the irregular exercise group (Marcus, Selby, Niaura, & Rossi, 1992). Self-efficacy in exercise was measured using the Exercise Self-Efficacy scale, which consists of five items that are scored on a 5-point scale, with higher total scores associated with higher self-efficacy (Marcus et al., 1992). The Cronbach's α was .82 at the time the instrument was developed and .855 in this study. Social support for physical activity was measured using a tool modified to suit Korean culture. The instrument is composed of seven items rated on a 5-point scale, with higher total scores indicating a higher level of social support for exercise (Choi, 2008). The Cronbach's α was .89 at the time the instrument was developed and .906 in this study. Exercise-related decision making was measured using the Decisional Balance Scale for Exercise, which consists of five items addressing factors that promote exercise and five items addressing factors that impede exercise (Nigg, Rossi, Norman, & Benisovich, 1998). At the time of instrument development, the Cronbach's α was .87 for exercise-promoting factors and .90 for exercise-impeding factors, and these values were .872 and .750 in this study, respectively. The extent to which participants managed their physical activity scheduling and planning was measured using the Exercise Planning Scale. This instrument consists of 10 items that are scored on a 5-point scale, with higher total scores indicating a higher level of physical activity planning adjustment (Rovniak, Anderson, Winett, & Stephens, 2002). The Cronbach's α was .87 at the time of instrument development and .760 in this study.

Statistical Analysis

Data were analyzed using SPSS Statistics 23.0 (IBM, Armonk, NY, USA). First, frequencies, percentages, means, and standard deviations were computed for the sociodemographic and physical activity characteristics of the participants according to their BP classification. Chi-square tests and analysis of variance were then performed to test homogeneity across these three groups. Second, multinomial logistic regression was performed to compute the odds ratios (*OR*s) and 95% confidence intervals for the BP classification of the participants, with the normal BP group used as the reference.

Results

Of the 403 subjects, 218 (54.1%) were categorized into the normal BP group, 147 (36.5%) were categorized into the prehypertensive group, and 38 (9.4%) were categorized into the hypertensive group (Table 1). Age, gender, economic status, smoking status, visceral fat level, and BMI classification differed significantly across the groups. Age was significantly higher in the prehypertensive and hypertensive groups than in the normal BP group ($F = 8.58, p < .001$). The proportion of men was significantly lower in the normal BP group than in the prehypertensive and hypertensive groups ($\chi^2 = 62.56$, $p < .001$). Moreover, economic status was significantly different across BP classification ($\chi^2 = 10.40$, $p = .034$). The prevalence of smoking was significantly higher in the hypertensive and prehypertensive groups than in the normal BP group, differing significantly across BP classification ($\chi^2 = 15.97$, $p < .001$). The rates of the borderline and visceral obese types of visceral fat level were significantly higher in the prehypertensive and hypertensive groups than in the normal BP group ($\chi^2 = 52.55$, $p < .001$). In terms of BMI, the percentage of people with a healthy weight was significantly higher in the normal BP group than in the prehypertensive and hypertensive groups ($\chi^2 = 51.81, p < .001$). Furthermore, stress, subjective health status, drinking status, and sleep duration did not differ significantly across BP classification.

In terms of physical activity characteristics, only those factors that impede exercise differed significantly across BP classification, with related scores higher in the normal BP group than in the prehypertensive group ($F = 3.65, p = .027$). Apart from factors that impede exercise, all other variables, including physical activity level, exercise habits, self-efficacy in exercise, social support for physical activity, beneficial exercise factors, and physical activity planning adjustment, showed no significant difference across BP classification.

The results of the logistic regression analysis, conducted using the normal BP group as the reference and used to identify the factors that influence the BP classification of the participants, are presented separately for the prehypertensive and hypertensive groups in Table 2. The prehypertensive group was significantly associated with gender, visceral fat level, and BMI. The odds of being male were significantly higher in the prehypertensive group than in the normal BP group ($OR = 3.34, p < .001$). In terms of visceral fat level, using the balanced type in the prehypertensive group as a reference, the odds of being in the subcutaneous type ($OR = 0.51$, $p = .031$) and borderline type ($OR = 0.34, p = .017$) category were significantly lower in the prehypertensive group than in the normal BP group. Finally, for BMI, using healthy weight in the prehypertensive group as a reference, the odds of being overweight were significantly higher in the prehypertensive group than in the normal BP group ($OR = 4.80, p = .001$). The odds of social support for physical activity and exercise habits differed significantly between the prehypertensive and normal BP groups. Using irregular exercise in the prehypertensive group as a reference, the odds of performing regular exercise for < 6 months and of having social support for physical activity were both significantly lower in the prehypertensive group than in the normal BP group ($OR = 0.41, p = .043$, and $OR = 0.94, p = .029$, respectively). No other physical activity variable was significantly related to prehypertensive BP.

Significant differences in the odds for gender and economic status were found between the hypertensive and normal BP groups. The odds of being male were significantly higher in the hypertensive group than in the normal BP group ($OR = 13.91, p < .001$). Using the middle economic status in the hypertensive group as the reference, the odds of having a high economic status were significantly higher ($OR = 7.95$, $p = .021$) and the odds of having a low economic status were significantly lower ($OR = 0.21, p = .050$) in the hypertensive group than in the normal BP group. In terms of the physical activity characteristics, the visceral fat level and BMI were significantly related to hypertension. Specifically, the odds of having the subcutaneous visceral fat type (vs. the balanced type) was significantly lower in the hypertensive group than in the normal BP group ($OR = 0.17, p = .042$). Moreover, the odds of being overweight (vs. healthy weight) were significantly greater in the hypertensive group ($OR = 16.03$, $p = .015$). Exercise habits, physical activity level, and having factors that impeded exercise in exercise-related decision making were all significantly related to hypertension. The odds of having a vigorous (vs. light) level of physical activity were significantly lower in the hypertensive group ($OR = 0.19$, $p = .040$), whereas the odds of having more factors that impede exercise were significantly higher in the hypertensive group ($OR = 1.15, p = .035$).

Discussion

Overall, 36.5% of the participants were prehypertensive and 9.4% were hypertensive. Although the prevalence of

TABLE 1.

Participant Sociodemographic and Physical Activity Characteristics, by Blood Pressure Group (N = 403)

	①Normal (*n* = 218)		②Prehypertension (*n* = 147)		③Hypertension (*n* = 38)		Total (*N* = 403)			
Variable	*n*	%	*n*	%	*n*	%	*n*	%	F/χ^2	*p*/Post hoc
Age (years; *M* and *SD*)	20.88	1.96	21.65	2.48	22.16	2.43	21.28	2.25	8.58	< .001 ① < ②, ③
Gender									62.56	< .001
Male	60	27.5	87	59.2	32	84.2	179	44.4		
Female	158	72.5	60	40.8	6	15.8	224	55.6		
Economic status									10.40	.034
Upper	32	14.7	21	14.3	3	7.9	56	13.9		
Middle	181	83.0	119	81.0	30	78.9	330	81.9		
Lower	5	2.3	7	4.8	5	13.2	17	4.2		
Stress (*M* and *SD*)	11.89	3.64	11.04	3.62	11.05	4.01	11.50	3.69	2.69	.069
Subjective health status (*M* and *SD*)	3.27	0.84	3.24	1.00	3.16	1.05	3.25	0.92	0.22	.799
Drinking									2.54	.281
Yes	170	78.0	110	74.8	33	86.8	313	77.7		
No	48	22.0	37	25.2	5	13.2	90	22.3		
Smoking									15.97	< .001
Yes	23	10.6	34	23.1	12	31.6	69	17.1		
No	195	89.4	113	76.9	26	68.4	334	82.9		
Sleep time, hours/day									2.70	.260
≥ 7–8	103	47.2	80	54.4	16	42.1	199	49.4		
< 7	115	52.8	67	45.6	22	57.9	204	50.6		
Visceral fat type									52.55	< .001
Subcutaneous	97	44.5	28	19.0	5	13.2	130	32.3		
Balanced	95	43.6	82	55.8	16	42.1	193	47.9		
Borderline	24	11.0	24	16.3	11	28.9	59	14.6		
Visceral obese	2	0.9	13	8.8	6	15.8	21	5.2		
BMI									51.81	< .001
Underweight	16	7.3	4	2.7	3	7.9	23	5.7		
Healthy weight	187	85.8	96	65.3	19	50.0	302	74.9		
≥ Overweight	15	6.9	47	32.0	16	42.1	78	19.4		
IPAQ									2.47	.650
Light	26	11.9	13	8.8	5	13.2	44	10.9		
Moderate	101	46.3	66	44.9	20	52.6	187	46.4		
Vigorous	91	41.7	68	46.3	13	34.2	172	42.7		
Exercise habits									2.32	.677
Regular (≥ 6 months)	33	15.1	26	17.7	8	21.1	67	16.6		
Regular (< 6 months)	18	8.3	12	8.2	5	13.2	35	8.7		
Irregular	167	76.6	109	74.1	22	65.8	301	74.7		
	M	*SD*	*M*	*SD*	*M*	*SD*	*M*	*SD*		
Self-efficacy in exercise	15.27	4.55	16.33	4.77	16.29	4.63	15.75	4.66	2.58	.077
Social support for physical activity	24.23	5.33	23.58	6.68	23.63	5.48	23.94	5.86	0.61	.546
Beneficial exercise factors	20.21	3.34	20.69	3.73	20.76	3.27	20.44	3.48	1.03	.360
Barrier exercise factors	10.97	3.65	9.97	3.57	10.08	3.69	10.52	3.65	3.65	.027 ① > ②
Physical activity planning adjustment	13.36	2.55	13.80	2.60	14.03	2.73	13.58	2.60	1.91	.149

Note. BMI = body mass index; IPAQ = International Physical Activity Questionnaire.

TABLE 2.

Multinomial Logistic Regression for Characteristics Influencing the Blood Pressure Classification of University Students (N = 403)

	Prehypertension						Hypertension					
Variable	*B*	*SE*	Wald	*OR*	95% CI	*p*	*B*	*SE*	Wald	*OR*	95% CI	*p*
Age	−0.01	0.06	0.05	0.99	[0.87, 1.12]	.818	0.08	0.10	0.65	1.08	[0.89, 1.31]	.421
Gender (male)	1.20	0.34	12.72	3.34	[1.72, 6.47]	< .001	2.63	0.62	18.01	13.91	[4.12, 46.94]	<.001
Economic status												
Upper	0.80	0.71	1.29	2.23	[0.56, 8.92]	.255	2.07	0.90	5.34	7.95	[1.37, 46.15]	.021
Lower	0.01	0.37	0.00	1.01	[0.49, 2.10]	.975	−1.55	0.79	3.84	0.21	[0.05, 1.00]	.050
Stress	−0.06	0.04	2.70	0.94	[0.88, 1.01]	.100	−0.08	0.07	1.33	0.93	[0.81, 1.05]	.248
Subjective health status	−0.09	0.16	0.30	0.92	[0.68, 1.25]	.582	−0.18	0.26	0.47	0.84	[0.51, 1.39]	.494
Drinking (yes)	−0.30	0.30	1.02	0.74	[0.41, 1.33]	.314	1.01	0.65	2.38	2.74	[0.76, 9.85]	.123
Smoking (yes)	0.40	0.38	1.10	1.49	[0.71, 3.13]	.295	0.33	0.53	0.40	1.39	[0.50, 3.91]	.528
Sleep time (≥ 7–8 hours/day)	−0.37	0.26	2.06	0.69	[0.41, 1.15]	.152	0.38	0.45	0.70	1.46	[0.60, 3.51]	.402
Visceral fat												
Subcutaneous type	−0.68	0.31	4.67	0.51	[0.27, 0.94]	.031	−1.75	0.86	4.13	0.17	[0.03, 0.94]	.042
Borderline	−1.07	0.45	5.68	0.34	[0.14, 0.83]	.017	−0.40	0.66	0.37	0.67	[0.18, 2.43]	.542
Visceral obese	0.72	0.93	0.61	2.05	[0.34, 12.60]	.436	2.06	1.14	3.28	7.83	[0.85, 72.51]	.070
BMI												
Underweight	−0.24	0.65	0.13	0.79	[0.22, 2.84]	.714	1.13	0.71	2.54	3.09	[0.77, 12.37]	.111
≥ Overweight	1.57	0.48	10.71	4.80	[1.88, 12.28]	.001	2.77	1.15	5.86	16.03	[1.70, 15.53]	.015
IPAQ												
Moderate	0.00	0.42	0.00	1.00	[0.44, 2.30]	.996	−0.33	0.69	0.24	0.72	[0.19, 2.74]	.626
Vigorous	0.00	0.46	0.00	1.00	[0.41, 2.45]	1.000	−1.65	0.80	4.24	0.19	[0.04, 0.92]	.040
Exercise habit												
Regular (≥ 6 months)	−0.90	0.44	4.11	0.41	[0.17, 0.97]	.043	0.32	0.73	0.19	1.38	[0.33, 5.73]	.660
Regular (< 6 months)	−0.09	0.49	0.04	0.91	[0.35, 2.36]	.850	1.25	0.75	2.77	3.49	[0.80, 15.53]	.096
Social support for physical activity	−0.06	0.03	4.74	0.94	[0.89, 0.99]	.029	−0.03	0.05	0.40	0.97	[0.88, 1.07]	.529
Self-efficacy in exercise	0.06	0.04	2.30	1.06	[0.98, 1.14]	.129	0.07	0.07	1.02	1.07	[0.94, 1.21]	.313
Beneficial exercise factors	0.02	0.04	0.14	1.02	[0.93, 1.11]	.706	0.05	0.07	0.39	1.05	[0.91, 1.21]	.531
Exercise-impeding factors	0.00	0.04	0.00	1.00	[0.93, 1.08]	.993	0.14	0.07	4.43	1.15	[1.01, 1.31]	.035
Physical activity planning adjustment	0.03	0.06	0.24	1.03	[0.92, 1.14]	.624	0.04	0.09	0.21	1.04	[0.87, 1.25]	.644

Note. Reference groups are as follows: normal BP: female, economic status: middle, drinking: no, smoking: no, sleep time: < 7–8 hours/day, visceral fat: balanced type, BMI: healthy weight, IPAQ: light, and exercise habit: irregular. BMI = body mass index; IPAQ = International Physical Activity Questionnaire.

hypertension in this study was similar to that among adults aged 18–44 years in the United States (9%; Ashman et al., 2016), it was less than that among adults aged 18–35 years in Italy (11%; Bruno et al., 2016). Although the mean age of the participants (21 years) in this study was much lower than that in previous studies, the prevalence of hypertension was similar. Moreover, considering the high prevalence of prehypertension, it is likely that hypertension will markedly increase among these Korean adults within 5 years.

This study found that BP increased with age, which aligns with the changes in physical condition and the number of concomitant diseases by age group (Bruno et al., 2016; Everett & Zajacova, 2015; Yoon et al., 2015). Moreover, the finding that the percentage of men was lower in the normal BP group than in the prehypertensive and hypertensive groups is consistent with that in previous studies, which showed that BP is higher in men than in women (Lee et al., 2014; Mucci et al., 2016). Although young men have a higher prevalence of hypertension than young women, they have lower levels of management and awareness of hypertension (Everett & Zajacova, 2015).

In the logistic regression analysis, the prehypertensive group showed significant relationships with gender, visceral fat level, and BMI. Compared with the normal BP group, the prehypertensive group had greater odds of being male, which is consistent with a previous study that found being male to be the factor that most strongly influenced the development of hypertension in young adults (Bruno et al., 2016; Mucci et al., 2016). In terms of visceral fat level, the prehypertension group had lower odds of being in the subcutaneous and borderline categories than being in the balanced category. In terms of BMI, the odds of being overweight were significantly greater in the prehypertensive group than in the normal BP group when healthy weight in the former group was used as the reference. Obesity impairs renal function, increases BP, and increases visceral fat (i.e., fat around the kidneys), which is characteristic of obesity-related hypertension (Hall, do Carmo, da Silva, Wang, & Hall, 2015). However, this study did not find a relationship between BP classification and either drinking or smoking. Rather than drinking and smoking per se, the quantity, frequency, and duration of drinking and smoking likely influence BP elevation (Núñez-Córdoba et al., 2009; Samadian, Dalili, & Jamalian, 2016). In addition, this study found no relationship between BP classification and stress, subjective health status, or sleep duration, likely because obesity and visceral fat are the most important causes of BP elevation (Zhang & Moran, 2017). Moreover, the prehypertension group showed significant associations with exercise habits and social support for physical activity. The odds of regular exercise for < 6 months and having social support for physical activity were significantly lower in the prehypertensive group. These findings suggest that social support or group interventions aimed at increasing motivation have the potential to change and help maintain exercise habits in young adults, whereas regular physical activity helps maintain normal BP (Molanorouzi, Khoo, & Morris, 2015; Patnode, Evans, Senger, Redmond, & Lin, 2017; Ramchand et al., 2017). Therefore, both social support and motivation should be considered when planning physical activities that are aimed at preventing and managing hypertension.

The hypertensive group showed significant associations with gender and economic status. As previously reported, being male was found to be the factor with the greatest impact on hypertension, with the *OR* in this study nearly four times that reported in past studies (Bruno et al., 2016; Mucci et al., 2016). This finding may be related to the high rate of binge drinking among Korean adults, especially men in their 20s, which may increase BP (Korea Centers for Disease Control & Prevention, 2017; Wellman et al., 2016; World Health Organization, 2014). Compared with the normal BP group, the hypertensive group faced significantly lower odds of being in the subcutaneous visceral fat category and significantly higher odds of being overweight. These findings are consistent with those of a prior study showing that obesity accounted for > 65% of the contribution to the causes of hypertension and that risk of BP is increased by obesity-related renal dysfunction (Rovniak et al., 2002). In terms of exercise-related characteristics, the hypertensive group had lower odds of engaging in vigorous physical activity than the normal BP group and had significantly more exercise-impeding factors. These findings may be related to the mean age of the participants in this study (21 years). At this age, individuals tend to be particularly sensitive about body image, which affects their levels of physical activity and dietary habits (Molanorouzi et al., 2015). Moreover, previous studies found exercise-impeding factors to be more prevalent at younger ages, which in turn may decrease physical activity, increase weight, and, ultimately, increase BP (Bruno et al., 2016; Butt, Weinberg, Breckon, & Claytor, 2011). It is thought that variables other than those mentioned above were not influential in this study because of the smaller number of hypertensive young adults than prehypertensive young adults in the study sample.

Limitations of the Study

This study focused on physical activity, which is regarded as an effective BP control intervention for young adults. This study was limited by the fact that the participants were given group assignments based on only one BP measurement and dietary habits and lifestyle were measured based only on drinking and smoking behaviors. Future research should include factors other than physical activity that may influence hypertension in young adults. Another limitation was the convenience sampling approach used. Future research should adopt a more broadly representative approach to sampling to expand the generalizability of the findings.

Conclusion and Implications

In this study, the prevalence of hypertension and prehypertension was higher and the mean age of participants was lower than reported in previous studies. The analyses of factors influencing BP classification in university students revealed that gender, being overweight or obese, visceral fat, social support for physical activity, and exercise-impeding factors all influenced the development of prehypertension and hypertension. University students are at a stage in life in which they are establishing their independence from their parents and forming an independent lifestyle. Failure to form healthy habits at this time will impact directly on the prevalence of hypertension during middle and older ages. Therefore, nurses must recognize the importance of healthy habits at this time and actively provide preventative interventions. Accordingly, hypertension in young adults should be prevented and managed to reduce the prevalence of hypertension in all age groups, and related physical exercise interventions should include components of social support and work to eliminate exercise-impeding factors.

References

Ashman, J. J., Rui, P., & Schappert, S. M. (2016). *Age differences in visits to office-based physicians by adults with hypertension: United States, 2013.* Retrieved from https://www.cdc.gov/nchs/data/databriefs/db263.pdf

Benjamin, E. J., Blaha, M. J., Chiuve, S. E., Cushman, M., Das, S. R., Deo, R., ... American Heart Association Statistics Committee and Stroke Statistics Subcommittee. (2017). Heart disease and stroke statistics—2017 update: A report from the American

Heart Association. *Circulation, 135*(10), e146–e603. https://doi.org/10.1161/CIR.0000000000000485

Bruno, R. M., Pucci, G., Rosticci, M., Guarino, L., Guglielmo, C., Agabiti Rosei, C., ... Pengo, M. F. (2016). Association between lifestyle and systemic arterial hypertension in young adults: A national, survey-based, cross-sectional study. *High Blood Pressure & Cardiovascular Prevention, 23*(1), 31–40. https://doi.org/10.1007/s40292-016-0135-6

Butt, J., Weinberg, R. S., Breckon, J. D., & Claytor, R. P. (2011). Adolescent physical activity participation and motivational determinants across gender, age, and race. *Journal of Physical Activity & Health, 8*(8), 1074–1083. https://doi.org/10.1123/jpah.8.8.1074

Cheng, H. L., Medlow, S., & Steinbeck, K. (2016). The health consequences of obesity in young adulthood. *Current Obesity Reports, 5*(1), 30–37. https://doi.org/10.1007/s13679-016-0190-2

Choi, J. A. (2008). Construction of leisure physical activity model of middle-aged women in urban area. *Korean Journal of Adult Nursing, 20*(4), 626–640. (Original work published in Korean).

De Venecia, T., Lu, M., & Figueredo, V. M. (2016). Hypertension in young adults. *Postgraduate Medicine, 128*(2), 201–207. https://doi.org/10.1080/00325481.2016.1147927

Egan, B. M., & Stevens-Fabry, S. (2015). Prehypertension—Prevalence, health risks, and management strategies. *Nature Reviews Cardiology, 12*(5), 289–300. https://doi.org/10.1038/nrcardio.2015.17

Everett, B., & Zajacova, A. (2015). Gender differences in hypertension and hypertension awareness among young adults. *Biodemography and Social Biology, 61*(1), 1–17. https://doi.org/10.1080/19485565.2014.929488

Gabb, G. M., Mangoni, A. A., Anderson, C. S., Cowley, D., Dowden, J. S., Golledge, J., ... Arnolda, L. (2016). Guideline for the diagnosis and management of hypertension in adults—2016. *The Medical Journal of Australia, 205*(2), 85–89.

Hall, J. E., do Carmo, J. M., da Silva, A. A., Wang, Z., & Hall, M. E. (2015). Obesity-induced hypertension: Interaction of neurohumoral and renal mechanisms. *Circulation Research, 116*(6), 991–1006. https://doi.org/10.1161/CIRCRESAHA.116.305697

Hur, B. R., Yim, J. H., Bae, J. M., Choi, S. S., Kim, S. W., & Whang, W. S. (1996). The validity of modified Korean-translated BEPSI (Brief Encounter Psychosocial Instrument) as instrument of stress measurement in outpatient clinic. *Korean Journal of Family Medicine, 17*(1), 42–49.

IPAQ Research Committee. (2005). *Guidelines for data processing and analysis of the International Physical Activity Questionnaire (IPAQ)–Short and long forms.* Retrieved from https://sites.google.com/site/theipaq/scoring-protocol

Korea Centers for Disease Control & Prevention. (2017). *2016 Health behavior and chronic disease statistics.* Retrieved from https://knhanes.cdc.go.kr/knhanes/eng/index.do (Original work published in Korean)

Lee, M. H., Kang, D. R., Kim, H. C., Ahn, S. V., Khaw, K. T., & Suh, I. (2014). A 24-year follow-up study of blood pressure tracking from childhood to adulthood in Korea: The Kangwha Study. *Yonsei Medical Journal, 55*(2), 360–366. https://doi.org/10.3349/ymj.2014.55.2.360

Marcus, B. H., Selby, V. C., Niaura, R. S., & Rossi, J. S. (1992). Self-efficacy and the stages of exercise behavior change. *Research Quarterly for Exercise and Sport, 63*(1), 60–66.

Molanorouzi, K., Khoo, S., & Morris, T. (2015). Motives for adult participation in physical activity: Type of activity, age, and gender. *BMC Public Health, 15*(1), 66. https://doi.org/10.1186/s12889-015-1429-7

Mucci, N., Giorgi, G., De Pasquale Ceratti, S., Fiz-Pérez, J., Mucci, F., & Arcangeli, G. (2016). Anxiety, stress-related factors, and blood pressure in young adults. *Frontiers in Psychology, 7*(1682). https://doi.org/10.3389/fpsyg.2016.01682

Nigg, C. R., Rossi, J. S., Norman, G. J., & Benisovich, S. V. (1998). Structure of decisional balance for exercise adaptation. *Annals of Behavioral Medicine, 20,* S211.

Núñez-Córdoba, J. M., Martínez-González, M. A., Bes-Rastrollo, M., Toledo, E., Beunza, J. J., & Alonso, A. (2009). Alcohol consumption and the incidence of hypertension in a Mediterranean cohort: The SUN study. *Revista Española de Cardiología, 62*(6), 633–641. https://doi.org/10.1016/S1885-5857(09)72227-3

Patnode, C. D., Evans, C. V., Senger, C. A., Redmond, N., & Lin, J. S. (2017). Behavioral counseling to promote a healthful diet and physical activity for cardiovascular disease prevention in adults without known cardiovascular disease risk factors: Updated evidence report and systematic review for the US Preventive Services Task Force. *JAMA, 318*(2), 175–193. https://doi.org/10.1001/jama.2017.3303

Ramchand, R., Ahluwalia, S. C., Xenakis, L., Apaydin, E., Raaen, L., & Grimm, G. (2017). A systematic review of peer-supported interventions for health promotion and disease prevention. *Preventive Medicine, 101,* 156–170. https://doi.org/10.1016/j.ypmed.2017.06.008

Rovniak, L. S., Anderson, E. S., Winett, R. A., & Stephens, R. S. (2002). Social cognitive determinants of physical activity in young adults: A prospective structural equation analysis. *Annals of Behavioral Medicine, 24*(2), 149–156. https://doi.org/10.1207/S15324796ABM2402_12

Samadian, F., Dalili, N., & Jamalian, A. (2016). Lifestyle modifications to prevent and control hypertension. *Iranian Journal of Kidney Diseases, 10*(5), 237–263.

Shin, Y. A., & Ok, J. S. (2012). Relationships between age, physical activity and obesity index in men. *Korean Society for Wellness, 7*(3), 199–208. (Original work published in Korean)

Viera, A. J., & Hawes, E. M. (2016). Management of mild hypertension in adults. *BMJ, 355,* i5719. https://doi.org/10.1136/bmj.i5719

Wang, J., Zhang, L., Wang, F., Liu, L., Wang, H., & China National Survey of Chronic Kidney Disease Working Group. (2014). Prevalence, awareness, treatment, and control of hypertension in China: Results from a national survey. *American Journal of Hypertension, 27*(11), 1355–1361. https://doi.org/10.1093/ajh/hpu053

Wellman, R. J., Vaughn, J. A., Sylvestre, M. P., O'Loughlin, E. K., Dugas, E. N., & O'Loughlin, J. L. (2016). Relationships between current and past binge drinking and systolic blood pressure in young adults. *The Journal of Adolescent Health, 58*(3), 352–357. https://doi.org/10.1016/j.jadohealth.2015.10.251

WHO Expert Consultation. (2004). Appropriate body-mass index for Asian populations and its implications for policy and intervention strategies. *The Lancet, 363*(9403), 157–163. https://doi.org/10.1016/S0140-6736(03)15268-3

World Health Organization. (2014). *Global status report on noncommunicable diseases 2014.* Geneva, Switzerland: Author.

Yoon, S. S., Carroll, M. D., & Fryar, C. D. (2015). Hypertension prevalence and control among adults: United States, 2011–2014. *National Center for Health Statistics Data Brief, 220,* 1–8.

Zhang, Y., & Moran, A. E. (2017). Trends in the prevalence, awareness, treatment, and control of hypertension among young adults in the United States, 1999 to 2014. *Hypertension, 70*(4), 736–742. https://doi.org/10.1161/HYPERTENSIONAHA.117.09801

Permissions

All chapters in this book were first published by Wolters Kluwer; hereby published with permission under the Creative Commons Attribution License or equivalent. Every chapter published in this book has been scrutinized by our experts. Their significance has been extensively debated. The topics covered herein carry significant findings which will fuel the growth of the discipline. They may even be implemented as practical applications or may be referred to as a beginning point for another development.

The contributors of this book come from diverse backgrounds, making this book a truly international effort. This book will bring forth new frontiers with its revolutionizing research information and detailed analysis of the nascent developments around the world.

We would like to thank all the contributing authors for lending their expertise to make the book truly unique. They have played a crucial role in the development of this book. Without their invaluable contributions this book wouldn't have been possible. They have made vital efforts to compile up to date information on the varied aspects of this subject to make this book a valuable addition to the collection of many professionals and students.

This book was conceptualized with the vision of imparting up-to-date information and advanced data in this field. To ensure the same, a matchless editorial board was set up. Every individual on the board went through rigorous rounds of assessment to prove their worth. After which they invested a large part of their time researching and compiling the most relevant data for our readers.

The editorial board has been involved in producing this book since its inception. They have spent rigorous hours researching and exploring the diverse topics which have resulted in the successful publishing of this book. They have passed on their knowledge of decades through this book. To expedite this challenging task, the publisher supported the team at every step. A small team of assistant editors was also appointed to further simplify the editing procedure and attain best results for the readers.

Apart from the editorial board, the designing team has also invested a significant amount of their time in understanding the subject and creating the most relevant covers. They scrutinized every image to scout for the most suitable representation of the subject and create an appropriate cover for the book.

The publishing team has been an ardent support to the editorial, designing and production team. Their endless efforts to recruit the best for this project, has resulted in the accomplishment of this book. They are a veteran in the field of academics and their pool of knowledge is as vast as their experience in printing. Their expertise and guidance has proved useful at every step. Their uncompromising quality standards have made this book an exceptional effort. Their encouragement from time to time has been an inspiration for everyone.

The publisher and the editorial board hope that this book will prove to be a valuable piece of knowledge for researchers, students, practitioners and scholars across the globe.

List of Contributors

Hsing-Ju LU
Department of Nursing, Chiayi Chang Gung Memorial Hospital, Taiwan

Hsiu-Mei HUANG
Tzu-Yuan Hospital, Taiwan

Tsai-Yun HSIAO
Chung-Jen Junior College of Nursing, Health Sciences and Management, Taiwan

Chang-Chiao HUNG
Department of Nursing, Chang Gung University of Science and Technology and Associate Research Fellow, Department of Nursing, Chiayi Chang Gung Memorial Hospital, Taiwan

Wei-Ting LIN
College of Nursing, Kaohsiung Medical University, Taiwan

Bih-O LEE
College of Nursing, Neuroscience Research Center, Kaohsiung Medical University, Taiwan

JiSun CHOI
College of Nursing Science, Kyung Hee University, Seoul, Republic of Korea

Da Eun KIM
College of Nursing, Research Institute of Nursing Science, Kyungpook National University, Daegu, Republic of Korea

Ju Young YOON
College of Nursing, Research Institute of Nursing Science, Seoul National University, Seoul, Republic of Korea

Hsiu-Ling PENG and Ren-Hau LI
Department of Psychology, Chung-Shan Medical University and Department of Psychiatry, Chung-Shan Medical University Hospital, Taichung, Taiwan, Republic of China

Hui-Wen HSUEH
Department of Clinical Psychology, National Cheng Kung University Hospital, Dou-Liou Branch, Yunlin, Taiwan, Republic of China

Yu-Hsing CHANG
Department of Anesthesiology and Pain Medicine, Boston Children's Hospital, Boston, MA, USA

Wan Ling LEE
Faculty of Medicine, Department of Nursing Science, University of Malaya, Kuala Lumpur, Malaysia

Khatijah LIM ABDULLAH
Department of Nursing, School of Healthcare and Medical Sciences, Sunway University, Kuala Lumpur, Malaysia

Karuthan CHINNA
Faculty of Health and Medical Sciences, School of Medicine, Taylor's University, Malaysia

Imran Z. ABIDIN
Faculty of Medicine, Department of Medicine, University of Malaya, Kuala Lumpur, Malaysia

Kuei-Hui CHU
Department of Nursing, Ching Kuo Institute of Management and Health, Taiwan

Sen-Wen TENG
Department of Obstetrics and Gynecology, Cardinal Tien Hospital-Hsintien and School of Medicine, College of Medicine, Fu Jen Catholic University, Taiwan

Chen-Jei TAI
Department of Obstetrics and Gynecology, School of Medicine, College of Medicine, Taipei Medical University and Attending Physician, Department of Traditional Chinese Medicine, Taipei Medical University Hospital, Taiwan

Ching-Mei CHANG
Department of Nursing, Hungkuang University, Taiwan

Li-Yin CHIEN
Institute of Community Health Care, School of Nursing, National Yang Ming Chiao Tung University and National Yang Ming University, Taiwan

Ibtisam M. AL-ZARU
Faculty of Nursing, Department of Adult Health, Jordan University of Science and Technology, Jordan

Fadwa ALHALAIQA and Abdul-Monim BATIHA
Faculty of Nursing, Philadelphia University, Jordan

Heyam Fawaz DALKY
Faculty of Nursing, Department of Community/ Mental Health, Jordan University of Science and Technology, Jordan

Kholoud Ali ARRAMADAN
Ministry of Health, Jordan

Mei-Hua HUANG
Department of Nursing, Jhong Jheng Spine & Orthopedic Hospital and College of Nursing, Kaohsiung Medical University

Ruey-Hsia WANG and Hsiu-Hung WANG
College of Nursing, Kaohsiung Medical University

Ilknur Munevver GÖNENÇ
Faculty of Nursing, Department of Midwifery, Ankara University, Ankara, Turkey

Füsun TERZIOĞLU
Faculty of Health Sciences, Department of Nursing, Atılım University, Ankara, Turkey

Jingjing LIU, Chen CHEN, Maojie LIU and Shumei ZHUANG
School of Nursing, Tianjin Medical University, China

Jin Yi CHOI and Heejung CHOI
Department of Nursing, Konkuk University, Chungju

GyeongAe SEOMUN
College of Nursing, Korea University, Seoul

Eun Jung KIM
Department of Nursing, Dongyang University, Yeongju

Ji-Yu CAI, Man-Li ZHA, Yi-Ping SONG and Hong-Lin CHEN
School of Nursing, Nantong University, Nantong City, Jiangsu, People's Republic of China

Elham AKHLAGHI
School of Nursing and Midwifery, Iran University of Medical Sciences, Tehran, Iran

Sima BABAEI
Nursing and Midwifery Care Research Center, Faculty of Nursing and Midwifery, Isfahan University of Medical Science, Isfahan, Iran

Abbas MARDANI
Nursing Care Research Center, School of Nursing and Midwifery, Iran University of Medical Sciences, Tehran, Iran

Fatemeh ESKANDARI
Psychiatric/Mental Health Nursing, Mental Health Community Making Life Better, Sydney, Australia

Hee-Kyung CHANG and Cho-Rong GIL
College of Nursing, Gerontological Health Research Center in Institute of Health Sciences, Gyeongsang National University, Jinju, South Korea

Hye-Jin KIM
Department of Nursing Science, Kyungsung University, Busan, South Korea
Department of Nursing, University of Ulsan, Ulsan

Han-Ju BEA
School of Nursing, Yeungnam University College, Nam-gu, Daegu, South Korea

Yelda CANDAN DÖNMEZ
Faculty of Nursing, Department of Surgical Nursing, Ege University, Izmir, Turkey

Arzu ASLAN
Faculty of Health Science, Department of Surgical Nursing, Manisa Celal Bayar University, Manisa, Turkey

Meryem YAVUZ VAN GIERSBERGEN
Faculty of Nursing, Department of Surgical Nursing, Ege University, Izmir, Turkey

Hee-Seung KIM and Yang-Sook YOO
College of Nursing, The Catholic University of Korea, Seoul, South Korea

Hye-Ryoung KIM
College of Nursing, Shinhan University, Dongducheon

Byung Joo SONG
Department of Surgery, College of Medicine, St. Mary's Hospital, The Catholic University of Korea, Bucheon

Hsuan-Man HUNG
Department of Nursing, Fooyin University, Kaohsiung, Taiwan

Ming-Fu CHEN
Department of Rheumatology, St. Joseph Hospital, Kaohsiung, Taiwan

Chung-Hey CHEN
Department of Nursing, Hungkuang University, Taichung and Adjunct Professor, Department of Nursing & Institute of Allied Health Sciences, National Cheng Kung University, Taiwan

Kübra Pınar GÜRKAN
Faculty of Nursing, Department of Public Health Nursing, Dokuz Eylül University, Izmir, Turkey

Zuhal BAHAR
Faculty of Nursing, Department of Public Health Nursing, Okan University, Istanbul, Turkey

Keisuke KUBOTA and Akihiro SUZUKI
Department of Gastroenterological Surgery, St. Luke's International Hospital, Tokyo, Japan

Sachiko OHDE
Center for Clinical Epidemiology, St. Luke's International University, Tokyo, Japan

Ui YAMADA
Department of Psychosomatic Medicine, St. Luke's International Hospital, Tokyo, Japan

Ikumi FUJITANI and Aya KOITABASHI
Nursing Department of Gastroenterological Surgery, St. Luke's International Hospital, Tokyo, Japan

Ya-Fang HO
School of Nursing & Graduate Institute of Nursing, China Medical University, Taiwan

Yu-Chi CHEN
Institute of Clinical Nursing, School of Nursing, National Yang-Ming University, Taiwan

Chiu-Chin HUANG
China Medical University Hospital, Taiwan

Wen-Yu HU
School and Graduate Institute of Nursing, College of Medicine, National Taiwan University and Director, Nursing Department, National Taiwan University Hospital, Taiwan

Kuan-Chia LIN
Institute of Hospital and Health Care Administration, Community Medicine Research Center, Preventive Medicine Research Center, National Yang-Ming University, Taiwan

I-Chuan LI
Professor, Institute of Community Health Care, National Yang-Ming University, Taiwan

Michelle CLEARY and Sancia WEST
School of Nursing, College of Health and Medicine, University of Tasmania, Sydney, NSW, Australia

Rachel KORNHABER
School of Nursing, College of Health and Medicine, University of Tasmania, Sydney, NSW, Australia

Deependra Kaji THAPA
School of Nursing, College of Health and Medicine, University of Tasmania, Sydney, NSW, Australia

Denis VISENTIN
School of Health Sciences, College of Health and Medicine, University of Tasmania, Sydney, NSW, Australia

Jufang LI
School of Nursing, Wenzhou Medical University, Wenzhou, Zhejiang, PRC

Linda Denise OAKLEY and Roger L. BROWN
School of Nursing, University of Wisconsin-Madison, Madison, Wisconsin, USA

Yun LI
Neurological Department, The First Affiliated Hospital of Wenzhou Medical University, Wenzhou, Zhejiang, PRC

Yong LUO
Neurological Department, The First Affiliated Hospital of Chongqing Medical University, Chongqing, China

Chinemerem ELEKE
Faculty of Clinical Sciences, Department of Nursing, University of Port Harcourt, Choba, Nigeria

Sabinah Obele NGBALA-OKPABI
Africa Centre of Excellence in Public Health and Toxicology Research, University of Port Harcourt, Choba, Nigeria

Daprim OGAJI
Africa Centre of Excellence in Public Health and Toxicology Research, University of Port Harcourt, Choba, Nigeria

Ifeyinwa S. AGU
Department of Nursing Sciences, Abia State University, Uturu, Nigeria

Esther N. BEMPONG-ELEKE
Home Health Services, Amedisys, Worcester, USA

Yung-Cheng LIAO
Department of Nursing, Buddhist Tzu Chi General Hospital, Chia-Yi, Taiwan

Li-Li CHEN
School of Nursing, College of Health Care, China Medical University, Taichung, Taiwan and Department of Nursing, China Medical University Hospital, Taichung, Taiwan

Hsiao-Chiao WANG
School of Nursing, College of Health Care, China Medical University, Taichung, Taiwan and Department of Nursing, China Medical University Hospital, Taichung, Taiwan

Jui-Shan LIN
Department of Chinese Medicine, Tri-Service General Hospital, Taipei, Taiwan

Tin-Kwang LIN
Department of Cardiology, Buddhist Tzu Chi General Hospital, Chia-Yi, Taiwan

Shu-Chuan Amy LIN
Department of Nursing, National Yang Ming Chiao Tung University Hospital, Yilan, Taiwan and Assistant Professor, School of Nursing, National Yang Ming Chiao Tung University, Taipei, Taiwan

Jing HAN, Xue-Ping ZHOU, Jun-E LIU, Peng YUE and Li GAO
School of Nursing, Capital Medical University, Beijing, China

Eun-Ju CHOI
Department of Physical Education, Daegu Catholic University, Gyeongsan, Republic of Korea

Ae Kyung CHANG
College of Nursing Science, Kyung Hee University, Seoul, Republic of Korea

Index

www.ingramcontent.com/pod-product-compliance
Lightning Source LLC
LaVergne TN
LVHW080952210926
848485LV00004B/825